PHARMACOLOGY OF AGING PROCESSES

METHODS OF ASSESSMENT AND POTENTIAL INTERVENTIONS

ANNALS OF THE NEW YORK ACADEMY OF SCIENCES
Volume 717

PHARMACOLOGY OF AGING PROCESSES
METHODS OF ASSESSMENT AND POTENTIAL INTERVENTIONS

Edited by Imre Zs.-Nagy, Denham Harman, and Kenichi Kitani

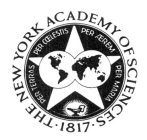

The New York Academy of Sciences
New York, New York
1994

The cover art is the image of the Prophet Jeremiah from the Sistine Chapel of the Vatican in Rome, painted by Michelangelo, symbolizing the wise old man.

Library of Congress Cataloging-in-Publication Data

Pharmacology of aging processes: methods of assessment and potential interventions / edited by Imre Zs.-Nagy, Denham Harman, and Kenichi Kitani.
    p.   cm. — (Annals of the New York Academy of Sciences, ISSN 0077-8923; v. 717)
    Papers from the 5th Congress of the International Association of Biomedical Gerontology, held on July 1–3, 1993 in Budapest, Hungary.
    Includes bibliographical references and index.
    ISBN 0-89766-880-4 (cloth: alk. paper). — ISBN 0-89766-881-2 (paper: alk. paper)
    1. Geriatric pharmacology—Congresses. 2. Aging—Molecular aspects—Congresses. 3. Nootropic agents—Congresses. 4. Longevity—Congresses. I. Zs.-Nagy, Imre. II. Harman, Denham. III. Kitani, Kenichi. IV. International Association of Biomedical Gerontology. International Congress (5th: 1993: Budapest, Hungary) V. Series.
    [DNLM: 1. Aging—drug effects—congresses. 2. Brain—drug effects—congresses. 3. Brain Diseases—drug therapy—congresses. 4. Longevity—drug effects—congresses. W1 AN626YL v. 717 1994 / WT 104 P536 1994]
Q11.N5 vol. 717
[RC953.7]
500 s—dc20
[615'.7'08460]
DNLM/DLC
for Library of Congress   94-15312
                                                 CIP

SP
Printed in the United States of America
ISBN 0-89766-880-4 (cloth)
ISBN 0-89766-881-2 (paper)
ISSN 0077-8923

ANNALS OF THE NEW YORK ACADEMY OF SCIENCES

Volume 717
June 30, 1994

PHARMACOLOGY OF AGING PROCESSES
METHODS OF ASSESSMENT AND POTENTIAL INTERVENTIONS[a]

Editors and Conference Organizers
IMRE ZS.-NAGY, DENHAM HARMAN, AND KENICHI KITANI

CONTENTS

[a]These papers are the result of a conference entitled 5th Congress of the International Association of Biomedical Gerontology (IABG), held on July 1–3, 1993 in Budapest, Hungary.

Financial assistance was received from:
- BIOGAL PHARMACEUTICAL WORKS, LTD., DEBRECEN, HUNGARY
- GLENN FOUNDATION FOR MEDICAL RESEARCH, SANTA BARBARA, CALIFORNIA
- SANDOZ FOUNDATION FOR GERONTOLOGICAL RESEARCH, BASEL, SWITZERLAND

Preface

The 5th Congress of the International Association of Biomedical Gerontology (IABG) took place at Budapest, Hungary, on 1–3 July, 1993. IABG was founded at New York in 1985 by Prof. Denham Harman (Omaha, Nebraska), and holds its Congresses biannually. The previous Congresses were organized in New York (1985), Hamburg (1987), Acapulco (1989), and Ancona (1991).

This volume contains a series of selected papers from the materials presented in the program of the 5th IABG Congress. The basis of selection was whether the papers were directly related to the central theme of the Congress being identical with the title of the present volume. The 34 submitted papers included in this volume most probably reflect the general trend present nowadays in experimental gerontology, namely, the existence of some hopes for a deeper understanding of the mechanisms of the aging processes, and the design of some useful and potential pharmacological interventions against those processes. The editors of this volume are convinced that some small steps forward are being achieved year by year in this field, and we are approaching well-established, scientifically solid ways of an antiaging therapy. This may be true independently from the actual situation in which these ways seem still to be closed.

The 5th IABG Congress of Budapest wishes to express its gratitude for the generous financial support offered by the sponsors listed in this volume. Their support rendered the organization possible.

I. Zs.-Nagy
D. Harman
K. Kitani

Free-Radical Theory of Aging

Increasing the Functional Life Span

DENHAM HARMAN

University of Nebraska
College of Medicine
Omaha, Nebraska 68198-4635

INTRODUCTION

Aging is the accumulation of diverse adverse changes[1,2]—aging changes—that increase the risk of death. These are responsible for both the commonly recognized sequential alterations that accompany advancing age beyond the early period of life and the progressive increases in the chance of disease and death associated with them. Aging changes can be attributed to development, genetic defects, the environment, disease, and an inborn process, the aging process. The chance of death—readily available from vital statistics data—serves as a measure of the number of accumulated aging changes, i.e., of physiologic age, and the rate of change of this parameter with time as the rate of aging.

Conventional means of decreasing the chance of death in a population are becoming increasingly futile. This is illustrated in FIGURE 1 by the curves of the logarithm of the chance of death versus age for Swedish females for various periods from 1751 to 1988; a straight line represents exponential increases with age. The chance of death[1–5] drops precipitously for a short period after birth, largely due to deaths related to development and birth, to reach a minimum around puberty. It then increases with age as deleterious effects of other contributors, e.g., environment and disease, to the chance of death increase. These adverse effects eventually give rise to the sequential changes associated with aging and the exponential increases in the chance of death; the latter ensures that few individuals reach 100 years and that none live beyond about 115 years.[6] As living conditions improved in Sweden, including better housing, nutrition, medical care, public health facilities and accident prevention, the chance of death decreased—more so in the young than in the old—while the straight terminal portion of the curve of the chance of death versus age moved essentially parallel to itself and started at progressively lower ages, reaching an age of about 28 today.

Today the chances for death for both sexes, in Sweden and the other developed countries, are near limiting values.[7–9] Only 2–3% of a cohort die before age 28, while average life expectancies at birth—determined by the chances for death—approach plateau values of around 75 years for males and 80 years females; this is exemplified in FIGURE 2 by Swedish data for 1950 to 1987.[7] Japan[10] is at present an exception to the other developed countries. Here, life expectancies rose rapidly from the fifties in 1950 so that by 1987 they had become the longest lived population. Japanese women in 1989 had a life expectancy of 81.8 years and males of 75.9 years; these figures are apparently still rising linearly at 0.38 year per year.

Thus, as living conditions in a population approach optimum, the curve of the logarithm of the chance of death versus age shifts towards a limit determined by the irreducible contributions to the chance of death of development, genetic defects, the environment, disease, and the aging process; the relative contributions of the aging

1

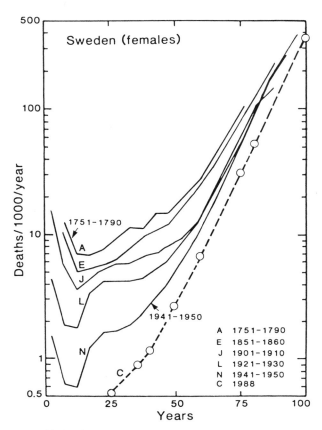

FIGURE 1. Age-specific death rates of Swedish females from 1751 to 1950 (adapted from H. R. Jones)[4] and for 1988.[7]

process to the chance of death increase as living conditions improve, and with advancing age. These contributions to the chance of death should differ between individuals and thus result in differences in the age of death and of the onset and rate of progression of disease. The aging process produces aging changes at an apparently unalterable exponentially increasing rate with advancing age. As chances for death approach limiting values, the associated life expectancy at birth rises toward a maximum value of about 85 years.[11-13] Average life expectancy at birth in the developed countries is today around 10 years less than the potential maximum, largely due to deaths from cancer and cardiovascular diseases.[14]

The contributions of the aging process to the chance of death are small early in life but rapidly increase with age due to the exponential nature of the process; this is illustrated in FIGURE 3. The aging process is now the major risk factor for disease and death after around age 28 in the developed countries. The importance of this process to our health and well-being is obscured by the protean nature of its contributions[2] to nonspecific change and to disease pathogenesis.

THE AGING PROCESS

The aging process may be common to all living things since the phenomena of aging and death are universal. It may also be the major determinant of the manifestations of aging for these occur even under optimal living conditions. Aging is under genetic control to some extent since the manifestations of aging and life span differ between species and individual members of a species. Aging is also subject to environmental influences like other chemical processes.

Many theories have been advanced to account for the aging process.[15-17] For example, it has been attributed to molecular cross-linking,[18] changes in immunologic function,[19] damage by free-radical reactions,[20] and to senescence genes in the DNA.[21] No single theory is generally accepted: "this remarkable process remains a mystery."[22] "It is doubtful that a single theory will explain all the mechanisms of aging."[23,24]

FREE-RADICAL THEORY OF AGING

The free-radical theory of aging[20,25-28] shows promise of application today. The theory arose in 1954 from a consideration of the aging phenomena from the premise[25] that a single common process, modifiable by genetic factors, was responsible for the aging and death of all living things. The theory postulates that aging is caused by free-radical reactions; it is based on the chemical nature of free-radical reactions[29,30] and their ubiquitous presence in living things.[31-33] In mammals, these reactions arise continuously, for the most part from oxygen in the course of normal metabolism,[34-39] and from nonenzymatic reactions.[40-42] The adverse effects of free radical reactions are countered in part by enzymatic, e.g., glutathione peroxidase[43] and catalase,[43] and by nonenzymatic means, such as the tocopherols[44] and ascorbic acid.[45] In general, tissue levels of these defenses vary from one tissue to another,

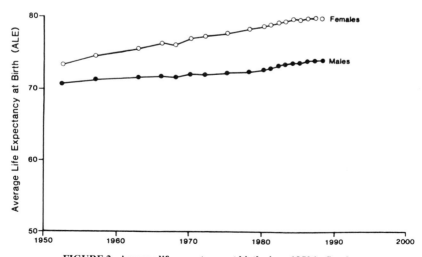

FIGURE 2. Average life expectancy at birth since 1950 in Sweden.

between species, and with age.[46–50] Changes in these defenses are probably not the major cause of the increases in free-radical reaction damage with age, as reflected by the exponential increases in protein oxidative changes[51] and hydrocarbon exhalation.[52] Rather, these increases are more likely due—as discussed below—largely to increased production of the superoxide radical and hydrogen peroxide, and decreased formation of ATP by the aging mitochondria.

Precisely how free-radical reactions cause aging and death is not known. The deleterious changes they produce throughout the body include alterations in membranes,[40,53,54] collagen,[55–57] DNA,[58] chromosomal material,[59,60] proteins and enzymes,[51] and molecules modulating Ca^{2+} levels in the intracellular compartments.[61,62] The latter may play a significant role in aging and cell death; increases in

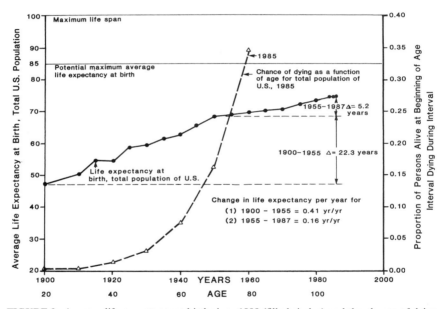

FIGURE 3. Average life expectancy at birth since 1900 (filled circles) and the chance of dying in 1985 as a function of age (triangles) for the total United States population.

oxidative stress can result in sustained elevations of cellular Ca^{2+} levels with subsequent disruption of the cytoskeleton and activation of calcium-dependent catabolic enzymes, including phospholipases, kinases, proteases, and endonucleases.

Oxidative changes in DNA and chromosomal material may shorten the life span, at least in part, by contributing to increases in improper gene expression with age, a process termed dysdifferentiation.[63]

Adverse effects of protein oxidation include memory impairment.[64,65] The free-radical reaction inhibitor N-tert-butyl-α-phenylnitrone (PBN)—a spin-trapping agent—gradually enhanced performance in a radial-arm maze test of old gerbils to near that of young gerbils over a two-week period of twice a day intraperitoneal injections of 32 mg/kg PBN (the threshold dose for protection against ischemia/reperfusion brain injury).[64] This was accompanied by increases in the brain of the ratio of unoxidized to oxidized protein and of the activities of glutamine synthetase and neutral protease. After the injections were stopped, these measures returned slowly over two weeks to their original values. These changes seem greater than those to be expected with inhibitors such as vitamin E, 2-mercaptoethylamine (2-MEA), butylated hydroxytoluene (BHT), etc.; apparently none have as yet been evaluated. If so, possible explanations include (1) the PBN–free radical adduct, or its decomposition products, e.g., NO, might act to increase endogenous free-radical defenses,[66] and (2) PBN may limit free-radical reaction damage by associating with mitochondria and/or other free-radical sources so as to depress free-radical release and/or shorten the chain lengths of released radicals.

Glycation is a common posttranslational modification resulting from the nonenzymatic reaction between sugars, e.g., glucose, and primary amino groups on proteins. These products undergo a slow peroxidation to form so-called advance glycosylation end products,[67] which are recognized by macrophages. Diabetic neuropathy may be due in part to formation of advanced glycosylation products on myelin followed by macrophage attack.[68,69]

INCREASING THE FUNCTIONAL LIFE SPAN

The functional life span is the period of healthy productive life. Future significant increases in this period in the developed countries will be achieved only by slowing the rate of production of aging changes by the aging process.[70] Average life expectancy at birth is employed as a rough measure of the functional life span because the average period of senescence is not known.

In view of the above discussion, it may be possible to increase the functional life span by decreasing endogenous free-radical reaction damage. Such efforts would include (1) nonspecific ones such as (a) caloric reduction, (b) decreasing intake of dietary components that tend to increase free radical reaction levels, e.g. copper, polyunsaturated lipids, or easily oxidized amino acids, while increasing those containing effective "natural" free radical reaction inhibitors, e.g., cabbage and cauliflower[71] or carrots,[72] (c) addition to the diet of one or more inhibitors, e.g., vitamin E, and (2) measures directed to minimizing the contributions of free-radical reactions to the pathogenesis of specific diseases.

It has been suggested that dietary antioxidant supplementation may depress endogenous antioxidant synthesis, so as to nullify the expected beneficial effect of the supplement.[73] Although supplementation may modulate endogenous synthesis to some extent, this can be overridden by an exogenous antioxidant as illustrated by the observations: (1) vitamin E decreases lipofuscin formation[74,75] and the exhalation of pentane,[76] (2) the beneficial effect of free-radical reaction inhibitors on life span and diseases—discussed below. It should be noted that an antioxidant capable of inhibiting essential free-radical reactions will become toxic beyond some level of intake, e.g., butylated hydroxytoluene (BHT) is toxic in the mouse when added to the diet at levels above about 0.5% by weight, presumably because it has a marked adverse effect on mitochondrial function.[77]

Studies are in accord with the above possibility that the functional life span can be increased by decreasing endogenous free-radical reactions, for example:

Caloric Reduction

Decreased caloric intake is associated with an increase in both average and maximum life spans. Thus, decreasing the caloric intake of rats by 40% while maintaining essential nutrients increased average life span by 40% and maximum life span by 47%.[78] This study demonstrated that caloric restriction slows production of aging changes by the inborn aging process: the slope of the curve of the log of the chance of death versus age for restricted animals is less than that of the controls.

The amount of oxygen utilized by control and restricted rats over the life span was essentially the same, as was the rate of oxygen consumption per average gram of body weight.[79] The latter observation probably indicates that a restricted animal contained more cells per average gram of body weight than that of a control.[80]

The beneficial effects of reduced calories, but with adequate essential nutrients, on both average and maximum life spans and disease processes may be due[80] to a decrease in the rate of production of more-or-less random free-radical damage throughout the cells and tissues, and in particular in the mitochondria where over 90% of the oxygen utilized by a mammal is consumed.

Although the life span can be extended beyond the "normal" maximum life span by food restriction in rodents—and most likely also in man—the goal for man is to increase our "normal" maximum life span while living a normal life. Efforts to achieve this goal will probably include some acceptable degree of food restriction.

Dietary Protein

Increasing the dietary content of easily oxidized amino acids might increase free-radical reaction damage and thereby decrease life expectancy. In accordance,[81] when 1% by weight of either histidine or lysine was added to a semisynthetic diet containing 20% by weight of casein as the sole source of protein, average life expectancy was decreased by 5 and 6% respectively. Conversely, replacing casein by a soybean protein containing a lesser amount of easily oxidized amino acids increased life expectancy by 13%.

Antioxidants

Many studies have shown that addition of one of a number of different antioxidants in the diet can increase the average life span: for example, of mice,[82–89] rats,[90] nematodes,[91] and rotifers,[92] as well as the "life span" of neurospora.[93]

In the case of mice, addition of 1.0% by weight of 2-mercaptoethylamine (2-MEA) to the diet of male LAF_1 mice,[82] starting shortly after weaning, increased the average life span by 30%. Corresponding increases produced by 0.5% ethoxyquin in the diet of male and female C3H mice[83] were 18 and 20% respectively.

The increases in average life expectancy of some groups of mice receiving one of a number of different free-radical reaction inhibitors were associated with lower body weights[82,83] of up to about 10% in some cases, but not all.[87] The reason for this is not clear. Possible contributing causes include decreased food consumption and/or assimilation, and deleterious effects on the mitochondria. If it is due to the former, the life span increases should have been less.[82] More likely, it is largely due to adverse effects on mitochondrial function: the antioxidants decrease ATP formation through partial uncoupling of mitochondrial respiration[77,94]—under these circumstances, superoxide radical and hydrogen peroxide formation is also decreased as the respiratory components are more oxidized.[95] Thus the effects of antioxidants on body weight and superoxide/hydrogen peroxide formation are somewhat similar to that of food restriction. ATP and superoxide/hydrogen peroxide formation are lowered in the latter case due to decreased mitochondrial substrates and in the former by a direct effect on mitochondrial function.

A study of the effect of 2-MEA and of BHT on the life span of female C57BL mice[96] led to the conclusion that the antioxidants did not increase the average life span, or the maximum life span, beyond values obtained for control mice surviving under optimal conditions. In contrast, BHT significantly increased the average life span of both male and female BALB/c mice under optimal living conditions.[87] The reason for the discrepancy between the results of the above C57BL mouse study and those of other mouse life span experiments with antioxidants is not clear.

The increases in average life expectancies of mice in studies such as the above that are not associated with increases in maximum life span—and, therefore, no apparent significant decreases in the rate of the inborn aging process—are attributed largely to inhibition by the antioxidants of nonspecific aging changes and those associated with the environment and disease.

Only three compounds have been reported to increase the maximum life span of mice: 2-mercaptoethanol[86] and two pyridine derivatives.[84,85] The study with 2-mercaptoethanol is the only antioxidant experiment reported in which food consumption and body weights of both control and treated mice were maintained the same; addition of 0.25% by weight of 2-mercaptoethanol to the diet of BC3F mice increased average life expectancy by 13% and maximum life span by 12%.

It is likely that the maximum life span of a species is largely determined by the rate of mitochondrial damage inflicted by free radicals arising in the mitochondria in the course of normal metabolism.[35,95,97–100] Such damage is associated with progressively higher rates of superoxide radical/hydrogen peroxide production and decreased formation of ATP. This leads to progressive increases in free-radical reaction levels, free-radical damage, i.e., aging changes, and the chance of death.

The general failure of antioxidants to increase the maximum life span may be largely because mitochondrial function is depressed by the compounds at concentrations below those needed to slow free-radical damage to the mitochondria.[35,94,97–100] It is reasonable to expect that suitable inhibitors will be found in the future; the role of mitochondria in aging and disease is now an active field of research.[93,99–105]

In contrast to mice, both the average and maximum life spans of *Drosophila*[88,89] and of nematodes[91] are increased by antioxidants. These effects, at least in *Drosophila,* are associated with decreased respiration[106] and, presumably, decreased oxidative phosphorylation. Increases in the maximum life span of these two poikilotherms by antioxidants is probably due largely to the same reason that these compounds increase the average life span of mice, coupled with a greater capacity than mice to live at reduced levels of ATP production. The greater longevity reported for a small fraction of a large cohort of medflies[107] may also be related to decreased respiration; aging changes in the tracheal oxygen delivery system[108] may progressively limit oxygen to the tissues.

THE "FREE-RADICAL" DISEASES

The reason for the increasing incidence of disease with advancing age has long been of interest. A disease is a combination of changes—usually forming a readily recognized pattern—that have detrimental effects on function, and in some cases may lead to death. A plausible explanation[109] for the association of age with disease is based on the observation that free-radical reactions are implicated[32,109-111] in the pathogenesis of a growing number of disorders: these include the two major causes of death, cancer and atherosclerosis, as well as the major cause of admission to nursing homes, senile dementia of the Alzheimer's type (SDAT).

The ubiquitous free-radical reactions would be expected to produce progressive adverse changes that accumulate with age throughout the body. The "normal" sequential alterations with age can be attributed to those changes more-or-less common to all persons. Superimposed on this common pattern of change are patterns that should differ from individual to individual owing to genetic, e.g., defective Cu/Zn superoxide dismutase in Lou Gehrig disease[112] and possible higher rates of formation of superoxide radicals in the vessel walls in essential hypertension,[113] and environmental differences that modulate free-radical reaction damage. The superimposed patterns of change may become progressively more discernable with time, and some may eventually be recognized as diseases at ages influenced by genetic and environmental risk factors. Aging may also be viewed as a disease, differing from others in that the aging pattern is universal.

The probability of developing any one of the "free-radical" diseases should be decreased by lowering the free-radical reaction level by any means, e.g., food restriction, antioxidants, and in the case of a specific disease, lowered further by decreases in contributing environmental factors—for example, cholesterol in atherosclerosis and carcinogens in cancer. In some instances, it may be necessary to "target" the inhibitor(s) in order to achieve effective inhibitor concentrations. For example, the blood pressure of spontaneously hypertensive rats is not lowered by intravenously injected Cu/Zn superoxide dismutase (SOD) but it is lowered when the enzyme is coupled with a basic peptide to form HB-SOD.[113] Unlike SOD, HB-SOD undergoes transendothelial transport and localizes within arterial cells.

Some of the data implicating free-radical reactions in cancer, atherosclerosis, essential hypertension, and senile dementia of the Alzheimer type, are presented briefly below.

Cancer

It is a reasonable possibility that some endogenous free radicals will result in tumor formation. Support for this possibility is extensive[80,114] and includes epidemiological studies[115] that indicate that free-radical inhibitors present in fruits and vegetables decrease the incidence of cancer.

Atherosclerosis

Atherosclerosis, the major cause of death in developed countries, can be initiated by substances capable of irritating the arterial wall.[116-118] A likely constant source of such compounds[80,116] is the reaction of molecular oxygen with the polyunsaturated substances present in serum and arterial wall lipids. The numerous studies[80,119] in accord with this possibility include the observation that men and women who supplemented their diets for two or more years with at least 100 mg of vitamin E per day had about a 40% reduction in the risk of coronary artery disease.[120,121]

Essential Hypertension

At any given age, increases in blood pressure over the "normal" for that age are associate with increased morbidity and mortality risks.[122] Based on a 50% or greater increase in mortality in adults, the following operational criteria have been proposed for hypertension:[123] men under 45 years, 130/90; men over 45 years, 140/95; women at any age, 160/95. About ninety % of cases of hypertension are due to unknown causes, i.e., essential hypertension.

The endothelium-derived superoxide radical—apparently formed by xanthine oxidase[113]—has been found to be a vasoconstricting factor.[124] This radical may play a significant role in essential hypertension.[113] Superoxide dismutase injected intravenously does not effect the blood pressure of either normal or spontaneously hypertensive rats (SHR). However, SOD coupled with a C-terminal basic peptide with a high affinity for the heparin sulfate on endothelial cells decreased the blood pressure of SHR but not that of normal rats.

The rise in blood pressure with age may reflect increases in conversion of xanthine dehydrogenase to the oxidase form due to the increasing level of free-radical reactions with advancing age.[125]

Senile Dementia of the Alzheimer's Type

SDAT is the major cause of dementia.[126] It is a spontaneous, i.e., sporadic, systemic disorder whose major manifestations are in the brain. It is hypothesized[110] that SDAT may be the result of one of a number of potential mutations in a mitochondrial DNA molecule, early in development and after germ cell segregation, that impairs oxidative phosphorylation and increases production of superoxide radical and hydrogen peroxide. Replicative segregation distributes the mutated mtDNA to the cells of the developing organism in such a manner that with advancing age significant cellular dysfunction occurs first in areas of the brain associated with Alzheimer's disease.

Neuronal cell damage and death are attributed to random free-radical damage secondary to falling ATP production and increasing formation of superoxide radical and hydrogen peroxide. The rising oxidative stress contributes to cell damage and eventual death, in part by impairing cellular control of calcium concentration; sustained increases in cellular $Ca2+$ disrupts the cytoskeleton and activates calcium-dependent catabolic enzymes.

COMMENT

Chronic disorders now decrease the quality of life of numerous older persons, while the need of many of them for services and medical care from society imposes a significant and growing burden on the remainder of the population. Amelioration of these two interrelated problems should be possible by applications of measures to slow the aging process.

Studies based on the free-radical theory of aging suggest that the functional life span may be increased by keeping body weight down, at a level compatible with a sense of well-being, while ingesting diets adequate in essential nutrients but designed to minimize random damaging free-radical reactions in the body. Such diets would contain minimal amounts of components prone to enhance free-radical damage, e.g., copper and polyunsaturated lipids, and increased amounts of those capable of decreasing such damage, e.g., the "natural" antioxidants present in some foods; the diets would also be supplemented with one or more synthetic antioxidants.

The maximum life span is apparently determined largely by the rate of aging of the mitochondria. Measures that slow initiation of damaging free-radical reactions by mitochondria and/or shorten their chain lengths without significantly depressing mitochondrial function may increase both the maximum and functional life spans. Prospects are good that such measures will be found.

REFERENCES

1. KOHN, R. R. 1985. Aging and age-related diseases: normal processes. *In* Relation between Normal Aging and Disease. H. A. Johnson, Ed.: 1–44. Raven Press. New York, N.Y.
2. UPTON, A. C. 1977. Pathobiology. *In* The Biology of Aging. C. E. Finch & L. Hayflick, Eds.: 513–535. Van Nostrand. New York, N.Y.
3. NATIONAL CENTER FOR HEALTH STATISTICS. 1988. Vital Statistics of the United States. 1985. Life Tables, Vol. 2 (6). Hyattsville, MD, (U.S. Dept. Health & Human Serv.) PHS Publ. No. 88-1104: 9.
4. JONES, H. R. 1955. The relation of human health to age, place and time. *In* Handbook of Aging and the Individual. J. E. Birren, Ed.: 333–363. Chicago University Press. Chicago, Ill.
5. DUBLIN, L. I., A. J. LOTHA & M. SPIEGEL. 1949. The contribution of medical and sanitary science to health and longevity. *In* Length of Life: 141–166. Ronald Press. New York, N.Y.
6. COMFORT, A. 1979. The Biology of Senescence. 3rd edit.: 81–86. Elsevier. New York, N.Y.
7. SVERIGES OFFICIELLA STATISTIK. 1988. Befolknings-forandringar. 1987. Statistiska centralbyran: 114–115. Stockholm, Sweden.
8. OFFICE FEDERAL DE LA STATISTIQUE. 1988. Suisse—Table de Mortalite 1986–1987. Swiss Government. Berne, Switzerland.
9. NATIONAL CENTER FOR HEALTH STATISTICS. 1989. Annual Summary of Births, Marriages, Divorces, and Deaths. United States. 1988. Monthly Vital Statistics 37: (13). Hyattsville, Md. (U.S. Dept. Health Human Ser.) PHS Publ. No. 89-1120:19.
10. STATISTICS AND INFORMATION DEPARTMENT. 1989. Average Life Expectancy 1948–1989. (Minister's Secretariat, Ministry Health Welfare, Japanese Government, Tokyo 162, Japan).
11. WOODHALL, B. & S. JOBLON. 1957. Prospects for future increases in average longevity. Geriatrics 12: 586–591.
12. FRIES, J. F. 1980. Aging, natural death, and the compression of morbidity. N. Engl. J. Med. 303: 130–135.
13. OLSHANSKY, S. J., B. A. CARNES & C. CASSEL. 1990. In search of Methuselah: estimating the upper limits to human longevity. Science 250: 634–640.
14. CURTIN, L. R. & R. J. ARMSTRONG. 1988. National Center for Health Statistics. United States life tables eliminating certain causes of death. U.S. Decennial Life Tables for 1979–1981. Vol. 1 (2) (U.S. Dept. Health Human Serv.) PHS Publ. No. 88-1150-2: 56.
15. ROCKSTEIN M., M. L. SUSSMAN & J. CHESKY, Eds. 1974. Theoretical Aspects of Aging. Academic Press. New York, N.Y.
16. WARNER, H. R., R. N. BUTLER, R. L. SPROTT & E. L. SCHNEIDER, Eds. 1987. Modern Biological Theories of Aging. Raven Press. New York, N.Y.
17. MEDVEDEV, Z. A. 1990. An attempt at a rational classification of theories of aging. Biol. Rev. 65: 375–398.
18. BJORKSTEN, J. 1968. The crosslinkage theory of aging. J. Am. Geriatr. Soc. 16: 408–427.
19. WALFORD, R. L. 1969. The Immunologic Theory of Aging. Munksgaard. Copenhagen, Denmark.

20. HARMAN, D. 1993. Free radical involvement in aging: pathophysiology and therapeutic implications. Drugs Aging **3:** 60–80.
21. HAYFLICK, L. 1987. Origins of longevity. *In* Modern Biological Theories of Aging. H. R. Warner, R. N. Butler, R. L. Sprott & E. L. Schneider, Eds.: 21–34. Raven Press. New York, N.Y.
22. ROTHSTEIN, M. 1986. Biochemical studies of aging. Chem. Eng. News **64**(32): 26.
23. SCHNEIDER, E. L. 1987. Theories of aging: a perspective. *In* Modern Biologic Theories of Aging. H. R. Warner, R. N. Butler, R. L. Sprott & E. Schneider, Eds.: 1–4. Raven Press. New York, N.Y.
24. VIJG, J. 1990. Searching for the molecular basis of aging: the need for life extension models. Aging **2:** 227–229.
25. HARMAN, D. 1956. Aging: a theory based on free radical and radiation chemistry. J. Gerontol. **11:** 298–300.
26. HARMAN, D. 1962. Role of free radicals in mutation, cancer, aging, and the maintenance of life. Rad. Res. **16:** 753–763.
27. HARMAN, D. 1981. The aging process. Proc. Natl. Acad. Sci. USA **78:** 7124–7128.
28. HARMAN, D. 1992. Free radical theory of aging: history. *In* Free Radicals and Aging. I. Emerit & B. Chance, Eds.: 1–10. Birkhauser. Basel, Switzerland.
29. NONHEBEL, D. C. & J. C. WALTON. 1974. Free Radical Chemistry. University Press. Cambridge, Mass.
30. PRYOR, W. A. 1966. Free Radicals. Raven Press. New York, N.Y.
31. FREEMAN, B. A. & J. D. CRAPO. 1982. Biology of disease: free radicals and tissue injury. Lab. Invest. **47:** 412–426.
32. HALLIWELL, B. & J. M. C. GUTTERIDGE. 1989. Free radicals in biology and medicine. 2nd edit. Clarendon Press. Oxford, England.
33. PRYOR, W. A., Ed. 1976–1984. Free Radicals in Biology **1–6.** Academic Press. New York, N.Y.
34. CHANCE, B., H. SIES & A. BOVERIS. 1979. Hydroperoxide metabolism in mammalian organs. Physiol. Rev. **59:** 527–605.
35. HARMAN, D. 1972. The biological clock: the mitochondria? J. Am. Geriatr. Soc. **20:** 145–147.
36. NOHL, H. & D. HEGNER. 1978. Do mitochondria produce oxygen radicals *in vivo?* Eur. J. Biochem. **82:** 863–867.
37. KLEBANOFF, S. J. 1980. Oxygen metabolism and the toxic properties of phagocytes. Ann. Intern. Med. **93:** 480–489.
38. PORTER, N. H. 1980. Prostaglandin endoperoxides. *In* Free Radicals in Biology, W. A. Pryor, Ed. **4:** 261–294. Academic Press. New York, N.Y.
39. SANTO, R. & T. OMURA, Eds. 1978. Cytochrome P-450. Academic Press. New York, N.Y.
40. MEAD, J. 1976. Free radical mechanisms of lipid damage and consequences for cellular membranes. *In* Free Radicals in Biology. W. A. Pryor, Ed. **1:** 51–68. Academic Press. New York, N.Y.
41. SCOTT, G. 1965. Atmospheric Oxidation and Antioxidants. Elsevier Press. New York, N.Y.
42. ALTMAN, K. I., G. B. GERBER & S. OKADA. 1970. Radiation Chemistry **1 & 2.** Academic Press. New York, N.Y.
43. FLOHE, L., W. A. GUNZIES & R. LANDENSTEIN. 1976. Glutathione peroxidases. *In* Glutathione: Metabolism and Function. I. M. Arias & U. B. Jakoby, Eds.: 115–138. Raven Press. New York, N.Y.
44. DE DUVE, C. & O. HAYAISHI, Eds. 1978. Tocopherol, Oxygen, and Biomembranes. Elsevier/North Holland. New York, N.Y.
45. FREI, B., L. ENGLAND & B. AMES. 1989. Ascorbate is an outstanding antioxidant in human blood plasma. Proc. Natl. Acad. Sci. USA **86:** 6377–6381.
46. PREZ-CAMPO, R., M. LOPEZ-TORRES, D. PATON, E. SEQUEROS & G. BARJA DE QUIROGA. 1990. Lung antioxidant enzymes, peroxidation, glutathione system and oxygen consumption in catalase inactivated young and old *Rana Perezi* frogs. Mech. Aging Dev. **56:** 281–292.

47. RAO, G., E. XIA & A. RICHARDSON. 1990. Effect of age on the expression of antioxidant enzymes in male Fischer F344 rats. Mech. Aging Dev. **53:** 49–60.
48. SEMSEI, I., G. RAO & A. RICHARDSON. 1991. Expression of superoxide dismutase and catalase in rat brain as a function of age. Mech. Aging Dev. **58:** 13–19.
49. SOHAL, R. S., L. H. ARNOLD & W. C. ORR. 1990. Effect of age on superoxide dismutase, catalase, glutathione reductase, inorganic peroxides, TBA-reactive material, GSH/GSSG, NADPH/NADP+ in *Drosophila melanogaster.* Mech. Aging Dev. **56:** 223–235.
50. SOHAL, R. S., L. A. ARNOLD & B. H. SOHAL. 1990. Age-related changes in antioxidant enzymes and peroxidant generation in tissues of the rat with special references to parameters in two insect species. Free Radical Biol. Med. **10:** 495–500.
51. STADTMAN, E. R. 1990. Metal ion–catalyzed oxidation of proteins: biochemical mechanisms and biological consequences. Free Radical Biol. Med. **9:** 315–325.
52. SAGAI, M. & T. ICHINOSE. 1980. Age-related changes in lipid peroxidation as measured by ethane, ethylene, butane and pentane in respired gases by rats. Life Sci. **27:** 731–738.
53. NOHL, H. & J. KRAMER. 1980. Molecular basis of age-dependent changes in the activity of adenine nucleotide translocase. Mech. Aging Dev. **14:** 137–144.
54. ZS.-NAGY, I. 1989. Functional consequences of free radical damage to cell membranes. *In* CRC Handbook of Free Radicals and Antioxidants in Biomedicine. J. Miquel, A. T. Quintanilha & H. Weber, Eds. **1:** 199–207. CRC Press. Boca Raton, Fla.
55. BAILEY, A. J., M. H. RANTA, A. C. NICHOLLS, S. M. PARTRIDGE & D. F. ELSDEN. 1977. Isolation of α-amino adipic acid from mature dermal collagen and elastin: evidence for an oxidative pathway in the maturation of collagen and elastin. Biochem. Biophys. Res. Commun. **78:** 1403–1410.
56. BAYNES, J. W. 1991. Role of oxidative stress in development of complications in diabetes. Diabetes **40:** 405–412.
57. DUNN, J. A., D. R. MCCHANCE, S. R. THROPE, T. J. LYONS & J. W. BAYNES. 1991. Age-dependent accumulation of N^ϵ-(carboxymethyl)lysine and N^ϵ-(carboxymethyl)hydroxylysine in human skin collagen. Biochemistry **30:** 1205–1210.
58. RICHTER, C., J. W. PARK & B. N. AMES. 1988. Normal oxidative damage to mitochondrial and nuclear-DNA is extensive. Proc. Natl. Acad. Sci. USA **85:** 6465–6467.
59. RATTAN, S. I. S. 1989. DNA damage and repair during cellular aging. Intern. Rev. Cytol. **116:** 47–48.
60. TAS, S. & R. L. WALFORD. 1982. Increased disulfide-mediated condensation of the nuclear DNA-protein complex in lymphocytes during postnatal development and aging. Mech. Aging Dev. **19:** 73–84.
61. ORRENIUS, S., D. S. MCCONKEY, G. BELLOMO & P. NICOTERA. 1989. Role of Ca^{2+} in toxic cell killing. Trends Pharmacol. Sci. **10:** 281–285.
62. ORRENIUS, S., D. S. MCCONKEY & P. NICOTERA. 1991. Role of calcium in toxic and programmed cell death. Adv. Exp. Med. Biol. **283:** 419–425.
63. CUTLER, R. G. 1991. Antioxidants and aging. Am. J. Clin. Nutr. **53**(Suppl. 1): 373S–379S.
64. CARNEY, J. M., P. E. STARKE-REED, C. N. OLIVER, R. W. LANDUM, M. S. CHENG, J. F. WU & R. A. FLOYD. 1991. Reversal of age-related increase in brain protein oxidation, decrease in enzyme activity, and loss in temporal and spatial memory by chronic administration of the spin-trapping compound *N*-tert-butyl-α-phenylnitrone. Proc. Natl. Acad. Sci. USA **88:** 3633–3636.
65. FLOYD, R. A. 1991. Oxidative damage to behavior during aging. Science **254:** 1597.
66. CHAMULITRAT, W., S. J. JORDAN, R. P. MASON, K. SAITO & R. G. CUTLER. 1993. Nitric oxide formation during light-induced decomposition of phenyl *N*-tert-butylnitrone. J. Biol. Chem. **268:** 11520–11527.
67. WOLFF, D. P., Z. Y. JIANG & J. V. HUNT. 1991. Protein glycation and oxidative stress in diabetes mellitus and ageing. Free Radical Biol. Med. **10:** 339–352.
68. VLASSARA, H., N. BROWNLEE & A. CERAMI. 1985. Recognition and uptake of human diabetic peripheral nerve myelin by macrophages. Diabetes **34:** 553–557.
69. VLASSARA, H., N. BROWNLEE & A. CERAMI. 1988. Specific macrophage receptor activity for advanced glycosylation end products inversely correlates with insulin levels *in vivo.* Diabetes **37:** 456–461.

70. HARMAN, D. 1991. The aging process: major risk factor for disease and death. Proc. Natl. Acad. Sci. USA **88:** 5360–5363.
71. STOHS, S., T. A. LAWSON, L. ANDERSON & E. BUEDING. 1986. Effect of oltipraz, BHA, ADT, and cabbage on glutathione metabolism, DNA damage and lipid peroxidation in old mice. Mech. Aging Dev. **37:** 137–145.
72. DIPLOCK, A. T. 1991. Antioxidant nutrients and disease prevention: an overview. Am. J. Clin. Nutr. **53**(Suppl. 1): 189S–193S.
73. CUTLER, R. G. 1984. Antioxidants, aging and longevity. *In* Free Radicals in Biology. W. A. Pryor, Ed. **6:** 371–428. Academic Press. New York, N.Y.
74. TAPPEL, A. L., B. FLETCHER & D. DEAMER. 1973. Effect of antioxidants and nutrients on lipid peroxidation fluorescent products and aging parameters in the mouse. J. Gerontol. **28:** 415–424.
75. BLACKETT, A. D. & D. A. HALL. 1981. Tissue vitamin E levels and lipofuscin accumulation with age in the mouse. J. Gerontol. **36:** 529–533.
76. LEMOYNE, M., A. VAN GOSSUM, R. KURIAN, M. OSTRO, J. AXLER, *et al.* 1987. Breath pentane analysis as an index of lipid peroxidation: a functional test of vitamin E status. Am. J. Clin. Nutr. **46:** 267–272.
77. HORRUM, M. A., D. HARMAN & R. B. TOBIN. 1987. Free radical theory of aging: effects of antioxidants on mitochondrial function. Age **10:** 58–61.
78. YU, B. P., E. J. MASORO, E. J. MURATA, H. A. BERTRAND & F. T. LYND. 1982. Life span study of SPF Fischer 344 male rats fed ad libitum or restricted diets: longevity, growth, lean body mass and disease. J. Gerontol **37:** 130–141.
79. MASORO, D. J., B. P. YU & H. A. BERTRAND. 1982. Action of food restriction in delaying the aging process. Proc. Natl. Acad. Sci. USA **79:** 4239–4241.
80. HARMAN, D. 1986. Free radical theory of aging: role of free radicals in the origination and evolution of life, aging, and disease processes. *In* Free Radicals, Aging, and Degenerative Diseases. J. E. Johnson, Jr., R. Walford, D. Harman & J. Miquel, Eds.: 3–49. Alan R. Liss. New York, N.Y.
81. HARMAN, D. 1978. Free radical theory of aging: nutritional implications. Age **1:** 145–152.
82. HARMAN, D. 1968. Free radical theory of aging: effect of free radical inhibitors on the mortality rate of male LAF$_1$ mice. J. Gerontol. **23:** 476–482.
83. COMFORT, A. 1971. Effect of ethoxyquin on the longevity of C3H mice. Nature **229:** 254–255.
84. EMANUEL, N. M. 1976. Free radicals and the action of inhibitors of radical processes under pathological states and aging in living organisms and man. Q. Rev. Biophys. **9:** 283–308.
85. EMANUEL, N. M., G. DUBURS, L. K. OBUKHOV & J. ULDRIKIS. 1981. Drug for prophylaxis of aging and prolongation of lifetime. Chem. Abstr. **94:** 9632a.
86. HEIDRICK, M. L., L. C. HENDRICKS & D. E. COOK. 1984. Effect of dietary 2-mercaptoethanol on the life span, immune system, tumor incidence and lipid peroxidation damage in spleen lymphocytes of aging BC3F$_1$ mice. Mech. Aging Dev. **27:** 341–358.
87. CLAPP, N. K., L. C. SATTERFIELD & N. D. BOWLES. 1979. Effects of the antioxidant butylated hydroxytoluene (BHT) on mortality in BALB/c mice. J. Gerontol. **34:** 497–501.
88. MIQUEL, J. & J. E. JOHNSON, JR. 1975. Effects of various antioxidants and radiation protectants on the life span and lipofuscin of *Drosophila* and C57BL/6J mice. Gerontologist **15**(3, part 2): 25.
89. MIQUEL, J., A. C. ECONOMOS, K. G. BENSCH, H. ATLAM & J. E. JOHNSON, JR. 1979. Review of cell aging in *Drosophila* and mouse. Age **2:** 78–88.
90. BUN-HOI, N. P. & A. R. RATSUNAMANGA. 1959. Age retardation in the rat by nordihydroguaiaretic acid. C. R. Soc. Biol. Paris **153:** 1180–1182.
91. EPSTEIN, J. & D. GERSHON. 1972. Studies on aging in nematodes. IV. The effect of antioxidants on cellular damage and life span. Mech. Aging Dev. **1:** 257–264.
92. ENESCO, H. E. & C. VERDONE-SMITH. 1980. α-Tocopherol increases life span in the rotifer *Philodina.* Exp. Gerontol. **15:** 335–338.
93. MUNKRES, K. D. & M. MINSSEN. 1976. Aging of *Neurospora crassa.* I. Evidence for the

free radical theory of aging from studies of a natural death mutant. Mech. Aging Dev. **5:** 790–798.

94. PARDINI, R. S., J. C. HEIDKER & D. C. FLETCHER. 1970. Inhibition of mitochondrial electron transport by nordihydroguaiaretic acid (NDGA). Biochem. Pharmacol. **19:** 2695–2699.

95. BANDY, B. & A. J. DAVISON. 1990. Mitochondrial mutations may increase oxidative stress: implications for carcinogenesis and aging? Free Radical Biol. Med. **8:** 523–539.

96. KOHN, R. R. 1971. Effect of antioxidants on life-span of C57BL mice. J. Gerontol. **26:** 376–380.

97. HARMAN, D. 1983. Free radical theory of aging: consequences of mitochondrial aging. Age **6:** 86–94.

98. HARMAN, D. 1992. Free radical theory of aging. Mutat. Res. **275:** 257–266.

99. FLEMING, J. E., J. MIQUEL, S. F. COTTRELL, L. S. YENGOYAN & A. C. ECONOMOS. 1982. Is cell aging caused by respiratory-dependent injury to the mitochondrial genome? Gerontology **28:** 44–53.

100. MIQUEL, J., A. C. ECONOMOS, J. FLEMING & J. E. JOHNSON, JR. 1980. Mitochondrial role in cell aging. Exp. Gerontol. **15:** 575–591.

101. YEN, T. C., Y. S. CHEN, K. L. KING, S. H. YEH & Y. H. WEI. 1989. Liver mitochondrial respiratory functions decline with age. Biochem. Biophys. Res. Commun. **165:** 995–1003.

102. HRUSZKEWYCZ, A. M. 1988. Evidence for mitochondrial DNA damage by lipid peroxidation. Biochem. Biophys. Res. Commun. **153:** 191–197.

103. LINNANE, A. W., S. MARZUKI, T. OZAWA & M. TANAKA. 1989. Mitochondrial DNA mutations as an important contributor to ageing and degenerative diseases. Lancet **1:** 642–645.

104. BYRNE, E., I. TROUNA & X. DENNETT. 1991. Mitochondrial theory of senescence: respiratory chain protein studies in human skeletal muscle. Mech. Aging Dev **60:** 295–302.

105. WALLACE, D. C. 1992. Mitochondrial genetics: a paradigm for aging and degenerative diseases? Science **256:** 628–632.

106. MIQUEL, J., J. FLEMING & A. C. ECONOMOS. 1982. Antioxidants, metabolic rate and aging in *Drosophila*. Arch. Gerontol. Geriatr. **1:** 159–165.

107. CAREY, J. R., P. LIEDO, D. OROZCO & J. W. VAUPEL. 1992. Slowing of mortality rates at older ages in large medfly cohorts. Science **258:** 457–463.

108. WIGGLESWORTH, V. B. 1965. The Principles of Insect Physiology. 6th edit.: 317–368. Methuen. London, England.

109. HARMAN, D. 1984. Free radical theory of aging: the "free radical" diseases. Age **7:** 111–131.

110. HARMAN, D. 1993. Free radical theory of aging: a hypothesis on pathogenesis of senile dementia of the Alzheimer's type. Age **16:** 23–30.

111. SLATER, T. F. & G. BLOCK, Eds. 1991. Antioxidant vitamins and β-carotene in disease prevention. Am. J. Clin. Nutr. **53**(Suppl. 1): 189S–396S.

112. ROSEN, D. R., T. SIDDIQUE, D. PATTERSON, *et al.* 1993. Mutations in Cu/Zn superoxide dismutase gene are associated with familial amyotrophic lateral sclerosis. Nature **362:** 59–62.

113. NAKAZONO, K., N. WATANABE, K. MATSUNO, J. SASAKI, T. SATO & M. INOUE. 1991. Does superoxide underlie the pathogenesis of hypertension? Proc. Natl. Acad. Sci. USA **88:** 10045–10049.

114. TOTTER, J. R. 1980. Spontaneous cancer and the possible relationship to oxygen metabolism. Proc. Natl. Acad. Sci. USA **77:** 1763–1767.

115. BLOCK, G., B. PATTERSON & A. SUBAR. 1992. Fruit, vegetables, and cancer prevention: a review of the epidemiological evidence. Nutr. Cancer **18:** 1–29.

116. HARMAN, D. 1957. Atherosclerosis: a hypothesis concerning initiating steps in pathogenesis. J. Gerontol. **12:** 199–202.

117. TEXON, M. 1980. Hemodynamic basis of atherosclerosis. Hemisphere Publishing Corp. New York, N.Y.

118. MINICK, C. R. 1981. Synergy of arterial injury and hypercholesterolemia in atherosclero-

sis. *In* Vascular Injury and Atherosclerosis. S. Moore, Ed.: 149–173. Marcel Dekker. New York, N.Y.

119. STEINBERG, D. 1990. Lipoproteins and atherogenesis: current concepts. JAMA **264:** 3047–3052.

120. STAMPFER, M. J., C. H. HENNEKENS, J. E. MASON, G. A. COLDITZ, B. ROSNER & W. C. WILLETT. 1993. Vitamin E consumption and the risk of coronary disease in women. N. Engl. J. Med. **328:** 1444–1449.

121. RIMM, E. B., M. J. STAMPHER, A. ASCHERIO, E. GIOVANNUCCI, G. A. COLDITZ & W. C. WILLETT. 1993. Vitamin E consumption and the risk of coronary heart disease in men. N. Engl. J. Med. **328:** 1450–1456.

122. MANGER, W. M. & I. M. PAGE. 1982. An overview of current concepts regarding the pathogenesis and pathophysiology of hypertension. *In* Arterial Hypertension. J. Rosenthal, Ed.: 1–40. Springer-Verlag. New York, N.Y.

123. KAPLAN, N. M. 1978. Clinical Hypertension. 2nd edit.: 7. Williams & Williams. Baltimore, Md.

124. KATUSIC, Z. S. & P. M. VANHOUTTE. 1989. Superoxide anion is an endothelium-derived contracting factor. Am. J. Physiol. **257:** H33–H37.

125. HARMAN, D. 1993. Free radicals and age-related diseases. *In* Free Radicals in Aging. B. P. Yu, Ed.: 205–222. CRC Press. Boca Raton, Fla.

126. KATZMAN, R. 1986. Alzheimer's disease. N. Engl. J. Med. **314:** 964–973.

New Pharmacological Strategies for Cognitive Enhancement Using a Rat Model of Age-Related Memory Impairment

DONALD K. INGRAM, EDWARD L. SPANGLER,
SETSU IIJIMA,[a] HUI KUO, ELAINE L. BRESNAHAN,[b]
NIGEL H. GREIG,[c] AND EDYTHE D. LONDON[d]

Molecular Physiology and Genetics Section
Nathan W. Shock Laboratories
Gerontology Research Center[e]
National Institute on Aging
National Institutes of Health
Bayview Research Campus
4940 Eastern Avenue
Baltimore, Maryland 21224

[b] Essex Community College
Baltimore, Maryland 21237

[c] Laboratory of Neurosciences
National Institute on Aging
National Institutes of Health
Bethesda, Maryland 20892

[d] Neuroimaging and Drug Action Section
Addiction Research Center
National Institute on Drug Abuse
National Institutes of Health
Bayview Research Campus
4940 Eastern Avenue
Baltimore, Maryland 21224

RATIONALE FOR USE OF RAT MAZE MODELS

The search for appropriate rodent models of memory dysfunction in normal aging and in Alzheimer's disease has developed along two parallel lines. First, there are subject-based considerations. Such questions concern which rodent species and strain to use and also whether to analyze memory dysfunction that is produced by pharmacological or surgical means or by normal aging.[1,2] The second consideration is paradigm based. Many different learning and memory tasks have been assessed.[2–4]

[a] Current address: Department of Geriatrics, University of Tokyo, 7-3-1 Hongo, Bunkyo-ku, Tokyo 113, Japan.
[e] Fully accredited by the American Association for the Accreditation of Laboratory Animal Care.

The selection is usually based on a mix of practical considerations, such as ease of obtaining data, matched against the inherent capabilities of the animal.

Both types of considerations have prompted the use of complex maze tasks in many studies of memory dysfunction. Laboratory rodents perform well in maze tasks likely because of the ecological relevance of this type of behavior. Additionally, the practical considerations of data collection in these tasks are not overly taxing for most laboratories. More important, however, is the appropriateness of the model to the human condition observed in normal aging or Alzheimer's disease. In this regard, complex maze tasks are particularly useful because they assess acquisition of new information by taxing *working* memory. It is this aspect of memory processing, *secondary* or *working* memory, that appears to be initially and primarily affected in age-associated memory impairment[5] and in the memory dysfunction associated with Alzheimer's disease.[6,7]

THE STONE 14-UNIT T-MAZE

Many complex maze tasks have been applied in this area of research, including the Olton radial arm maze,[8] the Morris water maze,[9] and the Barnes circular maze.[10] Each of these paradigms offers distinct advantages. For our research program, we have selected a classic maze paradigm, the Stone 14-unit T-maze. The history and development of this maze have been described previously.[11–13]

Several major beneficial features of the Stone maze paradigm can be summarized as follows: (1) it has great ecological relevance for rodent species; (2) it has an established history of use; (3) it manifests robust age differences in performance in several rodent species and under a variety of motivational manipulations, i.e., food, water, and shock avoidance; (5) vision is not required to perform the task as is the case in the aforementioned maze paradigms; (6) other possible sensorimotor confounds are avoided by submitting the animals to extensive pretraining prior to introducing them to the maze task; and (7) the procedure can be automated to enhance the reliability of scoring.

The configuration of the maze is shown in FIGURE 1. The task requires the animal to locomote through 14 left-right choice-points from the start box en route to the goal box. Movement along the pathway is tracked by a series of infrared photosensors connected to a microprocessor. Deviations from the correct pathway, whether they are movements into the cul-de-sacs or retracing along the goal path, are counted as errors by a computer program. Guillotine doors are used to divide the maze into five segments. When a rat enters into each successive segment, the door is closed to reduce the degree of retracing.

As mentioned above, laboratory rodents can be motivated to negotiate the maze by applying one of several reinforcement contingencies. The current paradigm involves shock avoidance. The floor of the maze is constructed with a grid floor wired to a shock generator. The animal has 10 s to move from each segment of the maze to avoid the onset of scrambled foot shock (0.3–0.8 mA). The shock is activated until the animal moves through the next door at which time the 10-s response contingency is reset. All animals receive extensive pretraining in learning to locomote down a 2-m straight runway within 10 s to avoid footshock. Nearly all rats meet this criterion within the 30-trial maximum limit imposed. Thus, the response contingency is already well established prior to initiating training in the 14-unit T-maze. Thus, use of the shock avoidance paradigm has two major advantages over food and water deprivation techniques for assessing age differences. First, pretraining and training time is reduced substantially, from weeks to days. Second, the issue of motivational

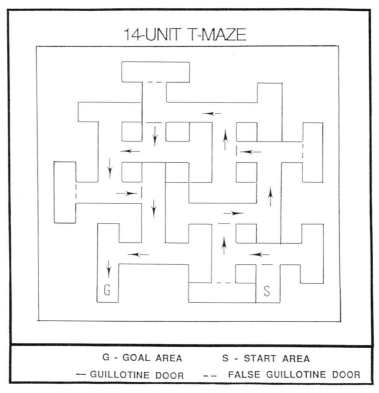

FIGURE 1. Configuration of Stone maze. Arrows denote correct pathway. Errors are scored as any deviation from this pathway.

differences is reduced because the pretraining procedure insures that only animals that have learned the avoidance contingency are subjected to maze training.[11]

AGE EFFECTS ON PERFORMANCE

By using the shock avoidance paradigm, age differences in performance in the Stone maze have been shown in many strains of rats and mice in our laboratory. TABLE 1 provides a listing of those strains that we have analyzed to date. With the exception of a study using the BNF344F$_1$ hybrid strain,[14] we have noted significant age-related decline in performance as measured by the number of errors made per trial in all other strains of mice and rats, including a hybrid strain of mice.[15] Most recently, we have also observed an age-related decline in the performance of gerbils in this maze task.[16] The rat strain that we have characterized most extensively is the inbred, male Fischer-344 (F-344) strain. This genotype performs well in avoidance paradigms, and its age-related neurobiological changes have been the subject of extensive investigation.

INVESTIGATIONS RELATED TO THE CHOLINERGIC HYPOTHESIS

An extensive list of studies performed during the 1980s provided strong evidence supporting the cholinergic hypothesis of geriatric memory dysfunction.[17,18] Parallel studies in humans and laboratory rodents suggested age-related decline in cholinergic neurotransmission. Biochemical studies demonstrated decrements in the levels of acetylcholine, in the activity of the synthetic enzyme, choline acetyltransferase, in concentrations of cholinergic receptors in brain, and in choline uptake. Morphological studies revealed losses or alterations in specific populations of cholinergic neurons.

Lesion Studies

Cholinergic involvement in the memory dysfunction observed in Alzheimer's disease was linked to the neuronal degeneration observed in the basal forebrain obtained from persons dying from this disease.[19] Consequently, attention was focused on the diffuse cholinergic innervation of the neocortex originating from the nucleus basalis magnocellularis (NBM), in which marked neuronal loss was observed in Alzheimer's disease.[20] Rodent models of NBM neuronal loss were used to show involvement of this nucleus and, thereby, of cholinergic innervation in memory performance and in cortical metabolism, but behavioral function and cortical metabolism showed recovery despite persistent cholinergic deficits.[21]

We focused our attention on the septohippocampal cholinergic system.[13] Neurons located in the medial septal area (MSA) provide cholinergic innervation to the hippocampus via the fimbria-fornix (FF) pathway. Neuronal alteration and loss in the MSA were observed in brains of persons with Alzheimer's disease as well as in aged rat brain.[22,23] Many studies using a variety of memory tasks had demonstrated that damage to the septohippocampal system would impair performance requiring working memory. Based on a series of studies, results from our laboratory showed that lesions of the MSA,[24] FF,[25] or the hippocampus[13,26] impaired learning performance of young F-344 rats in the Stone maze.

In such lesion studies, the assumption is made that it is the damage to the cholinergic system that accounts for the learning impairment. In the MSA study,[24] a correlation was observed between the number of errors made and the extent of loss in acetylcholinesterase staining in the hippocampi of the lesioned group. However, in all these studies, other neurotransmitter systems were damaged. Although these data identified neural systems likely involved in memory processing required in this task, it

TABLE 1. Rodent Strains that Have Been Examined for Age-Related Decline in Stone Maze Performance

Strain	Species	Sex	Age Range (mo)	Age Effects
Fischer-344	Rat	M	3–26	+++
Wistar	Rat	M	6–24	+++
Brown-Norway	Rat	M	7–24	+
F344BNF$_1$	Rat	M	7–31	−
A/J	Mouse	M	6–24	+++
C57BL/6J	Mouse	M	6–30	+
C3B10RF$_1$	Mouse	F	12–32	++

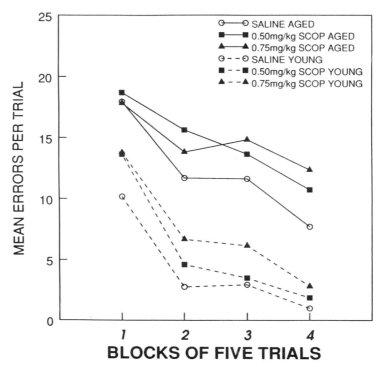

FIGURE 2. Error score performance [mean ± standard error of the mean (SEM)] in Stone maze for young (3 month) and aged (24–25 month) male F-344 rats ($n = 7$–11) according to scopolamine treatment (ip 30 min prior to training).

was necessary to consider the results of pharmacological studies to provide additional evidence for cholinergic involvement in the Stone maze performance.

Pharmacological Studies

In human studies, the use of the muscarinic cholinergic (mACh) antagonist scopolamine hydrochloride (SCOP) was suggested as a possible model of impaired memory acquisition as observed in Alzheimer's disease.[27] We have applied this pharmacological approach in several studies using the Stone maze to demonstrate that an intraperitoneal (ip) injection of SCOP 30 min prior to training impairs acquisition performance[28,29] but not retention performance[30] in young F-344 rats. The impairment of memory performance is presumably due to central effects on mACh receptors because treatment with methylscopolamine, which does not readily cross the blood barrier, has no effect on maze performance of rats given doses of SCOP that produce impairment.[28] FIGURE 2 presents the errors made as a function of training trials in young (3–6 mo) and aged (24 mo) F-344 rats subjected to SCOP treatment about 30 min prior to maze training. A dose-related increase in errors made is evident in both age groups.

The SCOP model can be used as an effective tool for screening drugs as cholinergic agonists. We have used this model most recently for assessing the effects of novel physostigmine derivatives, heptyl-physostigmine[31] and phenyl-physostigmine (phenserine),[32] on performance of young F-344 rats in the Stone maze. Both drugs are potent and long-acting inhibitors of acetylcholinesterase, which degrades ACh in the synaptic cleft. FIGURE 3 shows that treatment (ip) with phenserine 1 hour before training can attenuate the SCOP-induced impairment in maze learning at a wide range of doses in young rats. Currently we are investigating the effects of chronic treatment with phenserine (1–3 mg/kg ip) on performance of aged F-344 rats, and the preliminary results suggest marked efficacy of this new drug.

To date, we have no reliable success in using cholinergic agonists, both direct and indirect, to improve the performance of aged rats in the Stone maze.[13] This failure reflects the general lack of sustained success in applying cholinergic therapies for the treatment of memory dysfunction observed in Alzheimer's disease.[18,33,34] Evidence exists for limited success of some therapies, such as in the use of the anticholinesterase, tacrine.[34] However, despite the clear demonstration of cholinergic involvement in working memory in rodent models,[21] more current research has recognized the involvement of other neurotransmitter systems in memory processes in general and in the memory dysfunction observed in Alzheimer's disease.[33] In addition, increased emphasis is being placed on interactions between neurotransmitter systems.[33,35]

INVESTIGATIONS RELATED TO THE GLUTAMATE HYPOTHESIS

The glutamate system has been implicated in memory acquisition by several lines of evidence. First, the involvement of the *N*-methyl-D-aspartate (NMDA) subtype of the glutamate receptor has been demonstrated in formation of long-term potentiation,[36] which is considered the electrophysiological manifestation of memory forma-

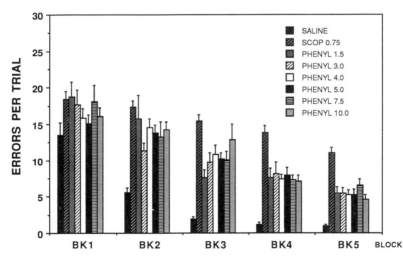

FIGURE 3. Error score performance (mean ± SEM) in Stone maze for young (3-month) male F-344 rats (*n* = 4–14) according to phenserine (phenyl) or saline treatment (ip 1 hour before training) followed by scopolamine treatment (0.75 mg/kg ip 30 min before training).

tion.[37,38] The NMDA receptor regulates a cationic channel, and the influx of calcium (Ca^{2+}) through this channel is involved in several intracellular signal transduction events.[39] Second, many pharmacological studies in rats have shown that antagonism of the NMDA receptor or its cationic channel will impair acquisition but not retention in a wide range of tasks.[40–44] Third, although the distribution of glutamate is ubiquitous in brain, high concentrations of NMDA receptors are particularly densely localized in hippocampus.[45]

A glutamate hypothesis of memory impairment in Alzheimer's disease has been proposed.[46] Indeed, the attraction of this hypothesis is that, in opposition to the normal function of glutamate in memory formation, overstimulation of glutamatergic systems has been implicated in neurodegenerative processes.[47,48] Cell death can be observed *in vitro* following addition of glutamate to neuronal cultures or *in vivo* following release of glutamate during an ischemic reperfusion event.[48] The sustained entry of calcium through the NMDA channel has been hypothesized to account for the resulting neuronal injury.[47,48] Thus, it has been hypothesized that in Alzheimer's disease, an overactive glutamate system may account for the reduced level of glutamate and NMDA receptors observed in brains of persons diagnosed with this neuropathology.[46] However, the involvement of glutamate in memory processing in general[49] and in Alzheimer's disease in particular[47,50] remains controversial.

The involvement of the NMDA receptor complex in Stone maze acquisition has been demonstrated by using a pharmacological probe, dizocilpine (DIZO). This drug is a noncompetitive antagonist which is thought to bind to sites within the cationic channel of the NMDA receptor. FIGURE 4 shows that when DIZO is administered subcutaneously (sc) to young F-344 rats 20 min prior to Stone maze acquisition, a dose-dependent increase in the number of errors is observed beginning at a dose of 0.05 mg/kg.[51] No effect on performance was observed when this dose was given prior to a retention test.[51]

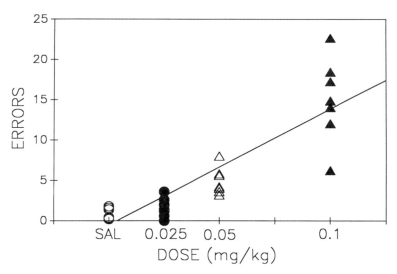

FIGURE 4. Scatterplot showing the dose response of individual young (3-month) male F-344 rats to dizocilpine treatment (sc 20 min prior to training) during the final 3-trial block within a 15-trial session.

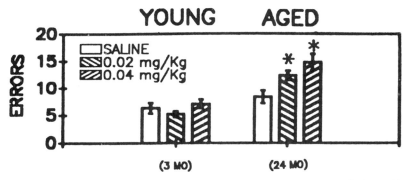

FIGURE 5. Error score performance (mean ± SEM) in Stone maze for young (3–4 month) and aged (24–25 month) male F-344 rats (*n* = 6–8) according to dizocilpine treatment (sc 20 min prior to training).

Compared to young counterparts, aged F-344 rats appear to be more sensitive to NMDA antagonism.[52] When given DIZO sc at doses lower than 0.05 mg/kg, aged rats (24–25 mo) exhibited impaired learning relative to controls as seen in FIGURE 5; whereas young rats (3–4 mo) were unimpaired following treatment at these doses. This increased sensitivity was associated with a marked age-related decline in hippocampal NMDA receptors as measured by [³H]glutamate binding.[52] This finding agreed with those reported in several previous studies in rats using a variety of ligands for the NMDA receptor.[9,53–55] Thus, we have developed evidence that the NMDA receptor complex was involved in acquisition performance in the Stone maze and that a loss of hippocampal NMDA receptors might be associated with the age-related impairment observed in this task.

Because of the potential neurotoxic effects that might result from overstimulating the NMDA receptor, direct pharmacological agonism might not be the safest strategy for augmenting neurotransmission in this neurochemical system, even though the use of monosodium glutamate has been investigated.[56] Therefore, other modulatory sites identified on the receptor complex have been suggested as reasonable alternatives. Because the amino acid glycine is a coagonist with glutamate at the NMDA receptor where it potentiates the response to NMDA,[57] the strychnine-insensitive glycine site on the NMDA receptor has received considerable attention in this regard.[58] Moreover, age-related decline in the binding site for glycine has been reported in rats.[54,59] Two glycine agonists that have been shown to enhance memory performance in rats are milacemide[60,61] and d-cycloserine.[62,63] Based on observations in our laboratory that milacemide could improve the learning performance of young mice in a swim maze,[64] we are currently assessing this compound for improving the performance of aged rats in the Stone maze. Although memory enhancement in normal humans is possible following acute treatment with this compound, results of early clinical trials of milacemide for improving memory performance of Alzheimer's patients have not been encouraging possibly because of tolerance.[65]

Electrophysiological and biochemical studies have demonstrated that poly-amines can also modulate the function of the NMDA receptor.[66,67] Moreover, specific binding sites for polyamines have been identified and characterized pharmacologically in brain. Thus, the polyamine site on the NMDA receptor complex can also be targeted for pharmacological manipulation to improve learning performance. Currently we are testing the efficacy of spermidine as a polyamine agonist to determine its effects on learning performance of young and aged rats in the Stone maze.

As an additional pharmacological strategy, we have considered manipulating both NMDA and ACh receptors simultaneously. Previous studies have demonstrated an interaction between these systems.[68] In a recent study in our laboratory,[69] we observed that combined doses of SCOP and DIZO impaired learning in the Stone maze while individual subthreshold doses of each compound did not. Therefore, an additional pharmacological strategy is to examine whether treatment with low doses of phenserine, acting as an acetylcholinesterase inhibitor, in combination with a glycine agonist, such as milacemide or d-cycloserine, or a polyamine agonist, such as spermidine, will enhance performance of aged rats in the Stone maze.

INVOLVEMENT OF NITRIC OXIDE

Our next direction explored in this rat model was stimulated by the hypothesis implicating NMDA receptor involvement in signal transduction events related to a new class of gaseous neurotransmitters.[70,71] Specifically, nitric oxide (NO) was hypothesized to be the retrograde messenger responsible for enhanced presynaptic glutamate release during stimulation required to establish LTP.[70,72] NO was known to act on endothelial cells as a potent vasodilator.[73] However, the neuronal hypothesis proposed that Ca^{2+} influx via NMDA receptor activation results in calmodulin binding to nitric oxide synthase (NOS) to produce NO from arginine.[70,71] As an oxygen radical, NO rapidly diffuses from the postsynaptic terminal to bind to heme in guanylyl cyclase in the presynaptic terminal. However, considering the issue of detrimental effects related to overstimulating the glutamate receptor, excess production of NO was implicated as the mechanism by which neurodegeneration occurs under these circumstances. Dawson et al. showed that glutamate toxicity in primary neuronal cultures could be attenuated when NO production was blocked by inhibiting NOS with nitro-arginine compounds or by scavaging NO with hemoglobin,[74] which binds the molecule to iron.

Using similar compounds to inhibit NOS, recent investigations in rats demonstrated that LTP formation could be blocked[75-77] and that learning performance in a swim maze could be impaired.[78] Thus, NO has emerged as a prime candidate of a molecule that was essential for normal function, e.g., learning and vasodilation, but potentially neurotoxic. This hypothesis was consistent with the long-standing free-radical theory of aging, which suggests that aging is caused by normal by-products of oxidative metabolism.[79]

Recently we have attempted to establish the involvement of NO in Stone maze acquisition by using N^{ω}-nitro-L-arginine (NARG) to inhibit NOS.[80] As presented in FIGURE 6, when NARG was administered ip 30 min prior to maze training, a dose-dependent increase in the number of errors was observed in young F-344 rats. Similar to the effects observed in SCOP and DIZO experiments, the NARG effect was specific to acquisition performance. When the 6.0-mg/kg dose of NARG was provided prior to a retention test, no impairment was observed. Thus, the impairment was related to cognitive factors and not to performance factors required for efficient maze performance.

No studies to date have attempted to examine age-related decline in NO production or NOS activity. Because of its short half-life (< 4 s), direct measurement of NO is difficult. Regarding NOS, monoclonal antibody to the enzyme is available,[72] but has not been used extensively in gerontological applications. An alternative means of assessing NOS concentration and activity is available by applying the histochemical technique for nicotinamide adenine dinucleotide phosphate diaphorase (NADPH). Work by Hope *et al.* indicated that NADPH-stained neurons were those that contained NOS.[81] Distinct NADPH-positive populations can be identified in several specific brain regions, including the cerebellum, cerebral cortex, striatum, tegmentum, and dentate gyrus of the hippocampus.[72] However, little distinctive NADPH staining of hippocampal pyramidal neurons has been noted. This observation might question the significance of NO in generation of LTP and in memory formation.

The use of the NADPH staining procedure was described in a recent study of brains at autopsy obtained from persons diagnosed with Alzheimer's disease.[82] Robeck and colleagues reported a significant loss of NADPH-containing neurons in the entorhinal cortex of these brains compared to those of age-matched controls. These neurons project via the perforant pathway to the dentate gyrus of the

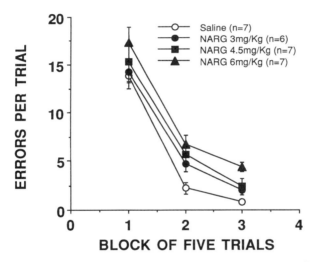

FIGURE 6. Error score performance (mean ± SEM) in Stone maze for young (3-month) male F-344 rats (n = 7–11) according to treatment with N^ω-nitro-L-arginine (ip 30 min prior to training).

hippocampus. These investigators also used densitometric analysis to show that there was less NADPH staining in the terminal fields of entorhinal neurons of brains from persons who died with Alzheimer's disease than in corresponding areas of control brains. Most analyses of NADPH staining patterns have focused on the somata of specific neuronal populations. Similar to the recent work of Robeck and colleagues, we are focusing more on the NADPH staining of neuronal fibers that can be seen in the neuropil as shown in FIGURE 7. Currently we are trying to determine if densitometric methods can quantitate NOS concentrations in specific brain regions in rats.[83]

If a link between NO production and memory performance can be established more firmly, then use of specific NO agonists can be explored. Among potential candidates would be sodium nitroprusside,[84] *S*-nitroso-*N*-acetylpenicillamine,[85] and molsidomine.[86] However, it will be difficult to distinguish the neuronal effects of such

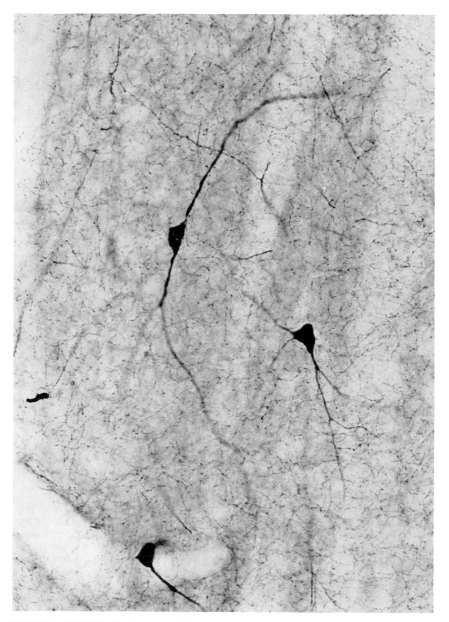

FIGURE 7. NADPH-diaphorase staining of corpus striatum of young (3-month) male F-344 rat. Note the dark staining of neurons but also the distinct staining of fibers. Magnification at 650×. (Reduced to 70%.)

compounds from their vascular effects and also to avoid potential neurotoxic effects resulting from overproduction of NO.[74] Other possibilities include spin trap compounds, like phenyl *N*-tert-butylnitrone (PBN). Treatment of aged gerbils with this compound has been observed to improve their performance in a radial arm maze with no evidence of toxic side effects.[87] Presumably this effect was due to the compound's ability to scavenge reactive oxygen species; however, a recent report suggested that the cognitive enhancing ability of PBN might be due to NO production as one of the metabolic products.[88] Thus, new research likely will reveal a wide range of therapeutic interventions for increasing NO generation safely.

SUMMARY

We have developed the Stone maze paradigm for use as a rat model of memory impairment observed in normal aging and in Alzheimer's disease. Evidence produced thus far clearly implicates both the cholinergic and glutamatergic systems in acquisition performance in this complex maze task. Although results have been very inconsistent regarding the cognitive enhancing abilities of cholinomimetics for use in Alzheimer's disease, new classes of cholinesterase inhibitors may offer greater therapeutic efficacy. The use of glycine and polyamine agonists appears to be a viable strategy for positive modulation of the NMDA receptor. In addition, an approach that combines stimulation both of cholinergic and glutamatergic systems may have greater potential than agonism of either separately.

Manipulation of signal transduction events might also have potential for cognitive enhancement. The influx of Ca^{2+} through the NMDA receptor stimulates production of NO via the action of NOS. By using NARG to block NOS activity, we have demonstrated in rats that NO production appears to influence learning in the Stone maze. We are currently exploring the age-related changes in NOS activity in specific brain regions of rats to determine if loss in the NO generating system is related to age-related memory impairment observed in the Stone maze. In addition, we are exploring pharmacological strategies for inducing NO production; however, because of the potential neurotoxicity for NO overstimulation, this strategy will present some obstacles. The identification of NO as a simple molecule serving vital physiological functions but representing potential for neurotoxicity presents an important unifying area for neurobiological investigations searching for mechanisms of normal brain aging and of age-related neuropathology, as observed in Alzheimer's disease.

ACKNOWLEDGMENTS

The authors recognize the valuable contributions of others on several of these projects as acknowledged in the references. We especially appreciate the contribution of J. Hengemihle, H. Kametani, I. Odano, C. Mantione, M. Chachich, A. Kimes, and D. Roberts. We also appreciated the valuable assistance in design and construction of the maze provided by R. Hiner, M. Zimmerman, G. Baartz, R. Zichos, and R. Bannar.

REFERENCES

1. BARTUS, R. T., C. FLICKER & R. L. DEAN. 1984. Logical principles for the development of animal models of age-related memory impairments. *In* Assessment in Geriatric Psycho-

pharmacology. T. Crook, S. Ferris & R. Bartus, Eds.: 263–269. M. Powley Associates. New York, N.Y.

2. DUNNETT, S. B. & M. BARTH. 1991. Animal models of Alzheimer's disease and dementia (with an emphasis on cortical cholinergic systems). *In* Behavioural Models in Psychopharmacology: Theoretical, Industrial, and Clinical Perspectives. P. Willner, Ed.: 359–418. Cambridge University Press. Cambridge, England.

3. BARNES, C. A. 1991. Memory changes with age: neurobiological correlates. *In* Learning and Memory: a Biological View. J. L. Martinez & R. P. Kesner, Eds.: 259–298. Academic Press. San Diego, Calif.

4. WOODRUFF-PAK, D. S. 1990. Mammalian models of learning, memory, and aging. *In* Handbook of the Psychology of Aging. J. E. Birren & K. W. Schaie, Eds.: 235–258. Academic Press. San Diego, Calif.

5. CRAIK, F. I. M., R. G. MORRIS & M. L. GICK. 1989. Adult age differences in working memory. *In* Neuropsychological Impairments of Short-Term Memory. G. Vallar & T. Shallice, Eds.: 231–245. Cambridge University Press. New York, N.Y.

6. KOPELMAN, M. D. 1985. Rates of forgetting in Alzheimer-type dementia and Korsakoff's syndrome. Neuropsychologia **23:** 623–638.

7. MORRIS, R. G. & M. D. KOPELMAN. 1986. The memory deficits in Alzheimer's-type dementia: a review. Q. J. Exp. Psychol. **38A:** 575–602.

8. INGRAM, D. K., E. D. LONDON & C. L. GOODRICK. 1981. Age and neurochemical correlates of radial maze performance in rats. Neurobiol. Aging **2:** 41–47.

9. PELLEYMOUNTER, M. A., G. BEATTY & M. GALLAGHER. 1990. Hippocampal [^{3}H]-CPP binding and spatial deficits in aged rats. Psychobiology **18:** 298–304.

10. BARNES, C. A. 1979. Memory deficits associated with senescence: a neurophysiological and behavioral study in the rat. J. Comp. Physiol. Psychol. **93:** 74–104.

11. INGRAM, D. K. 1985. Analysis of age-related impairments in learning and memory in rodent models. Ann. N.Y. Acad. Sci. **444:** 313–331.

12. INGRAM, D. K. 1988. Complex maze learning in rodents as a model of age-related memory impairment. Neurobiol. Aging **9:** 475–485.

13. INGRAM, D. K. 1990. Complex maze learning in rodents: progress and potential for modeling age-related memory dysfunction. *In* Biomedical Advances in Aging. A. L. Goldstein, Ed.: 451–467. Plenum Press. New York, N.Y.

14. SPANGLER, E. L., K. S. WAGGIE, J. HENGEMIHLE, D. ROBERTS, B. HESS & D. K. INGRAM. Behavioral characteristics of aging in male Fischer 344 and Brown Norway rat strains and their F_1 hybrid. Neurobiol. Aging. (In press.)

15. INGRAM, D. K., R. WEINDRUCH, E. L. SPANGLER, J. R. FREEMAN & R. L. WALFORD. 1987. Dietary restriction benefits learning and motor performance of aged mice. J. Gerontol. **42:** 78–91.

16. SPANGLER, E. L., J. HENGEMIHLE, G. BLANK, D. SPEAR, S. BRZOZOWSKI, N. PATEL & D. K. INGRAM. 1993. An assessment of behavioral aging in the gerbil. Neurosci. Abstr. **19:** 897.

17. BARTUS, R. T., R. L. DEAN, B. BEER & A. S. LIPPA. 1982. The cholinergic hypothesis of geriatric memory dysfunction. Science **217:** 408–412.

18. COLLERTON, D. 1986. Cholinergic function and intellectual decline in Alzheimer's disease. Neuroscience **19:** 1–28.

19. WHITEHOUSE, P. J., D. L. PRICE, R. G. STRUBLE, A. W. CLARK, J. T. COYLE & M. R. DELONG. 1982. Alzheimer's disease and senile dementia: loss of neurons in the basal forebrain. Science **215:** 1237–1239.

20. ETIENNE, P., Y. ROBITAILLE, P. WOOD, S. GAUTHIER, N. P. V. NAIR & R. QUIRION. 1986. Nucleus basalis neuronal loss, neuritic plaques and choline acetyltransferase activity in advanced Alzheimer's disease. Neuroscience **19:** 1279–1291.

21. OLTON, D. S. & G. WENK. 1987. Dementia: animal models of the cognitive impairments produced by degeneration of the basal forebrain cholinergic system. *In* Psychopharmacology: The Third Generation of Progress. H. Y. Meltzer, Ed.: 941–953. van Nostrand. New York, N.Y.

22. FISCHER, W., F. H. GAGE & A. BJORKLUND. 1989. Degenerative changes in forebrain

cholinergic nuclei correlate with cognitive impairments in aged rats. Eur. J. Neurosci. **1:** 34–45.

23. DECKER, M. W. 1987. The effects of aging on hippocampal and cortical projections of the forebrain cholinergic system. Brain Res. Rev. **12:** 423–438.
24. KAMETANI, H., E. L. SPANGLER, E. L. BRESNAHAN, S. KOBAYASHI, J. M. LONG & D. K. INGRAM. 1993. Impaired acquisition in a 14-unit maze following medial septal lesions in rats is correlated with lesion size and hippocampal acethylcholinesterase staining. Physiol. Behav. **53:** 221–228.
25. BRESNAHAN, E. L., H. KAMETANI, E. L. SPANGLER, M. E. CHACHICH, P. R. WISER & D. K. INGRAM. 1988. Fimbria-fornix lesions in young rats impair acquisition in a 14-unit T-maze similar to prior observed performance deficits in aged rats. Psychobiology **16:** 243–250.
26. JUCKER, M., H. KAMETANI, E. L. BRESNAHAN & D. K. INGRAM. 1990. Parietal cortex lesions do not impair retention performance of rats in a 14-unit T-maze unless hippocampal damage is present. Physiol. Behav. **47:** 207–212.
27. DRACHMAN, D. A. & J. LEAVITT. 1974. Human memory and the cholinergic system. Arch. Neurol. **30:** 113–121.
28. SPANGLER, E. L., P. RIGBY & D. K. INGRAM. 1986. Scopolamine impairs learning performance of rats in a 14-unit T-maze. Pharmacol. Biochem. Behav. **25:** 673–679.
29. SPANGLER, E. L., M. E. CHACHICH, N. J. CURTIS & D. K. INGRAM. 1989. Age-related impairment in complex maze learning in rats: relationship to neophobia and cholinergic antagonism. Neurobiol. Aging **10:** 133–141.
30. SPANGLER, E. L., M. E. CHACHICH & D. K. INGRAM. 1988. Scopolamine in rats impairs acquisition but not retention in a 14-unit T-maze. Pharmacol. Biochem. Behav. **30:** 949–955.
31. IIJIMA, S., N. H. GREIG, P. GAROFALO, E. L. SPANGLER, B. HELLER, A. BROSSI & D. K. INGRAM. 1992. The long-acting cholinesterase inhibitor heptyl-physostigmine attenuates the scopolamine-induced learning impairment of rats in a 14-unit T-maze. Neurosci. Lett. **144:** 79–83.
32. IIJIMA, S., N. H. GREIG, P. GAROFALO, E. L. SPANGLER, B. HELLER, A. BROSSI & D. K. INGRAM. Phenserine: a physostigmine derivative that is a long-acting inhibitor of cholinesterase and demonstrates a wide dose range for attenuating a scopolamine-induced learning impairment of rats in a 14-unit T-maze. Psychopharmacology. (In press.)
33. PALMER, A. M. & S. GERSHON. 1990. Is the neuronal basis of Alzheimer's disease cholinergic or glutamatergic? FASEB J. **4:** 2745–2752.
34. POMPONI, M., E. GIACOBINI & M. BRUFANI. 1990. Present state and future development of the therapy of Alzheimer disease. Aging **2:** 125–153.
35. DECKER, M. W. & J. L. McGAUGH. 1991. The role of interactions between the cholinergic system and other neuromodulatory systems in learning and memory. Synapse **7:** 151–168.
36. MULLER, D., M. JOLY & G. LYNCH. 1988. Contributions of quisqualate and NMDA receptors to the induction and expression of LTP. Science **242:** 1694–1697.
37. BARNES, C. A. 1988. Spatial learning and memory processes: the search for their neurobiological mechanisms in the rat. Trends Neurosci. **11:** 163–169.
38. GUSTAFSSON, F. & H. WINGSTROM. 1988. Physiological mechanisms underlying LTP. Trends Neurosci. **11:** 156–162.
39. COTMAN, C. W. & L. L. IVERSON. 1987. Excitatory amino acids in the brain—focus on NMDA receptors. Trends Neurosci. **10:** 263–265.
40. BUTELMAN, E. R. 1989. A novel NMDA antagonist, MK-801, impairs performance in a hippocampal-dependent spatial learning task. Pharmacol. Biochem. Behav. **34:** 13–16.
41. LYFORD, G. L. & L. E. JARRARD. 1991. Effects of the competitive NMDA antagonist CPP on performance of a place and cue radial maze task. Psychobiology **19:** 157–160.
42. MORRIS, R. G. M., E. ANDERSON, G. S. LYNCH & M. BAUDRY. 1986. Selective impairment of learning and blockade of long-term potentiation by an N-methyl-d-asparate receptor antagonist. Nature **319:** 774–776.
43. ROBINSON, G. S., G. B. CROOKS, P. G. SHRINKMAN & M. GALLAGHER. 1989. Behavioral

effects of MK-801 mimic deficits associated with hippocampal damage. Psychobiology **17:** 156–164.

44. SHAPIRO, M. L. & Z. CARAMANOS. 1990. NMDA antagonist MK-801 impairs acquisition but not performance of spatial working and reference memory. Psychobiology **18:** 231–243.

45. MONAGHAN, D. T. & C. W. COTMAN. 1985. Distribution of *N*-methyl-D-aspartate-sensitive L[³H]glutamate binding sites in rat brain. J. Neurosci. **5:** 2909–2919.

46. GREENAMYRE, J. T. & A. B. YOUNG. 1989. Excitatory amino acids and Alzheimer's disease. Neurobiol. Aging **10:** 593–602.

47. COTMAN, C. W. & D. MONAGHAN. 1988. Multiple excitatory amino acid receptor regulation of intracellular Ca^{2+}: implications for aging and Alzheimer's disease. Ann. N.Y. Acad. Sci. **522:** 138–148.

48. CHOI, D. W. & S. M. ROTHMAN. 1990. The role of glutamate neurotoxicity in hypoxic-ischemic neuronal death. Annu. Rev. Neurosci. **13:** 171–182.

49. KEITH, J. R. & J. W. RUDY. 1990. Why NMDA-receptor-dependent long-term potentiation may not be a mechanism of learning and memory: reappraisal of the NMDA-receptor blockade strategy. Psychobiology **18:** 251–257.

50. COTMAN, C. W., J. W. GEDDES, R. J. BRIDGES & D. T. MONAGHAN. 1989. *N*-Methyl-D-aspartate receptors and Alzheimer's disease. Neurobiol. Aging **10:** 603–605.

51. SPANGLER, E. L., P. GAROFALO, E. L. BRESNAHAN, N. J. MUTH, B. HELLER & D. K. INGRAM. 1991. NMDA receptor channel antagonism by dizocilpine (MK-801) impairs performance of rats in aversively-motivated complex maze tasks. Pharmacol. Biochem. Behav. **40:** 949–958.

52. INGRAM, D. K., P. GAROFALO, E. L. SPANGLER, C. R. MANTIONE, I. ODANO & E. D. LONDON. 1992. Reduced density of NMDA receptors and increased sensitivity to dizocilpine-induced learning impairment in aged rats. Brain Res. **580:** 273–280.

53. FIORE, L. & L. RAMPELLO. 1984. L-Acetylcarnitine attenuates the age-dependent decrease of NMDA-sensitive glutamate receptors in rat hippocampus. Acta Neurol. **11:** 346–350.

54. TAMARU, M., Y. YONEDA, K. OGITA, J. SHIMIZU & Y. NAGATA. 1990. Age-related decreases of the *N*-methyl-D-aspartate receptor complex in the rat cerebral cortex and hippocampus. Brain Res. **542:** 83–90.

55. WENK, G. L., L. C. WALKER, D. L. PRICE & L. CORK. 1991. Loss of NMDA, but not GABA-A, binding in the brains of aged rats and monkeys. Neurobiol. Aging **12:** 93–98.

56. WALLACE, D. R. & R. DAWSON, JR. 1990. Effect of age and monosodium-*l*-glutamate (MSG) treatment on neurotransmitter content in brain regions from male Fischer-344 rats. Neurochem. Res. **9:** 889–898.

57. JOHNSON, J. W. & P. ASCHER. 1987. Glycine potentiates the NMDA response in cultured mouse brain neurons. Nature **325:** 529–531.

58. BOWEN, D. M. 1990. Treatment of Alzheimer's disease: molecular pathology versus neurotransmitter-based therapy. Br. J. Psychiatr. **157:** 327–330.

59. MIYOSHI, R., S. KITO, N. DOUDOU & T. TOMOTO. 1990. Age-related changes of strychnine-insensitive glycine receptors in rat brain as studied by in vitro autoradiography. Synapse **6:** 338–345.

60. HANDELMANN, G. E., M. E. NEVINS, L. L. MUELLER, S. M. ARNOIDE & A. A. CORDI. 1989. Milacemide, a glycine prodrug, enhances performance of learning tasks in normal and amnestic rodents. Pharmacol. Biochem. Behav. **34:** 823–828.

61. QUARTERMAIN, D., T. NUYGEN, J. SHEU & R. L. HERTING. 1991. Milacemide enhances memory storage and alleviates spontaneous forgetting in mice. Pharmacol. Biochem. Behav. **39:** 31–35.

62. FLOOD, J. F., J. E. MORLEY & T. H. LANTHORN. 1992. Effect on memory processing by D-cycloserine, an agonist of the NMDA/glycine receptor. Eur. J. Pharmacol. **221:** 249–254.

63. MONAHAN, J. B., G. E. HANDELMANN, G. E. HOOD & A. A. CORDI. 1989. D-Cycloserine, a positive modulator of the *N*-methyl-D-aspartate receptor enhances performance of learning tasks in rats. Pharmacol. Biochem. Behav. **34:** 649–653.

64. FINKELSTEIN, J. E., J. M. HENGEMIHLE, D. K. INGRAM & H. L. PETRI. Milacemide

treatment in mice enhances acquisition of a Morris-type water maze task. Pharmacol. Biochem. Behav. (In press.)

65. HERTING, R. L. 1991. Milacemide and other drugs active at glutamate NMDA receptors as potential treatment for dementia. Ann. N.Y. Acad. Sci. **640:** 237–240.
66. LONDON, E. D., V. L. DAWSON & C. R. MANTIONE. 1990. Specific binding sites for polyamines in mammalian brain. *In* NMDA Receptor Related Agents: Biochemistry, Pharmacology, and Behavior. T. Kameyama, T. Nabeshima & E. F. Domino, Eds.: 71–78. NPP Books. Ann Arbor, Mich.
67. HASHIMOTO, E. D. & E. D. LONDON. Specific binding sites for polyamines in brain. *In* Neuropharmacology of Polyamines. C. J. Carter, Ed. Academic Press. New York, N.Y. (In press.)
68. MARKAM, H. & M. SEGAL. 1990. Acetylcholine potentiates responses to *N*-methyl-D-aspartate in the rat hippocampus. Neurosci. Let. **113:** 62–65.
69. GAROFALO, P., E. L. SPANGLER & D. K. INGRAM. Combined muscarinic and NMDA antagonism impairs complex maze learning in rats. Pharmacol. Biochem. Behav. (In press.)
70. GARTHWAITE, J. 1991. Glutamate, nitric oxide and cell-cell signalling in the nervous system. Trends Neurosci. **14:** 60–67.
71. SNYDER, S. H. & D. S. BREDT. 1992. Biological roles of nitric oxide. Sci. Am. (May): 68–77.
72. BREDT, D. S., P. M. HWANG & S. H. SNYDER. 1990. Localization of nitric oxide synthase indicating neural role for nitric oxide. Nature. **347:** 768–770.
73. FURCHGOTT, R. F. & J. V. ZAWADZKI. 1980. The obligatory role of endothelial cells in the relaxation of arterial smooth muscle by acetylcholine. Nature **288:** 373–376.
74. DAWSON, V. L., T. M. DAWSON, E. D. LONDON, D. S. BREDT & S. H. SNYDER. 1991. Nitric oxide mediates glutamate neurotoxicity in primary cortical cultures, Proc. Natl. Acad. Sci. USA **88:** 6368–6371.
75. BOHME, G. A., C. BON, J.-M. STUTZMANN, A. DOBLE & J. C. BLANCHARD. 1991. Possible involvement of nitric oxide in long-term potentiation. E. J. Pharmacol. **199:** 379–381.
76. HALEY, J. E., G. L. WILCOX & P. F. CHAPMAN. 1992. The role of nitric oxide in hippocampal long-term potentiation. Neuron **8:** 211–216.
77. MADISON, D. V. & E. M. SCHUMAN. 1991. A requirement for the intercellular messenger nitric oxide in long-term potentiation. Science **254:** 1503–1506.
78. CHAPMAN, P. F., C. M. ATKINS, M. T. ALLEN, J. E. HALEY & J. E. STEINMETZ. 1992. Inhibition of nitric oxide synthesis impairs two different forms of learning. Neuroreport **3:** 567–570.
79. HARMAN, D. 1987. Aging: a theory based on free radical and radiation chemistry. J. Gerontol. **11:** 298–300.
80. INGRAM, D. K., E. SPANGLER, D. ROBERTS, S. IIJIMA & E. D. LONDON. 1992. Nitric oxide synthase inhibition by N^ω-nitro-L-arginine impairs learning of rats in a 14-unit T-maze. Neurosci. Abstr. **18:** 1220.
81. HOPE, B. T., G. J. MICHAEL, K. M. KNIGGE & S. R. VINCENT. 1991. Neuronal NADPH-diaphorase is a nitric oxide synthase. Proc. Natl. Acad. Sci. USA **88:** 2811–2814.
82. ROBECK, G. W., K. MARZLOFF & B. T. HYMAN. The pattern of NADPH-diaphorase staining, a marker of nitric oxide synthase activity, is altered in the perforant pathway terminal zone in Alzheimer's disease. Neurosci. Lett. (In press.)
83. KUO, H., J. HENGEMIHLE, W. DELORIERS, S. GRANT & D. K. INGRAM. 1993. A quantitative analysis of the relationship between neuron counts and optical density of NADPH-diaphorase histochemistry in the rat striatum. Neurosci. Abstr. **19:** 1114.
84. FEELISH, M. & E. A. NOACK. 1987. Correlation between nitric oxide formation during degradation of organic nitrates and activation of guanylate cyclase. Eur. J. Pharmacol. **139:** 19–25.
85. SHAFFER, J. E. 1992. Lack of tolerance to a 24-hr infusion of *S*-nitroso-*N*-acetylpenicilla-mine in conscious rabbits. J. Pharmacol. Exp. Ther. **260:** 286–293.
86. NITZ, R. E. 1987. Molsidomine: alternative approaches to treat myocardial ischemia. Pharmacotherapy **7:** 28–37.
87. CARNEY, J. M., P. E. STARKE-REED, C. N. OLIVER, R. W. LANDUM, M. S. CHENG, J. F. WU & R. A. FLOYD. 1991. Reversal of age-related increase in brain protein oxidation,

decrease in enzyme activity, and loss in temporal and spatial memory by chronic administration of the spin-trapping compound N-tert-butyl-α-phenylnitrone. Proc. Natl. Acad. Sci. USA **88:** 3633–3636.

88. CHAMULITRAT, W., S. J. JORDAN, R. P. MASON, K. SAITO & R. G. CUTLER. 1993. Nitric oxide formation during light-induced decomposition of phenyl N-tert-butylnitrone. J. Biol. Chem. **268:** 11520–11527.

Neuroanatomy of Aging Brain

Influence of Treatment with L-Deprenyl[a]

FRANCESCO AMENTA, STEFANO BONGRANI,[b]
SANDRO CADEL,[b] ALBERTO RICCI,[c]
BRUNO VALSECCHI,[b] AND YONG-CHUN ZENG

Sezione di Anatomia Umana
Istituto di Farmacologia
Università di Camerino
Via Scalzino, 5
62032 Camerino, Italy

[b]*Chiesi Farmaceutici S.p.A.*
Parma, Italy

[c]*Dipartimento di Scienze Cardiovascolari e Respiratorie*
Università "La Sapienza"
Roma, Italy

INTRODUCTION

An age-dependent increase in monoamine oxidase (MAO) B activity has been observed in various areas of human and rat brain. These areas include primarily the nigrostriatal and the limbic systems and to a lesser extent the cerebral cortex and some portions of the brain stem.[1,2] The inhibition of the age-related increase in MAO-B activity could represent a therapeutic principle for treating age-related neurodegenerative diseases. In fact, it has been discovered that L-deprenyl (Selegiline), a MAO-B inhibitor, is able to increase both mean and maximum life span in the rat. It has also been reported that treatment with L-deprenyl improves learning and memory deficits associated with aging in rats,[3,4] and improves cognitive functions in patients suffering from Parkinson's disease or senile dementia of the Alzheimer's type (SDAT).[5,6]

The frontal cortex is the target of specific ascending projections (cholinergic, dopaminergic, noradrenergic, and serotonergic). An impairment of these pathways is probably involved in cognitive dysfunction associated with aging.[7-9] Although the occurrence of age-dependent alterations in the frontal cortex has been reported by several studies,[7] the senescent changes on the microanatomy of the frontal cortex received comparatively less attention than other cerebral areas. The hippocampus is a cerebral region involved in learning and memory processes which is particularly sensitive to aging. Age-dependent changes involving the hippocampal formation include cell loss, senile plaques and neurofibrillary tangles, granulovacuolar changes, and lipofuscin and amyloid accumulation.[7-9]

A variety of neuroanatomical changes occur both in "physiological" aging and in senile dementia,[7,8] and the mechanisms of age-dependent changes of the hippocampus and frontal cortex are still not clear. Moreover, as far as we know, only sparse information is available concerning the influence of L-deprenyl treatment on the

[a]Supported by a grant of Chiesi Farmaceutici (Parma, Italy).

age-related modifications in brain microanatomy. The present study was designed to assess whether long-term treatment with L-deprenyl has any effect on age-dependent microanatomical changes in the rat frontal cortex and hippocampus.

MATERIALS AND METHODS

Animals and Tissue Treatment

Male Sprague-Dawley rats were obtained from IFFA Credo (Lyon, France). Animals were kept under standardized humidity, temperature, and lighting conditions (07:00 AM–07:00 PM light-dark cycle). Twelve-month-old rats ($n = 15$), which were used as an adult reference group, were left untreated and considered as adult animals. Nineteen-month-old rats were randomly allotted to three groups. Rats of the first group received an oral daily dose of 1.25 mg/kg L-deprenyl ($n = 12$). The animals of the second group were treated with an oral daily dose of 5 mg/kg L-deprenyl ($n = 12$), whereas rats of the third group were left untreated and served as a control group ($n = 15$). Rats of the above three groups were allowed to survive for 5 months and were sacrificed by decapitation under ether anesthesia at 24 months of age. At this age they were considered to be old. Treatment with L-deprenyl was performed by adding the drug to the rat drinking water. Drug concentration was adjusted weekly in order to ensure the exposition to the established dose. Compound consumption was within 91–111% of the target dose level (mean values 100–101%). Rats had water consumption and body weight determined weekly. Furthermore, they were daily examined for clinical signs and mortality.

After sacrifice, the brain was removed, washed in ice-cold 0.9% NaCl solution, and weighed. The right and left hemispheres were separated and frontal coronal slices of each hemisphere corresponding to the sections A 7190 μm and A 3750 μm (according to the atlas of Konig and Klippel)[20] were obtained and processed as described below. Slices of the right frontal cortex were fixed in a 4% neutral formalin solution (derived from paraformaldehyde power), dehydrated in ethanol, and embedded in Historesin (Reichert-Jung, Vienna, Austria). Resin-embedded blocks were used for assessing the density of nerve cell profiles. Slices of the left hemisphere were embedded in a cryoprotectant medium (OCT, Ames, Iowa) and frozen in a dry ice-acetone mixture. OCT-embedded blocks were used for the immunohistochemical demonstration of glial fibrillary acidic protein (GFAP) immunoreactive astrocytes, for the histochemical analysis of sulfide silver staining, for the evaluation of lipofuscin deposition, and for the histochemical detection of MAO-B activity.

Density of Nerve Cell Profiles in the Rat Frontal Cortex and Hippocampus

The 1st, 4th, 7th, 10th, and 16th consecutive resin-embedded sections of the frontal cortex and hippocampus (20 μm apart, 3 μm thick) were mounted on microscope slides and stained with a 0.5% toluidine blue solution. Sections were viewed under a Zeiss Axiophot microscope at a final magnification of ×160. The different neuron profiles (identified by a clearly visible nucleolus) were then counted in an area of 1 mm² delineated with a Videoplan image analyzer (Kontron-Zeiss, Germany) connected via a TV camera to the microscope. Three different areas randomly selected were evaluated in each section. In total, 15 different 1 mm² wide areas of the frontal cortex were evaluated by image analysis. Hippocampal toluidine blue–stained sections were examined at a final ×200 magnification. The number of nerve cell profiles in the CA1 and CA3 fields of the hippocampus and in the dentate gyrus was then counted in a 1 mm^2 area of these different portions using the Videoplan image analyzer connected via a TV camera to the microscope. The maximal diameter of the nucleus and the area of pyramidal neurons of the frontal cortex and of the CA1 and CA3 fields of the hippocampus were evaluated as well. The number of nerve cell profiles of the consecutive sections of the frontal cortex and of the hippocampus was corrected by the method of Abercrombie.[10]

Astrocyte Profile Density

OCT-embedded blocks of the right hemisphere were cut with a microtome cryostat at −20°C. Serial 10 μm thick sections were mounted on gelatin-coated microscope slides. The 4th, 8th, 12th, 16th, and 21st consecutive sections 20 μm apart were fixed for 1 h in a 4% paraformaldehyde solution in 0.1 M phosphate buffer (pH 7.4). Sections were rinsed several times in the same buffer at 4°C to remove excess of fixative and then exposed to a 0.3% normal sheep serum dissolved in 2% 10 mM phosphate-buffered 0.9% (w/v) saline (PBS)–Triton X100 overnight. The sections were then incubated for 48 h at 4°C with anti–glial fibrillary acidic protein (GFAP) antiserum (Boehringer Mannheim, Mannheim, Germany. Cat. No. 814369) diluted 1:3 with 2% PBS-Triton X100. After rinsing several times with 2% PBS-Triton X100 at room temperature in a biotinylated rabbit IgG diluted 1:100 with the above PBS-Triton X100, sections were then rinsed and exposed to avidin-biotin complex. The immunohistochemical reaction was then revealed using 3,3'-diaminobenzidine as a chromogen. Sections were then rinsed, dehydrated, and mounted in Entellan.

The density of astrocyte profiles within the frontal cortex and the pyramidal neuron layer (including the stratum oriens) of CA1 field of the hippocampus was evaluated by counting the number of GFAP-immunoreactive cell profiles in a 1 mm^2 area of the section observed at a final ×200 magnification. This area was delimited with the same image analyzer system described above for nerve cell density evaluation. Analysis was done on the 5 consecutive sections of the frontal cortex or of the hippocampus sampled as above indicated.

Sulfide/Silver (Zinc) Histochemistry

The 1st, 5th, 9th, 15th, and 20th consecutive frozen sections 20 μm apart of the hippocampus were processed for the histochemical detection of tissue zinc stores by incubating for 15 min in a sulfide silver medium containing 20% arabic gum, 5% citric acid, 2% hydroquinone, and 10% silver nitrate. Sections were then mounted in Entellan and viewed under a light microscope.

The density of sulfide silver staining within the mossy fibers area was assessed microdensitometrically. Measurements were performed using a ×40/0.95 immersion objective and a ×10 ocular in a circular area 10 μm in diameter. Microdensitometric determinations were made in 5 different areas of the mossy fibers randomly selected per slide (e.g., 25 measurements per area per subject). The intensity of the sulfide silver staining within the white matter of the frontal cortex (area within positive staining) was also measured to use this value as covariate.

Lipofuscin Accumulation

The 2nd, 6th, 10th, 14th, and 18th 10 μm thick consecutive frozen sections 20 μm apart of the frontal cortex or of the hippocampus were air dried and mounted in Entellan. These sections were observed and photographed using a LeitzOrtholux microscope equipped with an epifluorescence system with a mercury lamp HBO 100W as a fluorescence source and 390–490 nm and 515 nm filters. Tissue autofluorescence passed as a yellow-orange autofluorescence. Under these conditions, we define lipopigment as a tissue pigment exhibiting yellow to yellow-orange autofluorescence.

Pyramidal neurons of the frontal cortex and of the CA3 field were photographed with a 400 ASA Fujichrome Color film, using a ×63/oil-immersion objective and a ×10 ocular to obtain a final magnification at the camera of ×400. Prints were enlarged to 18 × 24 cm. The pyramidal neuron borders were delineated using a magnetic pen connected to a Videoplan image analyzer. The same system was used to delineate the area occupied by lipofuscin granules present in the cytoplasm of pyramidal neurons. The percentage of the area of nerve cell body occupied by lipofuscin was then calculated.

MAO-B Activity

The 3rd, 7th, 11th, and 17th 10 μm thick 20 μm apart consecutive frozen sections of the frontal cortex or of the hippocampus were air dried and processed for the histochemical demonstration of MAO-B activity according to the tetranitroblue tetrazolium and coupled peroxidase technique using tyramine as a substrate and 0.1 μM clorgyline to inhibit MAO-A activity.[11] The specificity of the reaction was assessed by incubating some control sections in a medium from which tyramine has been omitted. Incubation was done at 37°C for 2 h.

The intensity of MAO-B activity within the neuropil of the frontal cortex or the pyramidal neurons layer of the CA1 and CA3 fields of the hippocampus was assessed microdensitometrically using the microphotometric system above described. Measurements were made on 5 different portions of the CA1 or CA3 fields and of the frontal cortex randomly selected per slide (e.g., 20 measurements per field of hippocampus per subject), using a ×40/0.95 immersion objective and a ×10 ocular. Microdensitometric analysis was done by measuring the intensity of MAO-B staining in a circular area 8 μm in diameter. The intensity of MAO-B staining within the corpus callosum (area without positive reaction) was measured as well and taken as a covariate.

Data Analysis

Values for the individual subjects within the 4 animal groups investigated were means of measurements of the different parameters studied as indicated above. Group means were then determined from these individual means. Statistical analysis was performed by analysis of variance (ANOVA) for body and brain weight, nerve cell and astrocyte profiles and lipofuscin density. Analysis of covariance (ANOCOVA) was used for sulfide silver and MAO-B stainings. In this latter analysis, the intensities of the corpus callosum or the white matter of the frontal cortex staining were taken as covariate. The significance of differences between means was assessed with Duncan's multiple range test.

RESULTS

During the 5-month treatment period, 13% (2/15) of the control animals and 8% (2/24) of the L-deprenyl-treated animals died due to spontaneous pathology. This mortality rate is in agreement with the expected fatality for aged rats of this strain, although a trend towards an increase of survival time appears for the L-deprenyl-treated animals (data not shown). Body weight was increased in 24-month-old in comparison with 11-month-old rats. The lower dose (1.25 mg/kg per day) of L-deprenyl did not affect the body weight of aged rats, whereas the higher dose (5 mg/kg per day) slightly reduced body weight. Brain weight was increased in aged rats and was unaffected by L-deprenyl treatment (data not shown).

TABLE 1. Density of Nerve Cell and Astrocyte Profiles in the Rat Frontal Cortex and Hippocampus[a]

Subjects	n	Frontal Cortex	CA1 Field	CA3 Field	Dentate Gyrus
Nerve cell profiles					
Adult	15	880 ± 30.5	4169 ± 259	2880 ± 129	6764 ± 455
Old	13	460 ± 25.6^b	2980 ± 134^b	1924 ± 119^b	5136 ± 341^b
Old + 1.25 mg/kg per day L-deprenyl	11	500 ± 22.8^b	3124 ± 141^b	2200 ± 186^b	5580 ± 244^b
Old + 5 mg/kg per day L-deprenyl	11	610 ± 26.7^c	3764 ± 258^c	2376 ± 121^c	5972 ± 324^c
Astrocyte profiles					
Adult	15	52 ± 3.4	90 ± 3.2		
Old	13	75 ± 2.7^b	151 ± 9.6^b		
Old + 1.25 mg/kg per day L-deprenyl	11	70 ± 1.9^b	136 ± 6.2^b		
Old + 5 mg/kg per day L-deprenyl	11	65 ± 3.1^c	114 ± 4.6^c		

[a]Values are means ± standard error (SE) and represent the number of nerve cell and GFAP-immunoreactive astrocyte profiles measured in a 1 mm^2 area of the frontal cortex and of the different portions of the hippocampus as described in the Materials and Methods section.
[b]$p < 0.001$ vs. adult.
[c]$p < 0.01$ vs. old or old + 1.25 mg/kg per day L-deprenyl.

TABLE 1 shows the density of nerve cell profiles in the frontal cortex of the 4 animal groups examined. The density of nerve cell profiles was significantly reduced in old in comparison with adult rats. The dose of 1.25 mg/kg per day of L-deprenyl did not induce significant changes in nerve cell profiles density, whereas rats treated with 5 mg/kg per day had a significantly higher density of nerve cell profiles than age-matched untreated control rats.

The structure of CA3 field of the hippocampus in the 4 animal groups examined is shown in FIGURE 1, whereas the values of the density of nerve cell profiles in the hippocampus are summarized in TABLE 1. The density of nerve cell profiles was decreased in the CA1 and CA3 fields and in the dentate gyrus of hippocampus of 24-month-old rats in comparison with 12-month-old ones. There were not significant differences in density of nerve cell profiles in CA1 and CA3 fields between the group of aged rats treated with 1.25 mg/kg per day L-deprenyl and untreated old rats. In the aged rats treated with 5 mg/kg per day L-deprenyl, the density of nerve cell profiles

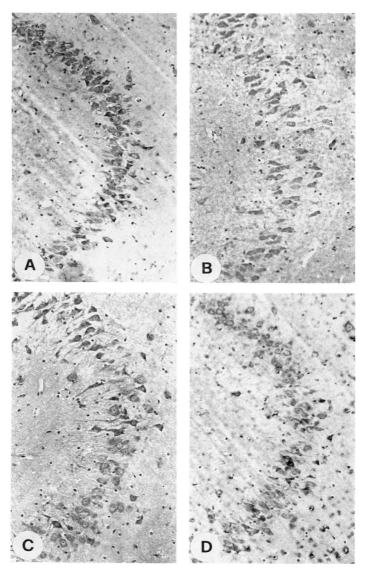

FIGURE 1. Micrographs of the CA3 field of the hippocampus of adult (A), old (B), old treated with 1.25 mg/kg per day L-deprenyl (C), and old treated with 5 mg/kg per day L-deprenyl (D). Toluidine blue. Note the decrease in the density of nerve cell profiles in old in comparison with adult rats. The density of nerve cell profiles is higher in old rats treated with 5 mg/kg per day L-deprenyl than in control old rats or in animals treated with the lower dose of L-deprenyl. (×85)

was significantly higher than in age-matched control rats. The area of the hippocampus most sensitive to L-deprenyl treatment was the CA1 field, while the least sensitive was the dentate gyrus (TABLE 1).

Immunoreactive astrocytes appeared as dark-brown cells primarily with a long and slender perikaryon with many different sized processes extending mainly vertically to the pial surface in the frontal cortex (FIGURE 2). The density of immunoreactive astroglial profiles is remarkably increased in old in comparison with adult rats (FIGURE 2). Moreover astrocytes of old rats develop thicker processes than those of adult animals (data not shown). In L-deprenyl-treated old rats, the density of astrocyte profiles is not changed in comparison with aged-matched control animals after administration of the 1.25 mg/kg per day dose, and is decreased after treatment with the 5 mg/kg per day dose (FIGURE 2). Similar findings were obtained in the hippocampus (TABLE 1).

Sections of rat hippocampus processed with the sulfide silver technique for the histochemical detection of tissue zinc stores developed a heavy dark-brown staining in the mossy fiber area. Aging is accompanied by a significant reduction of sulfide-silver staining within the mossy fibers (FIGURE 3). Treatment with both 1.25 and 5 mg/kg per day L-deprenyl countered in part the age-dependent decrease of sulfide silver staining in the mossy fibers (FIGURE 3). The effect was not dose related.

A faint yellow-orange lipopigment autofluorescence was observed in the cytoplasm of pyramidal neurons of the frontal cortex and of the CA3 field of adult rats (TABLE 2). A remarkable increase in lipofuscin deposition is noticeable in 24-month-old rats (TABLE 2). Treatment with 1.25 mg/kg per day or 5 mg/kg per day L-deprenyl reduced approximately to the same extent lipofuscin accumulation within the cytoplasm of pyramidal neurons of the frontal cortex or of the CA3 field of the hippocampus (TABLE 2).

Sections incubated for the histochemical detection of MAO-B activity developed a blue formazan staining within the frontal cortex and pyramidal neuron layers of the hippocampus. A significant increase of enzyme reactivity was observed in the frontal cortex and in the CA3 field of hippocampus of 24-month-old in comparison with 12-month-old rats (TABLE 2). Treatment with the 1.25 mg/kg per day dose of L-deprenyl was without significant effect on MAO-B reactivity both in the frontal cortex and in the CA3 field of the hippocampus, whereas the 5 mg/kg per day dose significantly decreased enzyme reactivity in the two cerebral areas.

DISCUSSION

A variety of age-dependent microanatomical changes occur in the mammalian frontal cortex and hippocampus in the process of aging. These changes include both regressive (nerve cell loss, dendritic spines reduction, mossy fiber impairment, microvascular changes) and progressive (lipofuscin accumulation, amyloid deposition, astrocyte hypertrophy, neurofibrillary tangles formation) alterations.[7,8] MAO-B is an enzyme involved in monoamine catabolism and selectively inhibited by low concentrations of L-deprenyl.[12] Experimental studies have reported that long-term treatment with L-deprenyl increased animal life span and improved sexual activity.[3] We have investigated consequently whether long-term treatment with L-deprenyl has any effect on some morphological changes occurring in frontal cortex and hippocampus of old rats. Two doses of L-deprenyl were used in the present study: the higher 5 mg/kg per day corresponding with the ED_{50} oral dose of L-deprenyl for cerebral MAO-B inhibition, and the lower (1.25 mg/kg per day) dose, which does not interfere with the cerebral enzyme.[13] The results of enzyme histochemical analysis

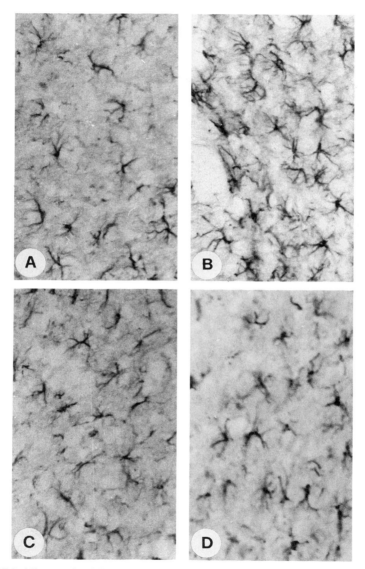

FIGURE 2. Micrographs of the frontal cortex of adult (A), old (B), old treated with 1.25 mg/kg per day L-deprenyl (C), and old treated with 5 mg/kg per day L-deprenyl (D). GFAP immunohistochemistry. GFAP-immunoreactive astrocyte profiles are more in old in comparison with adult rats. The higher dose of L-deprenyl causes a reduction in the density of GFAP-immunoreactive astrocyte profiles. (×120)

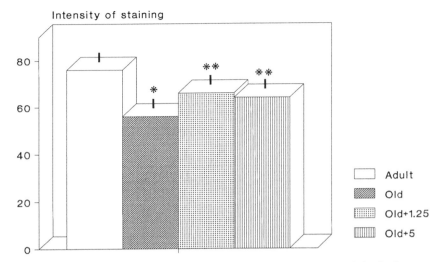

FIGURE 3. Microdensitometric analysis of the intensity of sulfide silver staining in the mossy fiber area in adult, old, and old rats treated with 1.25 mg/kg per day (Old + 1.25) or 5 mg/kg per day (Old + 5) L-deprenyl. Values are means ± standard error (SE) and are expressed in arbitrary units. *p < 0.001 vs. adult; **p < 0.01 vs. old.

performed on MAO-B reactivity in the rat frontal cortex and hippocampus confirmed that the two doses of L-deprenyl allow respectively inhibition of (5 mg/kg per day) and no effect on (1.25 mg/kg per day) MAO-B activity.

Both "physiologic" and "pathologic" aging are associated with nerve cell loss in brain. In this work, we have observed that the frontal cortex and CA1 and CA3 fields

TABLE 2. Surface Area of Pyramidal Neurons Occupied by Lipofuscin and Microdensitometry of MAO-B in the Frontal Cortex and in CA3 Field of the Hippocampus of Rats of Different Ages[a]

	n	Frontal Cortex	CA3 Field
Lipofuscin area			
Adult	15	17.8 ± 0.1	14.2 ± 0.6
Old	13	45.0 ± 1.3[c]	39.1 ± 1.5[c]
Old + 1.25 mg/kg per day L-deprenyl	11	31.6 ± 1.8[b]	29.2 ± 2.0[b]
Old + 5 mg/kg per day L-deprenyl	11	30.8 ± 1.8	25.3 ± 0.9
MAO-B			
Adult	15	16 ± 0.5	18 ± 1.3
Old	13	23 ± 1.5[c]	26 ± 0.5[c]
Old + 1.25 mg/kg per day L-deprenyl	11	24 ± 1.2[b]	23 ± 0.6[b]
Old + 5 mg/kg per day L-deprenyl	11	19 ± 0.7	20 ± 0.9

[a]Values are means ± SE and represent the percentage area of a neuron occupied by lipofuscin or the intensity of enzymatic of MAO-B (expressed in arbitrary units) in the frontal cortex and in CA3 field of the hippocampus. Results were obtained as described in the Material and Methods section.
[b]p < 0.01 vs. adult.
[c]p < 0.001 vs. adult.

of the hippocampus or the dentate gyrus lose nerve cells from the adult to old age in Sprague-Dawley rats. Similar findings were reported by other authors.[7] The density of nerve cell profiles in 3 key areas of hippocampal formation, the CA1 and CA3 fields and the dentate gyrus, represents one of the most extensively investigated topics in neurogerontological research. Although the subject of age-dependent neuroanatomical changes is debated, there is an agreement among investigators about the occurrence of a neuronal loss in hippocampus of mammalian species investigated including man.[7,14] The higher dose of L-deprenyl administration partially counters the neuron loss in rat frontal cortex and in hippocampus. This suggests that long-term treatment with a dosage of inhibition on MAO-B activity slows the age-dependent nerve cell loss in the frontal cortex and the hippocampus.

Parallel with decreased neuronal density, we have observed both hypertrophic and hyperplastic changes of GFAP-immunoreactive astroglial cells in the frontal cortex and hippocampus of aged rats. Hypertrophy of astrocytes has been reported in the hippocampus of aged memory-deficient rats,[15] and both astrocyte hypertrophy and hyperplasia were found in the rat hippocampus as a function of age.[16] This observation is also consistent with enzyme histochemistry data showing an increased expression of MAO-B, which is an enzyme located primarily in astrocytes,[17] in the frontal cortex and the hippocampus of the 24-month-old rat. Moreover, increases in GFAP-containing astrocytes and astrogliosis have been described in Alzheimer's disease and in other neurodegenerative disorders.[18] In our experiment, a higher dose L-deprenyl treatment, which inhibits MAO-B activity, attenuated hypertrophy and hyperplasia of astrocytes in old rats. The dose inactive on MAO-B activity was without effect.

The density of sulfide silver reactive fibers may have some relevance from a morphofunctional point of view. Sulfide silver technique stains primarily vesicular zinc stores in the intrahippocampal associative pathway of mossy fibers (see Reference 19), which are impaired in aging rats as well as passive avoidance responses (see Reference 19). The findings that doses of L-deprenyl affecting or not affecting MAO-B restore in part the density of sulfide silver staining in the mossy fiber area of hippocampus suggest that the compound "per se" may have some influence on the hippocampal circuitry involved in passive avoidance behavior. Along this line, our recent studies show that the compound reversed cognitive impairment in tasks exploring hippocampal function in aged rats.[4]

Intracytoplasmic lipofuscin accumulation probably is one of the best known age-related changes in postmitotic cells.[21] Several drugs or dietary factors have been claimed to have some influence on lipofuscin accumulation in nerve cells.[21] The main source of intracellular lipofuscin is probably represented by lysosomes. As to the nature and composition of lipofuscin, it is hypothesized that they derive from the peroxidative action of the free radicals on membrane lipids.[21] However, in spite of the extensive studies on the possible significance of lipofuscin deposition within neurons, the role of the lipopigment in the pathophysiology of the nerve cell has not been yet clarified.[21,22] L-Deprenyl administration at both dosages inhibiting and not inhibiting MAO-B reduced lipofuscin accumulation within the cytoplasm of pyramidal neurons of the hippocampus and frontal cortex in rats. This effect was not dose dependent, and is probably not related to the inhibition of MAO-B activity elicited by L-deprenyl.

Taken together, the above results obtained by neurohistological, immunocyto-chemical, and histochemical techniques suggest that long-term oral administration of L-deprenyl is able to counter some microanatomical changes of the aging frontal cortex and hippocampus in the rat. The improvement of the neuronal density and attenuation of the astroglial hyperplasia are probably related to the MAO-B inhibitory activity of L-deprenyl; whereas the effects on mossy fibers and lipofuscin accumulation do not seem to depend on inhibiting enzyme activity. The functional and clinical relevance of these observations should be clarified in future studies.

SUMMARY

The present study was designed to assess the influence of long term L-deprenyl treatment on some microanatomical parameters of aging rat frontal cortex and hippocampus. Male Sprague-Dawley rats of 19 months of age were divided into three groups. Rats of the first group received an oral daily dose of 1.25 mg/kg L-deprenyl; animals of the second group were treated with an oral daily dose of 5 mg/kg L-deprenyl, whereas rats of the third group were left untreated and used as control. Treatment lasted for 5 months, and rats were sacrificed at 24 months. At this age they were considered to be old. Another group of 11-month-old rats was used as an adult reference group. The density of nerve cell profiles and of glial fibrillary acidic protein (GFAP) immunoreactive astrocytes was decreased and increased respectively in the frontal cortex and in the different portions of the hippocampus in old in comparison with adult rats. A decrease in the intensity of sulfide silver staining in the mossy fibers of the hippocampus was also observed in old rats. Moreover, a cytoplasmatic accumulation of lipofuscin was noticeable in old rats as well as a significant increase of the monoamine-oxidase (MAO) B reactivity both in the frontal cortex and in the hippocampus. A higher density of nerve cell profiles, of sulfide silver staining, and fewer astrocyte profiles were noticeable in the frontal cortex and in the hippocampus of old rats treated with 5 mg/kg/day of L-deprenyl. This dose of the compound also significantly reduced lipofuscin accumulation and MAO-B reactivity in old rats. However, the lower dose of the compound did not cause any statistically significant effect on the microanatomical parameters investigated with the exception of sulfide silver staining and lipofuscin accumulation, which were increased and decreased respectively after 1.25 mg/kg per day of L-deprenyl. The above results suggest that long-term treatment with L-deprenyl is able to counter some microanatomical changes typical of the aging frontal cortex and hippocampus in the rat. These changes seem to be in part related to the MAO-B inhibitory activity of L-deprenyl.

ACKNOWLEDGMENTS

The authors are greatly indebted to Ms. S. Beatty for the critical revision of the manuscript and Mrs. T. Bolzoni and G. Bonelli for their expert technical assistance.

REFERENCES

1. GOTTFRIES, C. G., L. ORELAND, A. WIBERG & B. WINDBLAD. 1975. Lowered monoamine oxidase activity in brains from alcoholic suicides. J. Neurochem. **25:** 667–673.
2. STROLIN-BENEDETTI, M. & P. E. KEANE. 1980. Deferential changes in monoamine oxidase A and B activity in the aging rat brain. J. Neurochem. **35:** 1026–1032.
3. KNOLL, J., J. DALLO & T. T. YEN. 1989. Striatal dopamine, sexual activity and lifespan. Longevity of rats treated with (−) deprenyl. Life Sci. **45:** 525–531.
4. BRANDEIS, R., M. SAPIR, Y. KAPON, G. BORELLI, S. CADEL & B. VALSECCHI. 1991. Improvement of cognitive function by MAO-B inhibitor L-deprenyl in aged rats. Pharmacol. Biochem. Behav. **39:** 297–304.

5. TARIOT, P. N., T. SUNDERLAND, H. WEINGARTNER, D. L. MURPHY, J. A. WELKOWITZ, K. THOMPSON & R. M. COHEN. 1987. Cognitive effects of L-deprenyl in Alzeimer's disease. Psychopharmacology **91:** 489–495.
6. MANGONI, A., M. P. GRASSI, L. FRATTOLA, R. PIOLTI, A. MOTTA, A. MARCONE & S. SMIRNE. 1991. Effects of a MAO-B inhibitor in the treatment of Alzeimer disease. Eur. Neurol. **31:** 100–107.
7. FLOOD, D. G. & P. D. COLEMAN. 1988. Neuron numbers and sizes in ageing brain: comparisons of human, monkey and rodent data. Neurobiol. Aging **9:** 453–463.
8. BLACKWOOD, W. & J. A. N. CORSELLIS. 1976. Greenfield's Neuropathology. Arnold. London, England.
9. AMENTA, F., D. ZACCHEO & W. L. COLLIER. 1991. Neurotransmitters, neuroreceptors and aging. Mech. Aging Dev. **61:** 249–273.
10. ABERCROMBIE, M. 1946. Estimation of nuclear populations from microtome sections. Anat. Rec. **94:** 239–247.
11. UCHIDA, E. & G. B. KOELLE. 1984. Histochemical investigation of criteria for the distinction between monoamine oxidase A and B in various species. J. Histochem. Cytochem. **32:** 667–673.
12. GERLACH, M., P. RIEDERER & M. B. H. YOUDIM. 1992. The molecular pharmacology of L-deprenyl. Eur. J. Pharmacol. **226:** 97–108.
13. FOZARD, J. R., M. ZREIKA, M. ROBIN & M. G. PALFREYMAN. 1985. The functional consequences L-deprenyl and MDL 72145. Naunyn-Schmiedeberg's Arch. Pharmacol. **331:** 186–193.
14. NAPOLEONE, P., F. FERRANTE, O. GHIRARDI, M. T. RAMACCI & F. AMENTA. 1990. Age-dependent nerve cell loss in the brain of Sprague-Dawley rats. Effect of long term acetyl-L-carnitine treatment. Arch. Gerontol. Geriatr. **10:** 173–185.
15. LANDFIELD, P. W., G. ROSE, L. SANDLES, T. C. WOHLSTADTER & G. LYNCH. 1977. Patterns of astroglial hypertrophy and neuronal degeneration in the hippocampus of aged, memory-deficient rats. J. Gerontol. **12:** 3–12.
16. LOLOVA, I. 1991. Qualitative and quantitative glial changes in the hippocampus of aged rats. Anat. Anz. **172:** 263–271.
17. LEVITT, P., J. E. PINTAR & X. O. BREAKEFIELD. 1982. Immunocytochemical demonstration of monoamine oxidase B in brain astrocytes and serotonergic neurons. Proc. Natl. Acad. Sci. USA **79:** 6385–6389.
18. FREDERICKSON, R. C. A. 1992. Astroglia in Alzheimer's disease. Neurobiol. Aging **13:** 239–253.
19. RICCI, A., M. T. RAMACCI, O. GHIRARDI & F. AMENTA. 1989. Age-related changes of the mossy fibre system in rat hippocampus: effect of long term acetyl-L-carnitine treatment. Arch. Gerontol. Geriatr. **8:** 63–71.
20. KONIG, F. R. & R. H. KLIPPEL. 1963. The rat brain: a stereotoxic atlas. Krieger. New York, N.Y.
21. DOWSON, J. H. & H. WILTON-COX. 1988. The effect of drugs on neuronal lipopigment. *In* Lipofuscin-1987: State of the Art. I. Zs.-Nagy, Ed.: 271–288. Elsevier. Amsterdam, the Netherlands.
22. DORMANDY, T. L. 1982. Free radicals and lipopigments. *In* Ceroid Lipofuscinosis (Batten's Diseases). D. Armstron, N. Koppang & J. A. Rider, Eds.: 345–349. Elsevier. Amsterdam, the Netherlands.

Effects of L-Deprenyl on Manifestations of Aging in the Rat and Dog

GWEN O. IVY, JOHN T. RICK, M. PAUL MURPHY,
ELIZABETH HEAD, CHRIS REID, AND N. W. MILGRAM

Department of Psychology
University of Toronto
Scarborough Campus
1265 Military Trail
Scarborough, Ontario M1C 1A4 Canada

The possibility of extending average and maximum life span in experimental animals, with the eventual goal of applying these procedures to humans, has been studied extensively. Various drug strategies have been tried, the most notable being the administration of antioxidants such as vitamin E. However, as a whole, drug therapies to counteract aging have proved disappointing, with restriction of caloric intake remaining the only way to consistently prolong life.[1-4]

L-Deprenyl (DPR), a potent MAO-B inhibitor, has been shown to extend both mean and maximum life span in rats[5-9] and in patients in the early stages of Parkinson's disease receiving concurrent L-dopa therapy.[10,11] There is some evidence to suggest that DPR is capable of enhancing cognitive function in rats, particularly in tasks that show an age-related decline.[7,12,13] There has also been some suggestion of cognitive improvement in humans.[14,15]

This paper is a review of three separate long-term studies on the effects of chronic DPR administration on a number of survival, biochemical, and behavioral measures. Our first study (experiment I) examined the effects of subcutaneous (sc) injection of DPR on longevity, body weight, blood serum chemistry, and behavioral tests (open field, water maze) in aged (≥ 23 months) male Fischer 344 (F344) rats. Experiment II examined the effects of DPR on behavior in the open field and water maze and on various neurological tests at ages ≥ 17 months in both male and female F344 rats. These animals received the drug intragastrically, which more closely approximates the pattern of intake in humans. Biochemical measurements of rat brain and liver MAO-A and B activity indicated that the dose and mode of administration used in this study resulted in a level of MAO-B inhibition similar to that produced by sc injection in experiment I.[16] Our third study employed four male and female purebred beagle dogs (aged 8–10 years) and one pound-source dog (aged 1.5 years) to determine if orally administered DPR would improve short-term spatial memory, which is known to decline with age. The dog was chosen for the study because this species exhibits age-related neuroanatomical and behavioral changes similar to those seen in humans.

SUBJECTS AND DRUG ADMINISTRATION

All subjects in experiment I were male F344 rats for whom treatment began at 23–24 months and continued until the end of the experiment, and were equally divided amonge saline (SAL) and DPR groups ($n = 66$ each). Half of these animals received frequent tests in the open field beginning at 23 months. Water maze testing was carried out on a different group of animals at ages 26 and 29 months (3 and 6 months of treatment, respectively), with additional untreated control groups aged 7–8 and 23 months (n per group = 7–12). Drug subjects received 0.25 mg/kg DPR dissolved in 0.85% SAL (1 mg/ml) by sc injection three times per week, while controls were administered an equivalent volume of SAL.

Subjects in experiment II were F344 rats of both sexes, aged 14–15 months at the start of the experiment. The drug was administered by intragastric gavage three times per week at a dose of 1 mg/kg DPR in 0.85% SAL (0.25 mg/ml) until the end of the study. Controls received the same volume of SAL.

Dogs in experiment III received a single oral dose (0–1.5 mg/kg in 6 levels) of DPR in tablet form once each morning. As noted above, the subjects were 4 purebred beagles aged 8–10 years and one pound dog aged approximately 1.5 years (estimated from dentition). Other details relating to animal care have been published elsewhere.[17]

SURVIVAL, BODY WEIGHT, AND BLOOD CHEMISTRY (EXP. I)

Method

Half of the 132 subjects in this portion of the experiment had blood samples taken at age 24–25 months for serum chemistry analysis; the other half were tested monthly for sexual behavior (data not reported) and spontaneous activity in the open field beginning at about 23 months of age. No other tests were conducted with these subjects. Our procedures and data analysis methods have been published elsewhere.[8]

Results

The DPR-treated animals survived 16% longer than our controls (calculated from start of treatment), a significant increase in mean and maximum survival time that was not due to self-induced dietary restriction, as body weights remained significantly higher in DPR- than in SAL-treated rats.

The only blood serum measure that differed between the two groups after 3 months of drug administration was blood urea nitrogen, with values being significantly lower in the DPR group, possibly indicating greater maintenance of kidney function in old age. Although necropsies and histological analyses of tissues were performed, no differences in cause of death were found between the two groups.

Discussion

While the differences in survival due to DPR were not large, it should be noted that 24 months is approximately the mean survival time of this rat strain.[18] In addition, a number of our rats already had tumors, cataracts, and kidney problems at the beginning of the study. We suspected that starting drug administration at an earlier age might produce greater effects, and so these findings provided the rationale for using younger subjects in experiment II.

DEPRENYL AND SPONTANEOUS ACTIVITY IN THE OPEN FIELD (EXP. I)

Method

Subjects were the same male F344 rats as those used for survival, body weight, and blood chemistry. A 10-minute open field test was administered once per month beginning at 23 months of age and continuing until death or termination of the experiment (7 months later). Testing was conducted in an open-field arena (75 × 75 × 30 cm) constructed of unstained, sealed plywood and divided into 25 equal squares. The behavior of the animals was observed directly and recorded using an IBM PC–compatible computer and software developed in our lab. Testing was conducted in a normally lit room during the light phase of the animals' cycle. Variables measured included number of squares entered, number of rears and defecations, and total time spent in grooming behaviors.

Results

Analysis of variance revealed a main effect of age on all measures (confounded with time on drug and repeated testing). Activity decreased over the first 6 sessions, possibly as a result of habituation, then increased again after 7 months of testing, perhaps due to a handling effect. Time spent grooming and number of defecations decreased over the first 4 sessions then increased almost to baseline levels. DPR resulted in an increase in square crossings and number of rears, but only on the third test (at 26 months of age). The DPR-treated rats did not differ significantly on any other measure or test session.

Discussion

DPR-treated rats exhibited a temporary increase in spontaneous activity relative to SAL counterparts after 3 months of treatment (26 months of age). No other drug effects were noted. This suggests that DPR may have certain effects that take some time to manifest themselves yet that are transient in nature (one of the metabolites of DPR is L-amphetamine). This increase in activity in the DPR rats at 26 months of age may also be related to the impairment observed in the water maze at same age.

EFFECTS OF DEPRENYL ON MOTOR FUNCTION AND NOVELTY-INDUCED BEHAVIOR IN THE RAT (EXP. II)

In order to determine if chronic treatment with DPR attenuated the age-associated decline in motor function, a series of neurological tests (NTs) was administered, while spontaneous activity was evaluated in an open-field arena. Total distance and rearing behavior were used to assess locomotor/exploratory activity, while grooming and defecation were used as a behavioral assay of stress.[19,20]

Method

Male and female F344 rats (*n* = 40) were observed in an open-field as in experiment I. Testing lasted 10 minutes during the light phase of the animals' activity cycle (3 PM–8 PM) and was repeated over 3 consecutive days. After each open field session, the animals were given one of 3 NTs to assess overall motor function: wire suspension, horizontal bar, or inclined plane (adapted from References 21 and 22). Over the course of the 3 days of testing, each animal received all 3 tests in counterbalanced order.

Results

None of the three NTs revealed any significant effects of age, sex, or drug (data not shown). Neither did DPR have any effect on locomotor/exploratory activity under the conditions of this experiment. Normal habituation was obvious for both total distance (FIGURE 1A) and rearing (FIGURE 1B), measures that were highly correlated ($r = 0.83, p < 0.001$).

DPR did not affect defecation, but did influence grooming behavior, which increased significantly with age. The older animals groomed more on all three test sessions, while the mature animals exhibited clear habituation (FIGURE 2A). Overall, females groomed more than males. However, DPR differentially affected grooming in each sex, producing an increase in the males but having no effect on the females (FIGURE 2B).

Discussion

The NTs used here have been shown to detect the age-related decline in motor performance in both mice[23] and rats,[21,22] yet were unsuccessful in detecting any such differences in this experiment. However, these age differences are usually observed between fairly young (about 3 months) and relatively old (26+ months) animals. It is possible that either the age difference between the two groups was not large enough or the number of subjects was too small.

DPR has been shown to increase locomotor activity in rats,[12,24–26] dogs,[27] and man[28] using doses comparable to or lower than those used in this study. We have observed increases in locomotor/exploratory behavior in the rat at higher doses using this paradigm (10 mg/kg oral; unpublished observations). It may be that the dosing schedule (1.0 mg/kg oral, 3 times/week) minimized accumulation of DPR's amphetamine metabolites, which are the most likely source for any observed increases in activity.

Rats will often exhibit increased grooming when placed in a novel environment,[20] with older rats showing a greater increase than younger animals, possibly reflecting an elevated response to this form of mild stress.[29,30] The dopaminergic system is thought to be a critical regulator of grooming behavior in the rat.[20] DPR might affect grooming by altering the relative tone of the dopaminergic system in the rat either through elevated levels of DA[31,32] or 2-phenylethylamine.[33] Any such changes must be small, however, since we did not observe any increases in locomotor activity. The lack of a similar effect in the female rat may be related to DPR's differential effectiveness in the two sexes at this dose.[16]

EFFECTS OF DEPRENYL ON SPATIAL LEARNING IN THE WATER MAZE (EXP. I)

The Morris water maze (WM) is a common test of spatial learning in studies with aged rats. It consists of placing the subject into a tank of water containing a

1A

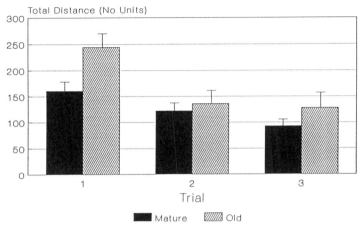

1B

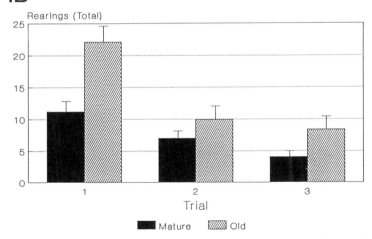

FIGURE 1. Habituation of activity over three consecutive testing days in the open field, as shown by (A) total distance traveled, and (B) total number of rearings. Both of these measures are highly correlated ($r = 0.83, p < 0.001$). Habituation effects are clear for both age groups in each case (distance and rearing; both $p < 0.001$). Mature (17–18 months) and old (24–25 months) animals were treated for 2 and 9 months, respectively.

2A

2B

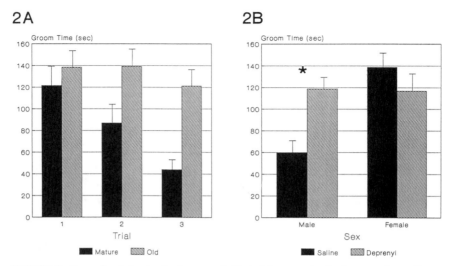

FIGURE 2. Grooming behavior in the open field. **A:** Mature animals show an almost linear habituation effect ($p < 0.001$), while older animals show either little or none ($p < 0.50$). **B:** Deprenyl increases grooming in male rats ($p < 0.0005$) but not females ($p < 0.15$). Females also groom more than males overall ($p < 0.05$).

submerged platform, which the animal must locate and climb onto in order to escape. As there are no intramaze cues, accurate performance on this test depends upon the rat's ability to orient itself relative to distal stimuli. It is generally preferable to active or passive avoidance or hunger-motivated tests as it does not require the use of stressful shocks or food deprivation.[34] A sizable literature indicates that aged animals may be impaired in acquisition, reversal, and/or retention of this task (e.g., References 35 and 36).

Method

Our version of the WM is a galvanized steel tank, 2 m in diameter and 1 m high, which is filled with water (25 ± 1 C) sufficient to submerge a 20 cm high Plexiglas® platform (20 cm diameter) by 2–3 cm. The rats are placed into the water at any one of 7 randomly determined starting locations spaced evenly along an arc approximately 1 m from the platform, which is located 0.375 m from the wall of the tank. The subjects have up to 90 s to locate and escape onto the platform (animals that fail to escape within the allotted time are guided to it) and then remain there for an additional 30 s. Upon completion of the trial, subjects are removed, toweled off, and then returned to their waiting cages under a heat lamp until the beginning of the next trial, 25–35 minutes after the start of the previous one.

SAL rats were tested in the water maze at 23 months ($n = 12$), 26 months ($n = 9$), and 29 months ($n = 7$) of age. Young untreated control subjects were obtained at 6–7 months of age ($n = 9$) and tested in the water maze one month later. The DPR subjects were tested in the water maze at 26 ($n = 9$) and 29 months ($n = 8$). Animals were given 10 trials per day for 3 days or until they reached a criterion of 4 out of 5 consecutive trials with escape latencies of 25 s or less. Five days later they received two 120 s free-swim (no platform) retention trials and then immediately began the next phase of acquisition, in which the platform was moved 120° around the tank. Three acquisition sessions were administered, each separated by five days, and five days after the last session the animals received two additional retention trials.

Results

The 29-month-old SAL rats showed significant deterioration in spatial learning ability relative to younger subjects as measured by trials to criterion (TTC), performing at near-asymptotic levels throughout the experiment (FIGURE 3). All other SAL

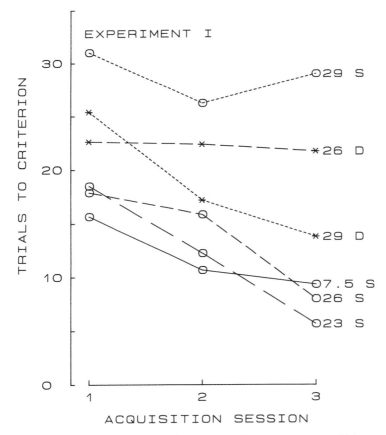

FIGURE 3. Trials to criterion scores on three consecutive water maze acquisition sessions (reversals) in experiment I. TTC scores for saline rats are labeled with circles and "S"; the Deprenyl animals' scores are labeled with asterisks and "D." Numbers to the right of each line indicate the age of the subjects. Error bars not shown for clarity.

rats demonstrated comparable declarative (location of the platform within an acquisition session) and procedural (improvement between sessions) learning. On the retention trials, the number of passes through the platform location was significantly affected by age, with older subjects making fewer such "contacts," but in general all animals improved with repeated testing. The DPR rats performed more poorly than SAL subjects at 26 months of age on both measures, but better at 29 months.

Swim speed on the retention trials also decreased with advancing age. In parallel with the TTC results, the DPR rats swam somewhat more slowly than did SAL animals at 26 months of age, but better at 29 months (though these differences were not statistically significant). Overall, swim speed was correlated with performance in the preceding acquisition session ($r = 0.52$–0.61, all $p < 0.01$), accounting for over one-third of the total variance in TTC. For the DPR animals, speed on the retention trials was only moderately correlated with TTC ($r = 0.06$–0.39, all $p > 0.10$), though this may be due in part to the higher percentage of animals performing at asymptotic levels in the DPR group.

Discussion

With this particular testing procedure, age-related impairments in spatial learning in the WM were not significant until approximately 29 months of age, well beyond the median life span (24–26 months) for this strain of rat,[18] though significant decreases in swim speed may begin to occur at 23–26 months of age. That swim speed on the SAL rats' retention trials accounts for approximately one-third of the variance in TTC on the preceding acquisition session suggests that this may be an important performance factor to control for in subsequent studies.

DPR produced fairly consistent, though minimal, effects. The DPR animals were slightly impaired at 26 months relative to SAL subjects on TTC and number of platform contacts. This suggests that chronic DPR treatment may produce some impairment in spatial learning. However, DPR rats at this age tested in the open field entered more squares and reared more often, suggesting that there is a difference in activity levels between SAL and DPR subjects (possibly due to elevated levels of the DPR metabolite amphetamine) that may be observed a few months after the start of drug treatment. The 29-month-old DPR animals, on the other hand, showed an *improvement* relative to their SAL counterparts, suggesting that the impairment, whatever its basis, was transient (with a duration of less than three months) and that DPR does have some beneficial effects on cognitive ability at advanced ages.

DEPRENYL AND SPATIAL LEARNING IN THE WATER MAZE (EXP. II)

Method

Our second experiment differed somewhat from the first in several respects. First, we tested both male and female rats, aged 17, 20, and 23 months ($n = 60$). The swim speed data from experiment I suggested to us that performance variables (such as reduced thermotolerance[36,37] and/or heightened swim stress[38]) might play a significant role in WM acquisition, and so we tested the subjects under two intertrial interval (ITI) conditions. The "massed" animals were tested 3–5 minutes after the start of the previous trial, while the "spaced" animals were subjected to our standard procedure of 25–35 minutes from the start of one trial to the beginning of the next. All animals were allowed at least one minute in their waiting cages between trials. We also gave each animal a fixed 30 trials at 5 trials per day for 6 days, rather than testing to a criterion, though we did calculate TTC for each subject in order to facilitate comparisons across experiments. As we did not actually test the subjects to a criterion, we did not administer any retention tests.

Results

The massed subjects had higher overall escape latencies than spaced animals at 20 and 23 months, but not at 17 months of age. The DPR rats were slightly impaired on this measure, though this seemed to be due to a tendency for these rats to have somewhat higher latencies on day 1 (significant only for trial 2). Female rats performed somewhat better than males, especially at more advanced ages. The TTC measure produced similar results, that is, the massed rats showed an age-related increase in TTC that was not seen in the spaced animals (FIGURE 4). DPR subjects had slightly higher TTC, though this is not surprising given that they had higher latencies on day 1, and TTC is essentially a latency-based measure.

The majority of the effects seen in the previous analyses were paralleled by results from the analysis of the swim speed measure. The correlation between swim speed and swim distance (a purer measure of spatial learning than TTC) ranges from −0.42 (SAL) to −0.50 (DPR). This similarity in the pattern of results for speed as well as measures of acquisition suggests that most of the observed effects may be attributable at least in part to differences in performance (as in experiment I).

Discussion

The TTC, latency, and distance measures were strongly affected by age and ITI. Older rats acquired the test more slowly, as did massed animals. Spaced subjects performed similarly at all ages tested, and at roughly the same level as the 7- to 8-month-old animals in experiment I. DPR appeared to have a slight effect on WM acquisition, though this could largely be accounted for by differences in latency on the first day of testing. The effects of DPR in this experiment were minimal, opposite to the predicted direction, and may be due to a reduction in swim speed relative to SAL animals.

In contrast to the results of experiment I, DPR had little or no effect on WM performance in experiment II. Our results with DPR in the WM are unclear, suggesting either no effect on spatial learning or a transient impairment followed by an improvement. Performance factors, such as swim speed and intertrial interval, may be important variables to control for in subsequent studies. Age at start of treatment may also be relevant. As well, the subjects in the two experiments received different doses of DPR by different methods, and since the doses in the two experiments were equated for amount of brain MAO inhibition, it is possible that route of administration may be a critical variable. Finally, the subjects in experiment II were younger than those in the first study, and it is therefore possible that significant effects of DPR on WM performance and/or learning might only be seen in very old animals.

EFFECTS OF ORAL ADMINISTRATION OF DEPRENYL ON SPATIAL MEMORY IN THE DOG (EXP. III)

Memory dysfunction is a well-known concomitant of aging in humans,[39] and as a result, there has been considerable interest in developing animal models to study both the phenomenon and possible interventions.[40] We have recently reported that

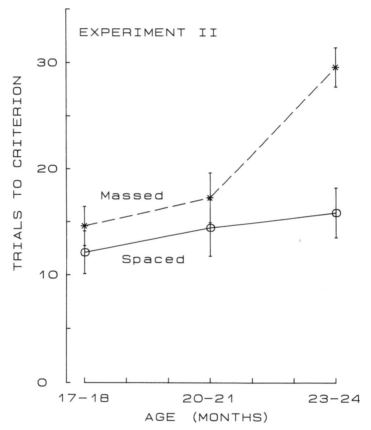

FIGURE 4. Water maze trials to criterion scores for massed (3–5 minute intertrial interval) and spaced (25–35 minute intertrial interval) rats in experiment II. Vertical bars denote standard error of the mean.

dogs can serve as a model of age-dependent cognitive deterioration based on performance in tests of object discrimination reversal and recognition memory. We have now extended these findings to age-dependent deficits in spatial learning,[17] and as part of this larger study, a pilot study was implemented to observe the effects of DPR on spatial short-term memory.

Spatial short-term memory is the ability to remember the location of an object in the environment for a restricted period of time. The most common techniques for measuring short-term spatial memory ability in the primate are the delayed matching or nonmatching to sample (DNMS) paradigms.[41-43] Animals are exposed to a sample presentation consisting of the "to be remembered" information, a delay interval, and then a test in which the animal is given the opportunity to demonstrate that it has recalled the information presented previously.

Method

All dogs had been previously tested on several nonspatial visual tasks including reward approach learning, object approach learning, discrimination learning, and reversal learning. These and subsequent spatial DNMS tests used a canine version of the Wisconsin General Test Apparatus. A detailed description of the subjects' previous experience, the apparatus, and the method of data collection has been published elsewhere.[17]

In the "sample" phase of the DNMS procedure, the subject was required to displace a red plastic Lego® block presented on either the left or right side of a tray in order to obtain a reward (approximately 1.5 g of lean ground beef rolled into a small ball). A delay interval followed, during which the tray was removed from sight of the dog and a meatball was placed in the well on the side opposite the location of the sample. Afterward, the tray was again presented, this time with identical red plastic Lego® blocks covering both the left and right wells. To obtain the reward, the dog had to recall the side which had been previously rewarded and choose the opposite side. Otherwise an error was recorded and the tray was withdrawn with no reward given. Dogs were initially trained on the DNMS task with a 10-second delay interval and were given 10 trials per day until they attained a criterion of 8/10 correct 2 days in a row or 9/10 correct in one day. Animals were then trained with a 20-second delay and, after criterion was reached in that condition, a 30-second delay.

Upon completion of the acquisition phase of the spatial memory task, the animals began the variable delay tests. The procedure was as previously outlined except that the delay between sample and test trials was varied randomly. The delays used in this phase were 20, 70, or 110 seconds, with each delay occurring four times in each daily session of 12 trials. Animals were tested for a minimum of two weeks on this phase prior to oral dosing with DPR.

Over the course of the experiment, the dogs received 6 doses of DPR ranging from 0 to 1.5 mg/kg orally, either in order of ascending or descending dose. Testing with variable delays was conducted for 5 days at each dose level, with each change in dose level preceded by a 2 day wash-in period. At the end of drug testing, a one week wash-out period was followed by one week of behavioral testing with a placebo. A placebo score (the average of baseline and wash-out scores combined) was calculated for each dog. The number of correct responses was divided by the number of trials completed for each delay and dose level. To determine the effect of DPR on spatial memory in the four old dogs, a score based on the percent change from baseline was used.

Results

On baseline tests, the performance of the four aged dogs decreased in accuracy with the increased memory demands. At the 20-second delay, all 4 dogs scored at least 85% correct. At the 70-second delay, accuracy ranged from 70 to 85% correct, while performance at the 110-second delay ranged from 50 to 70% correct. The young dog performed at less than 70% correct across all delays but appeared to have attentional difficulties (Head, personal observation).

DPR improved performance of the aged dogs at the longest delay interval (110 seconds) in a dose-dependent fashion (FIGURE 5). At the shortest delay, the effect of DPR was minimal, suggesting that DPR had no effect on the ability of the animals to

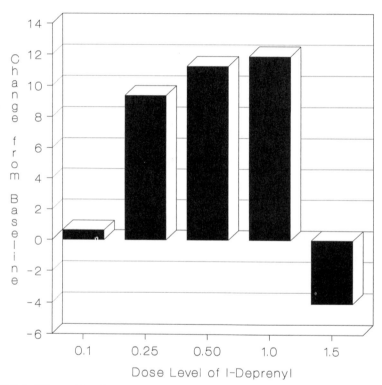

FIGURE 5. Effects of five doses of deprenyl on a spatial delayed nonmatch to sample memory test with a 110-second delay interval. The y-axis shows the average percent improvement of 4 dogs relative to performance in the placebo condition.

carry out the motor demands of the task. Performance at the intermediate delay was surprising in that in most cases there was a decrement in response accuracy. The young dog showed no improvement at any dose.

Discussion

DPR improved spatial short-term memory in a dose-dependent manner in four aged dogs, but had no effect on the performance of the single young dog. The drug improved performance at the longest delay (the most demanding), while the short delay (the least demanding) was relatively unaffected. The doses used were well below those previously shown to have an amphetamine-like effect on spontaneous behavior.[27]

Though the number of subjects used was too small for statistical analyses, there is a strong indication that DPR can improve short-term spatial memory in the aged animal and further studies are suggested.

SUMMARY AND GENERAL DISCUSSION

From these three studies, we draw several conclusions:

1. F344 rats treated with DPR as late as 24 months of age have significantly increased mean and maximum life spans relative to SAL-treated counterparts. This improvement is not a consequence of self-induced dietary restriction but may in part be due to maintenance of renal function.
2. While DPR did not affect performance on any of our three neurological tests, locomotor/exploratory activity was transiently increased in experiment I but not in experiment II. This is possibly related to the presence of metabolites such as amphetamine and/or to mode of drug administration. In addition, an increase in grooming behavior was observed in DPR-treated males in experiment II.
3. In experiment I, DPR-treated rats performed more poorly in the water maze after 3 months of treatment but performed significantly better than their SAL-treated counterparts after 6 months of treatment. It is possible that an adaptive period for the drug exists. In experiment II, we found that old rats performed much better in the water maze when given longer intertrial intervals. DPR treatment resulted in slight reductions in swim speed in both studies.
4. While the number of subjects in experiment III is too small for statistical analysis, our results thus far indicate that at least some elderly dogs can benefit greatly from DPR in performance of spatial tasks requiring short-term memory.

We conclude that, overall, DPR has some beneficial effects in both old rats and old dogs.

While the mechanisms of action of DPR are not totally understood, intriguing findings by Knoll's[6] and Kitani's[44–47] labs indicate that appropriate doses of DPR elevate levels of the free radical scavengers superoxide dismutase (SOD) and catalase (CAT) in certain brain regions. It is thus tempting to speculate that the elevated levels of free radical scavengers may be responsible for retarding some of the biochemical effects of aging and thus for prolonging life in both animals and in Parkinson's patients. However, Tatton[48,49] has recently found that levels of DPR that are too low to inhibit MAO B (or MAO A) or to increase free radical scavengers are sufficient to prevent neuronal death after various brain insults. He thus proposes that DPR may cause a release of trophic factors that promote neuron survival. It is possible that DPR may work via several mechanisms to promote neuronal survival and prolong life span. However, in future studies, it will be very important to clarify the age, sex, and strain differences in various physiological responses to different doses and modes of administration of DPR. Kitani's lab[44–47] has found these factors to be critical in elevating SOD and CAT levels in rats, and Tatton's lab has found at least dose level to be critical in promoting neuron survival in rats and mice.[48,49] Thus if either increased free radical scavengers or increased trophic factors are related to the life-prolonging effects of DPR, these factors must be strictly controlled in any life span study and may be responsible for much of the variability in the literature on the effects of DPR.

REFERENCES

1. BALIN, A. K. 1982. *In* Testing the Theories of Aging. R. C. Adelman & G. S. Roth, Eds.: 137–182. CRC Press. Boca Raton, Fla.
2. SCHNEIDER, E. L. & J. D. REED. 1985. *In* Handbook of the Biology of Aging. C. E. Finch & E. L. Schneider, Eds. 2nd Edit.: 45–76. Van Nostrand Reinhold Co. New York, N.Y.
3. MEHLHORN, R. J. 1988. *In* Physiological Basis of Geriatrics. P. S. Timiras, Ed.: 87–102. MacMillan. New York, N.Y.
4. WEINDRUCH, R. & R. L. WALFORD. 1988. The Retardation of Aging and Disease by Dietary Restriction. Charles C. Thomas. Springfield, Ill.
5. KNOLL, J. 1988. Mount Sinai J. Med. **55**(1): 67–744.
6. KNOLL, J. 1988. Mech. Ageing Dev. **46**: 237–262.
7. KNOLL, J. 1989. Acta Neurol. Scand. **126**: 83–91.
8. MILGRAM, N. W., R. J. RACINE, P. NELLIS, A. MENDONCA & G. O. IVY. 1990. Life Sci. **47**(5): 415–420.
9. BICKFORD, P. C., C. HERON, G. M. ROSE, N. MINICLIER, K. POTH, A. M.-Y. LIN, M. FRIEDEMANN & G. A. GERHARDT. 1992. Soc. Neurosci. Abstr. **18**(1): 904.
10. BIRKMAYER, W., J. KNOLL, P. RIEDERER, M. B. H. YOUDIM, V. HARS & J. MARTON. 1985. J. Neural Transm. **64**: 113–127.
11. THE PARKINSON STUDY GROUP. 1989. N. Engl. J. Med. **321**: 1364–1371.
12. DRAGO, F., G. CONTINELLA, *et al.* 1986. Funct. Neurol. **1**(2): 165–174.
13. BRANDEIS, R., M. SAPIR, Y. KAPON, G. BORELLI, S. CADEL & B. VALSECCHI. 1991. Pharmacol. Biochem. Behav. **39**: 297–304.
14. HEITANEN, M. H. 1991. Acta Neurol. Scand. **84**: 407–410.
15. LEES, A. J. 1991. Acta Neurol. Scand. **84**(Suppl. 136): 91–94.
16. MURPHY, M. P., P. H. WU, N. W. MILGRAM & G. O. IVY. 1993. Neurochem. Res. **18**: 1299–1304.
17. MILGRAM, N. W., E. HEAD, E. WEINER & E. THOMAS. Behav. Neurosci. (In press.)
18. YU, B. P., E. J. MASORO & C. A. MCMAHAN. 1985. J. Gerontol. **40**: 657–670.
19. WERBOFF, J. & J. HAVLENA. 1962. Psychol. Rep. **10**: 395–398.
20. GISPEN, W. H. & R. L. ISAACSON. 1981. Pharmacol. Ther. **12**: 209–246.
21. JÄNICKE, B., G. SCHULZE & H. COPER. 1983. Exp. Gerontol. **18**: 393–407.
22. JÄNICKE, B., D. WROBEL & G. SCHULZE. 1985. Pharmacopsychiatry **18**: 136–137.
23. DEAN, R. L., J. SCOZZAFAVA, *et al.* 1981. Exp. Aging Res. **7**: 427–451.
24. BRAESTRUP, C., H. ANDERSEN & A. RANDRUP. 1975. Eur. J. Pharmacol. **34**: 181–187.
25. WALDMEIER, P. C., A. DELINI-STULA & L. MAÎTRE. 1976. Naunyn-Schmiedeberg's Arch. Pharmacol. **292**: 9–14.
26. TURKISH, S., P. H. YU & A. J. GREENSHAW. 1988. J. Neural Transm. **74**: 141–148.
27. HEAD, E. & N. W. MILGRAM. 1992. Pharmacol. Biochem. Behav. **43**: 749–757.
28. TARIOT, P. N., R. M. COHEN, *et al.* 1987. Arch. Gen. Psychiatr. **44**: 427–433.
29. CONTINELLA, G., F. DRAGO, *et al.* 1985. Physiol. Behav. **35**: 839–841.
30. KAMETANI, H., H. OSADA & K. INOUE. 1984. Behav. Neural Biol. **42**: 73–80.
31. DLUZEN, D. E. & J. L. MCDERMOTT. 1992. J. Neural Transm. **85**: 145–146.
32. SAVASTA, M., M. CHRITIN, *et al.* 1992. Soc. Neurosci. Abstr. **18**(2): 1170.
33. GREENSHAW, A. J., A. V. JUORIO & A. A. BOULTON. 1985. Brain Res. Bull. **15**: 183–189.
34. MORRIS, R. 1984. J. Neurosci. Methods **11**: 47–60.
35. RAPP, P. R., R. A. ROSENBERG & M. GALLAGHER. 1987. Behav. Neurosci. **101**: 3–12.
36. GALLAGHER, M. & R. D. BURWELL. 1989. Neurobiol. Aging **10**: 691–708.
37. PANAKHOVA, E., O. BUREŠOVÁ & J. BUREŠ. 1984. Behav. Neural Biol. **42**: 191–196.
38. STONE, E. A. 1970. Life Sci. **9**: 877–888.
39. KUBANIS, P. & S. F. ZORNETZER. 1981. Behav. Neural Biol. **31**: 115–172.

40. DEAN, R. L. & R. T. BARTUS. 1988. *In* Handbook of Psychopharmacology, Psychopharmacology of the Aging Nervous System. L. L. Iversen, S. D. Iversen & S. H. Snyder, Eds. **20.** Plenum Press. New York, N.Y.
41. BARTUS, R. T., D. FLEMING & H. R. JOHNSON. 1978. J. Gerontol. **33:** 858–871.
42. WALKER, L. C., C. A. KITT, R. G. STRUBLE, M. V. WAGSTER, D. L. PRICE & L. C. CORK. 1988. Neurobiol. Aging **9:** 657–666.
43. RAPP, P. R. & D. G. AMARAL. 1989. J. Neurosci. **9:** 3568–3576.
44. CARRILLO, M.-C., S. KANAI, M. NOKUBO, G. O. IVY & K. KITANI. 1992. Exp. Neurol. **116:** 286–294.
45. CARRILLO, M.-C., K. KITANI, S. KANAI, Y. SATO & G. O. IVY. 1992. Life Sci. **50:** 1985–1992.
46. CARRILLO, M.-C., S. KANAI, Y. SATO, G. O. IVY & K. KITANI. 1992. Biochem. Pharmacol. **44:** 2185–2189.
47. KITANI, K., S. KANAI, M.-C. CARRILLO & G. O. IVY. Arch. Gerontol. Geriatr. (In press.)
48. TATTON, W. G. & C. E. GREENWOOD. 1991. J. Neurosci. Res. **30:** 666–672.
49. TATTON, W. G., C. E. GREENWOOD, N. A. SENINH & P. T. SALO. 1992. Can. J. Neurol. Sci. **19:** 124–133.

(−)Deprenyl Increases the Life Span as Well as Activities of Superoxide Dismutase and Catalase but Not of Glutathione Peroxidase in Selective Brain Regions in Fischer Rats

KENICHI KITANI,[a] SETSUKO KANAI,[b]
MARIA CRISTINA CARRILLO,[b] AND GWEN O. IVY[c]

[a]Radioisotope Research Institute
Faculty of Medicine
University of Tokyo
7-3-1, Hongo
Bunkyo-ku
Tokyo 113, Japan

[b]Tokyo Metropolitan Institute of Gerontology
35-2, Sakaecho
Itabashi-ku
Tokyo, Japan

[c]Division of Life Sciences
University of Toronto
1265 Military Trail
Scarborough, Ontario M1C 1A4, Canada

(−)Deprenyl was developed in Hungary about 30 years ago as a monoamine oxidase inhibitor[1] and was reported to be effective for Parkinson's disease.[2] Recently, the efficacy of the drug in the early stages of Parkinson's disease has been confirmed by several double-blind controlled studies.[3,4] Furthermore, Knoll reported that the drug, when first administered at the age of 24 months in male rats, increased the remaining life expectancy twofold compared with that of saline-treated control rats.[5] Since old rats do not develop a disease corresponding to human Parkinson's disease, the mechanism(s) for the life span extention, if real, may be different from those working in Parkinson's disease. Furthermore, if deprenyl really does extend life span, this fact should have a significant impact on experimental gerontology, since no other chemicals or pharmaceuticals have been reproducibly demonstrated to prolong the life span of animals. It is still the general consensus in experimental gerontology that the only means of prolonging the life span of animals (rodents in particular) is dietary restriction.[6–8]

More recently, Milgram *et al.* reported that the remaining life expectancy of male Fischer-344 (F-344) rats that began treatment at 24 months increased by only 16%,[9] while Knoll reported a more than 100% increase in 24 month-old rats of the Logan-Wistar strain.[5] This (16%) increase of life span found in the Canadian study was only marginally significant ($p = 0.048$, one-tailed t-test).[9] Thus, it appears that a more extensive study is necessary to draw a definite conclusion with regard to the life-prolonging effect of the drug.

Knoll further reported that when animals were treated with deprenyl for 21 successive days, activities of superoxide dismutase (SOD) in striatum of brain were significantly increased in both male and female rats.[5] In contrast, increases in activities of catalase (CAT) and glutathione peroxidase (GSH Px) were not statistically significant.[5] Knoll suggested that the increase in SOD activity in striatum may be causally related to the life-prolonging effect of the drug.[5]

In the present report, we will summarize the results of our own life span study as well as of a series of recent studies on the effect of deprenyl on antioxidant enzyme activities, primarily in the rat brain.

MATERIALS AND METHODS

Animals

F-344 rats of both sexes raised in the aging farm of the Tokyo Metropolitan Institute of Gerontology were used throughout. Husbandry conditions, life spans, and pathologies that appear in the later periods of the animals' lives were reported elsewhere.[10]

Life Span Study

Male F-344 rats that had been raised in the aging farm of the Tokyo Metropolitan Institute of Gerontology began to be administered with deprenyl at the age of 18 months. Animals of experimental groups were injected subcutaneously (sc) with deprenyl 3 times a week at a dose of 0.5 mg/kg per day. Control groups were given isovolumetric saline solution injections. Each 35 animals of three different cohorts (15, 10, 10 animals) constituted control and experimental animal groups. During the drug treatment, they were raised with 3 animals in one cage in a clean conventional facility of the institute. Other husbandry conditions were identical to those in the SPF aging farm. Details of the study have been reported elsewhere.[11] Animals were observed until natural death. No intervention was made except for the measurement of body weight once a month.

Antioxidant Enzyme Activity Studies

Animals of both sexes and of different ages were treated with sc injection or infusion of deprenyl solution primarily for 21 successive days. Some animals were treated longer, up to 4 weeks. Animals were sacrificed by decapitation and several brain regions such as striatum, s. nigra, three different parts of cerebral cortex (frontal, parietotemporal, and occipital), hippocampus, and cerebellum were dissected on an ice-cold plate. The liver was also removed in some experiments. Tissue preparations for enzyme activity measurements are described in detail in our previous publications.[12–15]

Enzyme Activity Measurements

Superoxide Dismutase (SOD)

The activity of SOD was assayed by the method of Elster and Heupel[16] based on the inhibition of nitrite formation from hydroxylammonium in the presence of O_2^- generators. Differentiation of the two different types of SOD (Cu, Zn-SOD and Mn-SOD) was performed by the addition of potassium cyanide (5×10^{-4} M) to the incubation medium. Cu, Zn-SOD activities were defined as those inhibited by potassium cyanide. The difference between total and KCN inhibited enzyme activities was defined as Mn-SOD activity.

Catalase (CAT)

CAT activity was assayed by the method described by Beers and Sizer.[17]

Glutathione Peroxidase (GSH Px)

Activities of GSH Px were determined by the method described by Paglia and Valentine.[18] Two different types of GSH Px (selenium dependent and nonselenium dependent) were assayed using two different substrates, hydroperoxide and cumene-hydroperoxide. Details of procedures for these enzyme activities are described elsewhere.[12-15]

Statistical Analysis

Average life spans of three different cohorts in the same group were analyzed by means of one-way analysis of variance (ANOVA). Since no significant difference could be noted in either the control or the experimental group among three different cohorts, all data were pooled into one group (35 rats each) and the comparisons between control and deprenyl-treated animals were made by using the Student t-test for unpaired values (two-tailed test). Enzyme activities among different groups were primarily analyzed by means of one-way ANOVA. When values were judged to be significantly different with respect to deprenyl treatment, values of any set of two groups were analyzed by Scheffe's test. When only a control group and an experimental group were compared, the Student t-test for the unpaired values (two-tailed test) was applied. p values lower than 0.05 were judged to be significant for these analyses.

RESULTS

TABLE 1 summarizes the average life expectancies of both control and experimental groups calculated from day 0, 18 months (the start of treatment), and 24 months of age. For the calculation of the average survival after 24 months, 3 animals that died before 24 months were included by using minus days in age. Details of this study have been published elsewhere.[11] The increases in mean survival in deprenyl-treated animals compared to respective values in control animals were 5.6%, 15.0%, and

33.8% for survivals from 0 days, 18 months, and 24 months, respectively, and these increases were all statistically significant. Only the 10% longest survivals did not differ significantly between the two groups.

FIGURE 1 illustrates the results of our first experiments on the enzyme assays on the striatum of young male[12] F-344 rats as well as young and old female rats.[14] As is clearly shown, an sc injection of deprenyl at a dose of 2.0 mg/kg per day for 21 successive days yielded a nearly threefold increase in activities of both types of SOD enzymes as well as a 60% (significant) increase in CAT (but not of GSH Px) activities in the striatum of the young male rats. However, in young female rats, the same treatment caused a threefold decrease in SOD activities,[14] while in old female rats activities remained unchanged.[14] Subsequently, we found that the effect of deprenyl on antioxidant enzyme activities is not specific to the striatum, but is also selective to certain brain regions such as s. nigra and cerebral cortex, while there was no effect on enzyme activities in hippocampus or cerebellum, or the liver (FIGURE 2).[13]

The reason(s) why we observed three different results (i.e., an increase, a decrease, and no change) in three different rat groups (FIGURE 1) has been explained by our subsequent studies. FIGURE 3 summarizes some of our recent studies[14,19] using different doses of deprenyl. The duration of treatment was again 21

TABLE 1. Mean Survival Times (Days) of Two Different Rat Groups[a]

	Control Rats (n = 35)	Deprenyl-Treated Rats (n = 35)	Increase (%)	P
From 0 days	876.7 ± 108.7	926.3 ± 97.4	5.6	<0.05
From 18 months	328.7 ± 108.8	378.3 ± 97.4	15.0	<0.05
From 24 months[b]	146.7 ± 108.7	196.3 ± 97.4	33.8	<0.05
Ten percent longest survivals (each n = 4)	1057.5 ± 27.0	1074.8 ± 22.0	1.0	>0.05

[a]Reproduced from Reference 19 with the permission of the publisher.
[b]Survival of animals that died before 24 months were included as age in negative days.

successive days. All values in treated animals are expressed in FIGURE 3 as a percent of respective control values obtained from saline-treated animals.

The discrepant results obtained in our study (FIGURE 1) turned out to be due to differences in the optimal dose of the drug for increasing antioxidant enzyme activities among different animal groups. For example, in young male rats, an optimal dosage appears to be 2.0 mg/kg per day or even greater because higher doses were not tested, while in young female rats, an optimal dosage is around 0.2 mg/kg per day, which is at least 10 times lower than that of young male rats. The reason why the optimal dose for young male rats (2.0 mg/kg per day) decreased SOD activities in young female rats appears to be due to an actual overdose of the drug, since as the dose was increased above the optimal dose, it tended to lose its effect, and as the dose increased up to 2.0 mg/kg per day, it reversed the effect. Similarly, the reason why 2.0 mg/kg per day did not change SOD activities in old female rats is that this dose is just between an optimal dose (1.0 mg/kg per day) and an excessive dose to reduce activities. From FIGURE 3, it is clear that in female rats, aging increased an optimal dose fivefold, while aging reduced the optimal dose fourfold in male rats, the optimal dose in old male rats being 0.5 mg/kg per day (FIGURE 3). The reason for the variability of an optimal dose caused by sex and aging will be discussed later.

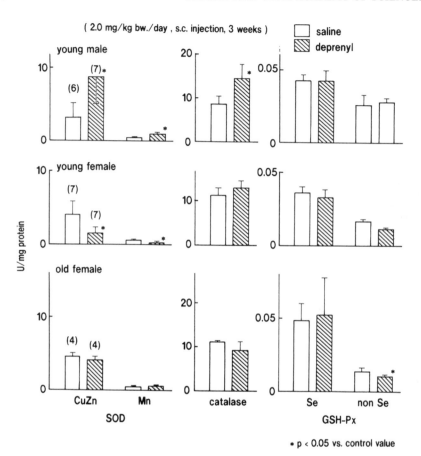

FIGURE 1. Enzyme activities of SOD, CAT, and GSH Px in the striatum of control rats (white column) and rats treated with sc injection of deprenyl for successive 21 days at a dose of 2.0 mg/kg per day (shadowed column). Redrawn from data previously reported by the authors for young male rats[12] and young and old female rats[14] with the permission of the publisher. Numbers in parentheses indicate the number of rats of each group. *Significantly different from corresponding control calues ($p < 0.05$, t-test).

FIGURE 4 summarizes the results of our recent study which examined sequential changes in SOD and CAT activities during the full 4 weeks of deprenyl infusion.[15] SOD activities in s. nigra and striatum started to increase 1 week after the start of infusion and continued to increase up to 4 weeks. In contrast, CAT activity remained unchanged after 1 week of deprenyl infusion and started to increase only after 2 weeks of infusion. Interestingly, unlike SOD activities, CAT activities peaked at 3 weeks and tended to decrease slightly at 4 weeks. This tendency is more clearly seen for CAT activities in frontal and parietotemporal cortices and for SOD activities in parietotemporal cortex, where a 4-week treatment lost its effect for increasing enzyme activities in this brain region.

DISCUSSION

Life Prolongation by Deprenyl

As previously discussed, the prolongation of the life span of animals by means of chemicals or pharmaceuticals has been claimed in a number of past studies. Thus far, however, none of these studies has been reproducible. The only reproducible way to prolong the life span of animals (especially rodents) is by dietary restriction.[6–8] However, with this paradigm, so many biochemical and physiological parameters are altered that we cannot discriminate which factors play a causal role in prolonging the life span of the animals. It is likely that most parameters that have been claimed to be altered by dietary restriction are all the result of the life prolongation, but not the cause. The twofold increase in the remaining life span of rats reported by Knoll[5] when deprenyl treatment was begun at 24 months is therefore an astonishing observation, if it is reproducible. Indeed, the first animal of the treated group died after all control rats died.[5] However, a subsequent study reported from Canada in this regard has cast doubt on the effect of the drug, although it was reported as a positive result.[9] A 16% increase of the remaining life span in this study after 24 months was only marginally significant with the *p* value of 0.048 by using one-tailed *t*-test. If an ordinary two-tailed test is applied, it easily loses its significance. Since the results of these studies differ so greatly, it is difficult to draw a simple conclusion about the effects of deprenyl. However, it should be noted that different rat strains were used in the two studies.

Our study design is somewhat different from the previous two studies.[5,9] Although we also used male F-344 rats as were used in the second (Canadian) study, we started to administer the drug at the age of 18 months, instead of 24 months as was

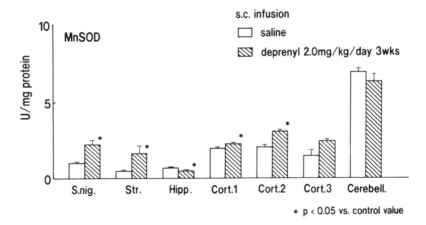

FIGURE 2. Mn-SOD activities in different brain regions in young male rats treated with saline solution (white column, *n* = 6) and rats treated with deprenyl infusion at a rate of 2.0 mg/kg per day for 21 days (shadowed column, *n* = 4). *Significantly different from corresponding control values (*p* < 0.05, *t*-test). (S. nig., substantia nigra; Str., striatum; Hipp., hippocampus; Cort 1, frontal cortex; Cort 2, parietotemporal cortex; Cort 3, occipital cortex; Cerebell., cerebellum). (Reproduced from Reference 13 with the permission of the publisher.)

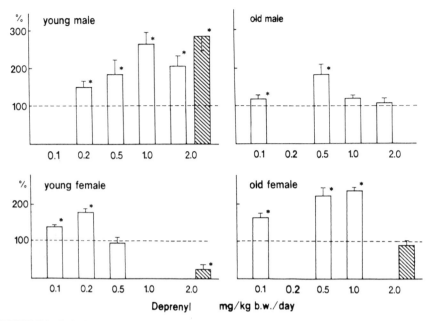

FIGURE 3. Relative enzyme activities of Cu Zn-SOD in striata from young and old rats of both sexes treated with different doses of deprenyl. All values are expressed as percentages of respective control values. White columns indicate values in rats given 21 day sc infusion, and shadowed columns represent values in rats given 21 day sc injection. *Significantly different from respective control values ($p < 0.05$). The number of rats studied in each group is 3 to 7 (mostly 4–5). (Reproduced from Reference 19 with the permission of the publisher.)

done in the previous two studies. Further, we used twice the dose (0.5 mg/kg per day) that was used previously (0.25 mg/kg per day).[5,9] Some quantitative differences between our study and that of the Canadian group may be explained by these differences in experimental design. The 34% increase obtained in our study was statistically significant ($p < 0.05$) as analyzed by means of two-tailed t test despite the fact that the number of animals in each group was almost one half (each 35) those used in the previous two studies (66).[5,9]

Our results, therefore, could be taken as clear evidence that the effect of deprenyl in prolonging the life span of rats is real. However, our results also suggest that such a robust effect as was originally reported by Knoll[5] is not always obtainable. It is possible, however, that if a more proper dosage is used, we can improve the results in terms of the percent increase of the remaining life span. If the real mechanism(s) underlying this phenomenon becomes clear, it will be a remarkable advance in our understanding of the mechanisms of aging. At the moment, however, nothing is known on the mechanism of deprenyl's action(s) except for an inhibition of MAO B and the alteration of antioxidant enzyme activities as will be discussed later.

The possibility that the life prolongation was obtained indirectly through the lower food intake of animals administered deprenyl could be ruled out, since the average body weights were almost identical for both groups throughout the observation period.[11] This also agrees with the observation by the Canadian group.[9] Interestingly, the standard deviation of body weight of the control group started to become greater after 24 months of age compared to the deprenyl-treated group. Although there was no specific comment on this observation, it was also true in the Canadian study.[9] This means that although the average body weight is the same at corresponding ages for both groups, some control animals lost body weights more quickly than did deprenyl-treated animals, while some others gained or lost body weight more slowly. The major reason why some control animals were heavier in their later lives was that many animals started to bear skin tumors after 24 months, some of them weighing more than 200 g in tumor weight alone.[11] Thus, it appears that deprenyl in some way retarded the growth of these skin tumors as well as the natural body weight loss that is known to occur in this animal strain in their later lives.

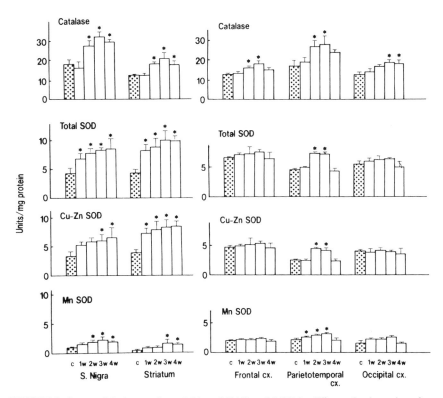

FIGURE 4. Sequential changes in activities of CAT and SOD in different brain regions from young male control rats (c) and rats treated with deprenyl for different time intervals. Deprenyl was continuously infused sc by osmotic minipumps. *Significantly different from corresponding control values (ANOVA + Scheffe's test, $p < 0.05$). Number of animals in each group was 4 except for the group treated with deprenyl for 2 wks ($n = 3$). (Reproduced from Reference 15 with the permission of the publisher.)

Increase in Antioxidant Enzyme Activities

At present, there is no direct proof that increases in antioxidant enzyme activities such as SOD and CAT in certain brain regions, especially the striatum and the s. nigra, are at least a partial cause for the life prolongation obtained by the administration of the (−)deprenyl. However, this phenomenon was demonstrated for all rat groups examined, if appropriate dosages were chosen.[14,19] Further, we have confirmed that it occurs in mice as well as in dogs (unpublished observations). Thus, this effect of the drug appeared to be a phenomenon not only in rats but also in a variety of animal species. Thus far, however, there are no life-prolongation studies in primate species, to the knowledge of the authors.

The question of why an optimal dose of deprenyl for increasing SOD and CAT activities varies so widely depending on sexes and ages has plausible explanations. First, the 10 times lower optimal dosage in young female than in male rats and the reduction of the optimal dose in male rats with aging can be at least partly explained by the possible differences in the metabolic rate for deprenyl among different animal groups. Deprenyl is known to be metabolized by N-demethylation or depropargylation, yielding nordeprenyl and depropargyl-deprenyl (methamphetamine), respectively, both eventually being further metabolized to (−)amphetamine.[20,21] These reactions are mediated mainly by the microsomal monooxygenase system in the liver.[20,21] In most rat strains, many of the reactions mediated by the monooxygenase system are known to be much faster in males than in females. Furthermore metabolic rates of these reactions are known to decline drastically during aging in male (but not in female) rat livers[22,23] (for review, see Reference 24). If we assume that young female rats have a 10 times lower metabolic rate than male rats, the 10 times lower optimal dose in the former can be accepted without any other explanation. In fact, Yoshida *et al.*[25] reported that the formation of amphetamine from deprenyl (the major metabolic pathway in rat liver), was 2-, 6-, and 11-fold lower in livers of female rats of Wistar, SD, and Donryu strains respectively than in males. With the known quantitative strain differences in regard to sex differences of drug metabolism in rat livers, it is not surprizing if we find a 10 times lower metabolic rate in females of the F-344 strain as was previously observed for Donryu rats.[25]

Since our group has repeatedly shown that, in general, drug metabolism in the livers of young male rats declines rapidly with age, approaching values in young (and old) female rats[22,23] (for review, see Reference 24), the reduction of an optimal dose in old male rats has a reasonable explanation as discussed above on the basis of difference in the metabolism of deprenyl. The increase in an optimal dose in female rats with aging, however, cannot be explained on the basis of metabolic rate differences, since hepatic drug metabolisms in female rats essentially stay unchanged during the whole aging process.[22,23] However, it has been well documented that not only in rats[26] but in humans[27] also, aging causes an increase in MAO B activity in many different tissues, such as brain and heart. Since deprenyl is irreversibly bound to the MAO B enzyme molecule and inactivates its enzyme activity, greater amounts of deprenyl may be required in old animals to block these enzymes. Consequently, the amounts of deprenyl that are used for increasing SOD (and CAT) activities may become more limited in old animals, if the same dose is used. This may be at least a partial cause for the increase in an optimal dose in old female rats compared with young ones. The same mechanism for increasing an optimal dose with age should also be operative in old males rats. However, the reduction of metabolic rate appears to have worked more strongly, actually decreasing an optimal dose in old male rats. Thus, we must recognize that sex and age are both strong determinants for an optimal dose in this animal strain.

As is shown in FIGURE 4, for some enzyme activities, a 4-wk treatment appears to be less effective than a 3-wk treatment. In this particular study,[15] however, we were not certain of this observation or of its interpretation. However, we have recently realized that the longer we treat animals, the smaller the optimal dose becomes. In old female rats treated for 6 months, 3 times a week, the results suggest that 0.25 (0.5 mg at largest) per mg/day is most appropriate.[28] An optimal dose of 1.0 mg/kg per day obtained in the study shown in FIGURE 3 for old female rats was the one obtained with 21 successive days of treatment. Therefore the dose of 1.0 mg/kg per day in this study is greater as a weekly dose than 2.0 mg/kg per day in a study where deprenyl was given only 3 times a week. It means that an optimal dose in a long-term study for increasing antioxidant enzyme activities should be at least 4 times lower (and probably less) than the one that was found in our initial short-term study. Our recent studies in progress in male rats, as well as in mice, have increasingly supported this contention. As is shown in FIGURE 1, an excessive dose of deprenyl not only becomes less effective in increasing activities of antioxidant enzymes but can eventually reduce these activities below physiological levels. From these observations, we suggest that a dose of deprenyl used for a long-term study, such as a life span study, must be planned very carefully, keeping in mind that an optimal dose varies widely depending on the sex, age, and, more importantly, the duration of drug treatment, at least in rats.

CONCLUSIONS

Although the underlying mechanism(s) remains unknown, it appears certain that deprenyl can prolong the life span of rats, when an appropriate dose is administered. The drug also increases SOD and CAT activities in selective brain regions, such as s. nigra, striatum, and cerebral cortex. However, an optimal dose for this effect varies widely depending on the sex and age and even the duration and mode of administration of the drug to the animal. Accordingly, the dosage of deprenyl used may considerably influence the results of long-term studies such as a life span study using this drug, if the effect on antioxidant enzyme activities is causally related to its effect on rat life span. Future studies, therefore, must be done with the caution in mind that the proper selection of an optimal dose of deprenyl is a critically important factor for studies evaluating the long-term effects of this drug.

SUMMARY

(−)Deprenyl, a MAO-B inhibitor that is also known to be effective for symptoms of Parkinson's disease, when injected subcutaneously (sc) in male Fischer-344 rats at a dose of 0.5 mg/kg per day (3 times a week) from 18 months of age, significantly increased the remaining life expectancy. The average life span after 24 months was 34% greater in treated rats than in saline-treated control animals. Furthermore, a short-term (3 wk) continuous sc infusion of deprenyl significantly increased activities of superoxide dismutase and catalase but not of glutathione peroxidase in selective brain regions such as s. nigra, striatum, and cerebral cortex, but not in hippocampus or cerebellum, or the liver. The optimal dose for increasing these activities, however, differed greatly depending on the sex and age of animals, with a 10-fold lower value for young female than male rats. Interestingly, aging caused an increase and a decrease in the optimal dose in female and male rats, respectively. In addition, treatment for a longer term tended to reduce the optimal dosage in the same animal group. The results clearly demonstrate that deprenyl increases antioxidant enzyme activities in selective brain regions. If this effect of deprenyl is causally related to its life-prolonging effect, the dosage to be used for any life span study would be a critical factor, with the dosage differing widely depending on sex, age of animal, and mode and duration of drug administration.

ACKNOWLEDGMENT

Skillful secretarial work by Mrs. Ohara is gratefully appreciated.

REFERENCES

1. KNOLL, J., Z. ECSERI, K. KELEMEN, J. NIEVEL & B. KNOLL. 1965. Phenylisopropylmethyl-propinylamine (E-250), a new spectrum psychic energizer. Arch. Int. Pharmacodyn. Ther. **155:** 154–164.
2. BIRKMAYER, W., J. KNOLL, P. RIEDER, M. B. H. YOUDIM, V. HARS & J. MARTON. 1985. Increased life expectancy resulting from L-deprenyl addition to Madopar treatment in Parkinson's disease: a long-term study. J. Neurol. Transm. **64:** 113–127.
3. THE PARKINSON STUDY GROUP. 1989. Effect of deprenyl on the progression of disability in early Parkinson's disease. N. Eng. J. Med. **321:** 1364–1371.
4. TETRUD, J. W. & J. W. LANGSTON. 1989. Effect of deprenyl on the progression of disability in early Parkinson's disease. Science **245:** 519–521.
5. KNOLL, J. 1988. The striatal dopamine dependency of life span in male rats. Longevity study with (−)deprenyl. Mech. Ageing Dev. **46:** 237–262.
6. WEINBRUCK, R. & R. L. WALFORD. 1988. The Retardation of Aging and Disease by Dietary Restriction. Charles C. Thomas. Springfield, Ill.
7. YU, B. Y., E. J. MASARO & E. MCMAHON. 1985. Nutritional influences on aging of Fischer 344 rats. I. Physical, metabolic and longevity characteristics. J. Gerontol. **40:** 657–670.
8. YU, B. Y., E. J. MASORO, I. MURATA, H. A. BERTRAND & F. T. LYND. 1982. Life span study of SPF Fischer 344 male rats fed ad libitum or restricted diets: longevity, growth, lean body maxs and disease. J. Gerontol. **37:** 130–141.
9. MILGRAM, N. W., R. J. RACINE, P. NELLIS, A. MENDONCA & G. O. IVY. 1990. Maintenance of L-deprenyl prolongs life in aged male rats. Life Sci. **47:** 415–420.
10. NOKUBO, M. 1985. Physical-chemical and biochemical differences in liver plasma membranes in aging F-344 rats. J. Gerontol. **40:** 409–414.
11. KITANI, K., S. KANAI, Y. SATO, M. OHTA, G. O. IVY & M. C. CARRILLO. 1993. Chronic treatment of (−)deprenyl prolongs the life span of male Fischer 344 rats. Further evidence. Life Sci. **52:** 281–288.
12. CARRILLO, M. C., S. KANAI, M. NOKUBO & K. KITANI. 1991. (−)Deprenyl induces activities of both superoxide dismutase and catalase but not of glutathione peroxidase in the striatum of young male rats. Life Sci. **48:** 517–521.
13. CARRILLO, M. C., K. KITANI, S. KANAI, Y. SATO & G. O. IVY. 1992. The ability of (−)deprenyl to increase superoxide dismutase activities in the rat is tissue and brain region selective. Life Sci. **50:** 1985–1992.
14. CARRILLO, M. C., S. KANAI, M. NOKUBO, G. O. IVY, Y. SATO & K. KITANI. 1992. (−)Deprenyl increases activities of superoxide dismutase and catalase in striatum but not in hippocampus: the sex and age-related differences in the optimal dose in the rat. Exp. Neurol. **116:** 286–294.
15. CARRILLO, M. C., S. KANAI, Y. SATO, G. O. IVY & K. KITANI. 1992. Sequential changes in activities of superoxide dismutase and catalase in brain regions and liver during (−)deprenyl infusion in male rats. Biochem. Pharmacol. **44:** 2185–2189.
16. ELSTNER, E. F. & A. HEUPEL. 1976. Inhibition of nitrite formation from hydroxylammoniumchloride: a simple assay for superoxide dismutase. Anal. Biochem. **70:** 616–620.

17. BEERS, R. F., JR. & I. W. SIZER. 1952. A specrophotometric method for measuring the breakdown of hydrogen peroxide by catalase. J. Biol. Chem. **195**: 133–140.
18. PAGLIA, D. E. & W. N. VALENTINE. 1967. Studies on the quantitative and qualitative characterization of erythrocyte glutathione peroxidase. J. Lab. Clin. Med. **70**: 158–169.
19. CARRILLO, M. C., S. KANAI, Y. SATO, M. NOKUBO, G. O. IVY & K. KITANI. 1993. The optimal dosage of (−)deprenyl for increasing superoxide dismutase activities in several brain regions decreases with age in male Fischer 344 rats. Life Sci. **52**: 1925–1934.
20. KAROUMS, F., L. W. CHUANG, T. EISLER, D. CALNE, M. R. LIEBOWITZ, F. M. QUOTKIN, D. F. KLEIN & R. J. WYATT. 1982. Metabolism of (−)deprenyl to amphetamine and methamphetamine may be responsible for deprenyl's therapeutic benefit; a biochemical assessment. Neurology (Ny) **32**: 503–509.
21. YOSHIDA, T., Y. YAMADA, T. YAMAMOTO & Y. KUROIWA. 1986. Metabolism of deprenyl, a selective monoamine oxidase (MAO) B inhibitor in rat: relationship of metabolism to MAO-B inhibitory potency. Xenobiotica **16**: 129–136.
22. FUJITA, S., H. KITAGAWA, M. CHIBA, T. SUZUKI, M. OHTA & K. KITANI. 1985. Age and sex associated differences in the relative abundance of multiple species of cytochrome P-450 in rat liver microsomes—a separation by HPLC of hepatic microsomal cytochrome P-450 species. Biochem. Pharmacol. **34**: 1861–1864.
23. KAMATAKI, T., K. MAEDA, M. SHIMADA, K. KITANI, T. NAGAI & R. KATO. 1985. Age-related alteration in the activities of drug-metabolizing enzymes and contents of sex-specific forms of cytochrome P-450 in liver microsomes from male and female rats. J. Pharmacol. Exp. Ther. **233**: 222–228.
24. KITANI, K. 1988. Drugs and the ageing liver. Life Chem. Rep. **6**: 143–230.
25. YOSHIDA, T., T. OGURO & Y. KUROIWA. 1987. Hepatic and extrahepatic metabolism of deprenyl, a selective monoamine oxidase (MAO) B inhibitor of amphetamines in rats: sex and strain differences. Xenobiotica **8**: 957–963.
26. STROLIN, B. M. & P. E. KEANE. 1980. Differential changes in monoamine oxidase-A and -B activity in the aging rat brain. J. Neurochem. **35**: 1026–1032.
27. ORELAND, L. & C. J. FOWLER. 1979. The activity of human brain and thrombocyte monoamine oxidase (MAO) in relation to various psychiatric disorders. The nature of the changed MAO activity. *In* Monoamine Oxidase: Structure, Functions and Altered Functions. T. P. Singer, *et al.,* Eds.: 389–396. Academic Press. New York, N.Y.
28. CARRILLO, M. C., K. KITANI, S. KANAI, Y. SATO, K. MIYASAKA & G. O. IVY. The effect of a long term (6 months) treatment with (−)deprenyl on antioxidant enzyme activities in selective brain regions in old female Fischer 344 rats. Biochem. Pharmacol. (In press.)

Influence of L-Deprenyl Treatment on Mouse Survival Kinetics

L. PIANTANELLI, A. ZAIA, G. ROSSOLINI, C. VITICCHI,
R. TESTA, A. BASSO, AND A. ANTOGNINI

Center of Biochemistry
Gerontological Research Department
Italian National Research Centers on Aging (INRCA)
Via Birarelli 8
I-60121 Ancona, Italy

INTRODUCTION

The study of the mechanisms of aging received an important momentum from the use of animal models whose life span can be modified by definite controlled interventions. These models present, however, their limits when the interpretation of the results is attempted. At present, in fact, there is no agreement about how to measure the aging rate of a population or the biological age of an individual.[1] Even when the findings seem clear-cut as happens in caloric restricted rats, caution is necessary in extrapolating results to animals living in unrestricted conditions.

Despite the limitation that any model may have, manipulations able to prolong life span, and maximal life span in particular, remain among the most powerful tools to gain insights into basic aging processes. Thus, any new way of extending life is welcome, as from a multifaceted view a more complete and understandable picture can stem. In this framework, the observations of some authors on the effects of the monoamine oxidase inhibitor L-deprenyl on aged animals sound very interesting.[2–4]

It has been observed that this drug can prolong the life span of treated rats and improve their sexual activity at the same time.[5,6] Interestingly, the treatment was effective when started at the end of the second year of life.[5,7] It is also worth stressing that L-deprenyl can be considered a safe drug, thus very useful in long-term experiments.[4,6] In addition to the interest due to these characteristics, our attention was drawn by the possible relationships of its mechanism of action with that at the basis of our previous findings in old mice: age-related alterations of the adrenergic system in different tissues of aging animals.[8–11] These changes were demonstrated to be not definitive, being corrected by endocrine manipulation exerted just a little before two years of age.[12–14]

Since our previous experimental work on aging was done on mice, first of all a survival experiment was planned with the strain of mice of our own laboratory. The drug was administered to 22-month-old mice, as one of the most interesting characteristic to verify was the efficacy of a treatment starting late in life.

MATERIALS AND METHODS

Animals

Animals were taken from our own colony of Balb/c-nu mice. The term "nu" refers to the recessive nude mutation introduced into inbred Balb/c mice by crossing

72

them with nude mutants. Three animal groups of different ages (a two month difference from each other) were used, each one further subdivided into L-deprenyl-treated and control ones. The animals (D mice) of the three treated subgroups ($n = 62$) were injected subcutaneously with 0.25 mg/kg bw L-deprenyl three times a week until time of natural death. The animals (C mice) of the three control subgroups ($n = 46$) received saline using the same schedule. Treatments started when animals of each subgroup were 22 months old. Survivals were checked daily, while body weights were assayed individually once a week. At the end of the experiment, data from subgroups were collected together. L-Deprenyl was kindly donated by Chiesi Farmaceutici S.p.A., Parma, Italy.

Survival Analysis

Survival data were analyzed using both the nonparametric test of Kolmogorov-Smirnov (SPSS package) and a parametric mathematical model of survivorships proposed recently.[15] An outline of the parametric model is given as follows. It is based on two aspects of survival kinetics: the deterministic component of aging rate and the statistical distribution of vitality among the subjects of a population. Vitality is used with the meaning of an index of comprehensive biological efficiency which allows the organism to survive.[16] Let $Z(v,t)dv$ be the probability that an individual of age t has vitality in the range $v - v + dv$:

$$Z(v, t) = \text{Fc}^{-1}[Z_1(v, t) - Z_2(v, t)]; \quad v < 1$$

where $Z_1(v,t)$ represents a normal distribution with mean $\mu(t)$ and standard deviation $S(t)$. $Z_2(v,t)$ only differs from $Z_1(v,t)$ in having its mean shifted of an amount equal to $2S(t)$; in this way, the resulting distribution of the positive vitality values has the upper boundary $v = 1$. Fc is a correcting factor which gives $l(0) = 1$:

$$\text{Fc} = \int [Z_1(v, t) - Z_2(v, t)]dv \quad \text{for } t = 0$$

If we assume unity as an upper bound for v, that is, $Z(v,t) = 0$ for all $v > 1$, the probability $l(t)$ that an individual survives to age t is given by

$$l(t) = \int_0^1 Z(v, t)dv;$$

The function $\mu(t)$ is linked to $S(t)$ as

$$\mu(t) + S(t) = 1$$

and has the following structure:

$$\mu(t) = 1 - S_0 + S_0^{10} - S_0^{10} \exp \frac{\omega t}{S_0}$$

Sometimes it can be more useful to represent the survival function reporting the absolute number of subjects $L(t)$ alive at any age t instead of the survivorship probability $l(t)$. Thus

$$L(t) = N_0 l(t)$$

where N_0 is representative of the initial number of individuals present in the cohort at birth.

Thus, the model here outlined contains only two parameters, ω and S_0, whose values can be determined fitting specific survivorship curves. The parameters are related to deterministic and stochastic factors: ω, a deterministic component describing the environmental and genetic influence on physiological functions, also used as an index of the aging rate of the population;[1] S_0, a stochastic component representing the fluctuating interaction of the living organism and its environment. Roughly, the deterministic parameter ω is related to the maximal life span of the population studied, while the stochastic parameter S_0 is linked to the shape of the curve.

The fitting of the model to experimental data was performed by Newton-Gauss nonlinear regression analysis, as described by Snedecor and Cochran.[17] Mean body weight (mbw) data were fitted by nonlinear regression analysis using Fig. P package, Biosoft.

RESULTS

Survival data are reported in FIGURE 1A. No dramatic changes took place in D mice with respect to the C ones, although in the middle period of the treatment, D mouse survival kinetics are slightly slower when compared with those from controls. The expected deprenyl-induced increase in maximum life span does not occur in our strain of Balb/c-nu mice. As a matter of fact, according to the nonparametric test of Kolmogorov-Smirnov, the two curves show no statistically significant differences. Since nonparametric tests are safe but often lack of power and do not give any information about the possible interpretation of the differences eventually observed,[1,18] the same data have been analyzed using the model outlined in the section Materials and Methods. The resulting fitting curves are shown in FIGURE 1B, while the goodness of the fit can be seen in FIGURES 1C and 1D. As expected, the two curves are very close to each other; the values of their estimated parameters together with their standard errors are given in the legend. While the difference between the two values of the parameter ω is extremely small, so that it hardly has any biological meaning, the difference found between S_0 values, although not dramatic, may deserve some attention.

Data on mbw of C and D mice are reported in FIGURE 2A. At first glance, the two patterns seem to present no differences. Both groups of mice show a slow progressive decrease in mbw with advancing age. However, a more thorough analysis shows that the two kinetics are different even from a qualitative point of view. While D mice present a roughly linear decrease of mbw, controls show a faster, nonlinear decreasing trend. When both sets of empirical data are fitted using a second-degree polynomial function, the two resulting curves are those shown in FIGURE 2B. The goodness of fit of C and D mouse data can be seen in FIGURE 2C and 2D, respectively. It is worth noting that D mice show a lesser degree of variability in mbw than C ones.

DISCUSSION

One of the most fruitful approaches to investigating the mechanisms of aging processes is the study of the animals with modified life span. Particularly important are the experimental models of extended maximal life span. At present, the caloric restricted rat is the best studied animal model, and many interesting data have recently been collected.[19] The efficacy of other treatments, such as antioxidant supplementation, is still questionable. In fact, some positive findings on survival

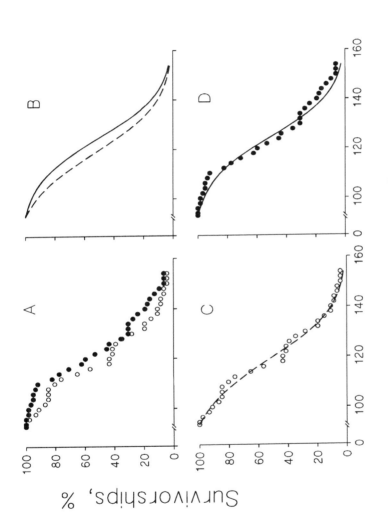

FIGURE 1. Survival data of C (open circles) and D (filled circles) mice. Data from both groups (A) are fitted using the mathematical model outlined in the section Materials and Methods. The two best fits are compared in B. They are also reported separately in C and D together with empirical data to better see the goodness of the fit. The values of the parameters ± SE for the best fits are given as follows: C mice, $\omega = 0.0275 \pm 0.0002$, $S_0 = 0.418 \pm 0.005$; D mice, $\omega = 0.268 \pm 0.0002$, $S_0 = 0.374 \pm 0.007$. D mice show a 10.5% decrease in S_0 value, which is statistically significant ($p < 0.01$).

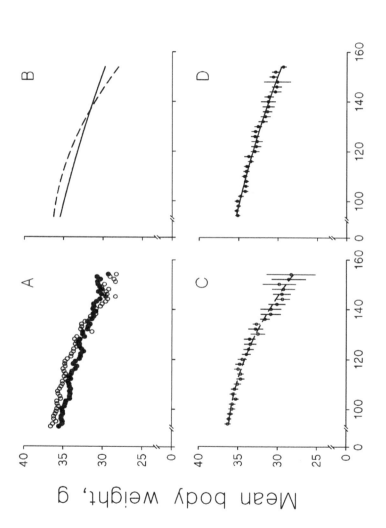

FIGURE 2. Data on mbw from C (open circles) and D (filled circles) mice are reported in A while their fitting curves are shown in B. Both C and D data and their own fittings are reported in the figures C and D, respectively. In order to avoid confusion, figures C and D report only every other point ± SEM, but all data were considered in the fitting procedure. Fits were first performed using linear functions. However, only D mouse data gave a good fit, thus the procedure was repeated with the equation $y = mx^2 + nx + p$. This function improves the goodness of the fit of C mouse data only, eliciting a qualitative difference in the kinetics of the two sets of data. The figures report the parabolic fits in order to make the comparison easier.

could be due to indirect underfeeding as a result of the bad taste of antioxidants given orally. As regards the caloric restriction itself, some basic questions cast some doubts on its use as a model of natural aging. On the one hand, we wonder whether restricted rats may live longer than ad libitum fed controls as a result of life shortening of controls due to their overeating. On the other hand, other important aspects to be taken into account are those concerning the survival capacity of restricted animals in nonprotected natural environments, or the interspecies differences in treatment efficacy.[20]

Interspecies differences have also to be taken into account in the analysis of present results, as L-deprenyl effects on survival obtained by other authors on rats differ from that found on our strain of mice. In fact, we did not observe any influence on maximal life span, while in other authors' experiments on rats, a life-prolonging effect was shown.[5-7] Since considerations about maximal life span are not reliable,[1,20] the aging rate of the population is often estimated. Even in this case, hardly any difference can be shown as the parameter ω entering our model is just an index of the aging rate. It seems safe to conclude that the schedule used in treating Balb/c-nu mice with L-deprenyl does not have any influence on the mechanisms that may control the pace of "physiological" aging.

Some feeble positive effects seem nevertheless to be present in treated mice when compared with their controls. The rate of mortality was slightly lower in the middle part of the survival curve, that is, a sort of mild rectangularization of survivorship was obtained. The very small difference between the two curves, which is not statistically significant according to the Kolmogorov-Smirnov test, would hardly have any interest per se. However, when a more sensitive tool such as a parametric model[15] is used, the slight changes induced in D mouse survival kinetics may reveal some interesting aspects. While the difference in ω values has not much biological meaning, that observed in S_0 deserves some attention, despite being as small as about 10%. Since S_0 is assumed to represent the stochastic component of the survival kinetics, its decrease can be representative of a narrower range of variability in the physiological functions of the D mouse population. Moreover, since maximal life span is not affected, the treatment is likely to influence most individuals with less physiological capacity. These considerations on individual function variability are supported by findings on mbw. D mice show lower standard error of the mean (SEM) of mbw than controls, a fact that is self-evident when the tails of the two curves are compared. Further support comes from the different kinetics of mbw: D mice show a decrease in mbw with age that is linear and slower than the parabolic one of their controls. The slowing down of the usual age-related decrease in D mouse mbw, already reported by other authors in rats,[7] also allows us to exclude an indirect undernourishment as the cause of the slightly different survival kinetics.

It is likely that this paper raises new questions instead of solving some. Certainly, many factors can be involved in and modulate any drug treatment. Species, duration of treatment, age at start, and breeding conditions are among the most important ones. The few data available until now on L-deprenyl survival effects might suggest that the same treatment induces a deep influence on basic processes of aging in rats prolonging their maximal life span, while it has no effect on maximal survival in mice, where it seems to have a beneficial influence on some pathological conditions, reflected in the mild rectangularization of their survival kinetics. It is not known, however, whether a more precocious beginning of treatment or different doses may be more effective even on mice. It may also be worth noting that from an applicative point of view, a strategy devoted to rectangularizing the survival curves may be more fruitful than one trying to prolong maximal life span, at its own turn more useful in studying basic aging processes.

ACKNOWLEDGMENTS

We thank Dr. A. Tibaldi for assistance in animal care and Ms. Giovanna Pennesi and Mr. F. Marchegiani for technical assistance.

REFERENCES

1. PIANTANELLI, L., A. BASSO & G. ROSSOLINI. Ann. N.Y. Acad. Sci. (In press.)
2. KNOLL, J. 1982. *In* Strategy in Drug Research. G. A. B. Buisman, Ed.: 107–135. Elsevier. Amsterdam, the Netherlands.
3. KNOLL, J. 1985. Mech. Ageing Dev. **30:** 109–122.
4. BURCHINSKY, S. G. & S. M. KUZNETSOVA. 1992. Arch. Gerontol. Geriatr. **14:** 1–15.
5. KNOLL, J. 1988. Mech. Ageing Dev. **46:** 237–262.
6. KNOLL, J., J. DALLO & T. T. YEN. 1989. Life Sci. **45:** 525–531.
7. MILGRAM, N. W., R. J. RACINE, P. NELLIS, A. MENDONCA & G. O. IVY. 1990. Life Sci. **47:** 415–420.
8. PIANTANELLI, L., R. BROGLI, P. BEVILACOUA & N. FABRIS. 1978. Mech. Ageing Dev. **7**(3): 163–169.
9. PIANTANELLI, L., P. FATTORETTI & C. VITICCHI. 1980. Mech. Ageing Dev. **14:** 155–164.
10. VITICCHI, C., R. GRINTA & L. PIANTANELLI. 1990. Gerontology **36:** 286–292.
11. PIANTANELLI, L., S. GENTILE, P. FATTORETTI & C. VITICCHI. 1985. Arch. Gerontol. Geriatr. **4:** 179–185.
12. PIANTANELLI, L., A. BASSO, M. MUZZIOLI & N. FABRIS. 1978. Mech. Ageing Dev. **7**(3): 171–182.
13. ROSSOLINI, G., C. VITICCHI, A. BASSO & L. PIANTANELLI. 1991. Int. J. Neurosci. **59:** 143–150.
14. VITICCHI, C., S. GENTILE & L. PIANTANELLI. 1989. Arch. Gerontol. Geriatr. **8:** 13–20.
15. PIANTANELLI, L., G. ROSSOLINI & R. NISBET. 1992. Gerontology **38:** 30–40.
16. PIANTANELLI, L. 1986. Arch. Gerontol. Geriatr. **5:** 107–118.
17. SNEDECOR, G. W. & W. G. COCHRAN. 1989. Statistical Methods. Iowa State University Press. Ames, Iowa.
18. MODE, C. J., R. D. ASHLEIGH, A. ZAVODNIAK & G. T. BAKER. 1984. J. Gerontol. **39:** 36–42.
19. YU, B. P. 1990. *In* Review of Biological Research in Aging. M. Rothstein, Ed. **4:** 349–371. Wiley-Liss. New York, N.Y.
20. GAVRILOV, L. A. & N. S. GAVRILOVA. 1991. The Biology of Life Span: A Quantitative Approach. Harwood Academic Publisher. London, England.

Aging, Stress, and Cognitive Function[a]

A. LEVY, S. DACHIR, I. ARBEL, AND T. KADAR

Department of Pharmacology
Israel Institute for Biological Research
Ness-Ziona 70450, Israel

INTRODUCTION

Landfield *et al.* have shown that brain hippocampal aging correlated with plasma levels of corticosteroids,[1] the hormones whose secretion is increased under stress. Their findings were summarized under the "glucocorticoid hypothesis of brain aging."[2] Sapolsky and his colleagues have demonstrated glucocorticoid toxicity both *in vitro*, in primary cultures of fetal hippocampal neurons,[3] and *in vivo*, in rats[4] and in primates,[5] and formulated the "glucocorticoid cascade hypothesis."[6] Sapolsky also suggested that the mechanism of the toxic effects of glucocorticoids (GC) in the hippocampus was associated with increased neuronal vulnerability to metabolic insults.[7]

The hippocampus is a brain structure well known for its role in cognitive functions such as memory, learning, and spatial orientation.[8,9] Its function in the feedback regulation of the hypothalamic-pituitary-adrenocortical (HPA) axis is still not completely clear.[10] Cognitive functions deteriorate in pathological[11] as well as in normal aging processes.[12–14] Recently, we have shown that the extent of the behavioral deficits in aging Wistar rats correlated well with the extent of morphological changes measured in the brain, especially in hippocampal regions.[15] The neurological damage found in the hippocampus following chronic stress or prolonged corticosterone (COR) exposure had not been associated with a defined behavioral deficit. The initial objective of our research was to establish a more complete animal model, one that will also exhibit the behavioral changes related to the long-term COR treatment. Instead of the repeated daily injection method,[4] which could not lead to steady circulating levels of corticosterone, we introduced the more consistent method of using COR sustained-release (SR) pellets, aiming at COR blood concentrations associated with mild stress (150–300 ng/ml).

In the first study, such SR pellets were implanted subcutaneously in young (3 months old) Fischer-344 rats, for the duration of 9 weeks.[16] One week following termination of the drug treatment, these rats were tested in the eight-arm radial maze. COR-treated rats exhibited cognitive deficits only during the initial acquisition stage of the maze. Preliminary histological examination of the hippocampal region revealed specific damage, mainly to pyramidal cells at the CA1 and CA4 subfields.[17]

In order to enhance the cognitive effect, COR treatment in young rats was prolonged in the present study from 63 to 90 days. In parallel, a nine-week COR treatment, similar to the previous treatment, was tested in middle-aged (12 months old) rats, assuming that older rats might be more sensitive to the long-term COR treatment.

It is well documented, based on our own research[15] as well as on other studies (e.g., References 18–21), that during aging, rat populations become more heterogenous, consisting of increasing numbers of cognitively impaired animals. In most

[a]The support of Bayer AG for this study is gratefully acknowledged.

79

strains, this process is clearly evident already at the age of 12 months. Middle-aged rats, which were selected for this study, were therefore initially screened for their cognitive performance using the Morris water maze. By selecting "nonimpaired" middle-aged rats, we attempted to investigate whether aging increased their vulnerability to the long-term COR treatment, and tried to separate COR effect on cognitive performance from the normal age-dependent performance decrements. The purpose of using the young group was to discover whether prolongation of the treatment from 63 to 90 days might also augment the cognitive impairment.

One of the main concerns in aging research, especially in the study of age-related cognitive effects, is the preferred animal model and behavioral paradigm. Aging animals are often affected by various diseases and partial physical incapacitation. In behavioral testing, when comparing the performance of aged animals to young ones, this issue is frequently addressed. The possibility of using long-term COR treatment to create aging-like cognitive deficits in middle-aged rats that are otherwise physically fit might be a new approach to deal with this problem.

ANIMALS, MATERIALS, AND METHODS

Animals

Twenty-four young (3 months old upon arrival) male Fischer 344 rats (Charles River, United Kingdom) were used for the prolonged 90 days COR treatment. Sixty-five rats, 12 months old, were used for the middle-aged experimental group. All rats were housed in individual cages in a temperature-controlled environment ($22 \pm 1°C$) with lights on from 5 AM to 6 PM, and *ad libitum* access to food (Altromin, Lage, Germany) and water. Their weight was monitored by daily weighing following implantation.

Drug Treatment

Placebo and COR SR pellets (produced by Innovative Research of America, Toledo, Ohio) were implanted under general anesthesia, induced by a mixture of halothane and oxygen. In the young rats group, four pellets (each containing 200 mg, released over 90 days; approximately 9 mg COR per day) or four placebo pellets were implanted subcutaneously approximately 4 cm lateral off the median line. In the middle-aged group, one 200 mg COR pellet, released over 21 days (around an average of 9 mg COR per day), was implanted subcutaneously in each rat every three weeks, three times in a row, similarly to an identical procedure used in the previous study carried out in young rats.[16]

To determine the hormone concentration in the blood, samples were collected from the tail vein into heparinized glass capillaries. Special care was taken to insure that all blood samples were collected within two minutes after approaching the rat's cage, so that stress would not affect the measurement. Plasma samples were stored at $-20°C$ until analyzed for COR concentration using a radioimmunoassay kit (ICN Biomedicals Inc, Costa Mesa, Calif.). According to the manufacturer, typical intraassay variation was around 4–7% and typical interassay variation around 7%.

Radial Arm Maze (RAM) Procedure

The apparatus and the basic training procedure were previously described.[8,16] The task involved a successive selection of arms, radiating from the center of the maze, in order to obtain a food reward, and the acquisition of the task was monitored daily over two weeks. Each animal was placed in the center of the maze and was allowed to visit all arms, while each arm was baited with one food pellet. Each trial (one per day) lasted until the animal had either visited all 8 arms or until 15 min had elapsed. Reentry into an arm that was visited before was scored as an error.

Morris Water Maze (MWM) Procedure

The MWM task enables the testing of rats for their spatial reference memory performance by following their ability to learn the location of an escape platform, submerged in opaque water. This behavioral paradigm was used to rank the performance of the middle-aged rats. Rats were trained and tested in a white circular metal water maze measuring 140 cm in diameter and 50 cm high, filled to a depth of 25 cm with water (26°C). Milk powder was dissolved in the water in order to make it opaque. A white metal platform was placed 2 cm beneath the water. The pool surface was divided into four imaginary quadrants of equal area and four equally spaced points around the edge of the pool were used as starting positions. Performance in the maze was monitored by a tracking system consisting of an overhead video camera linked to a computerized analysis system (Galai, Israel).

Each rat was given four training trials per day (up to 120 sec each) on four consecutive days, and escape latencies (time to find the platform) were recorded. For each rat, the platform position remained constant throughout the four training days.

Statistical Analysis

All the data were subjected to statistical analysis using ANOVA software for repeated measures, in order to determine the statistical significance of the results. The chi-square test for frequency data was used whenever needed.

RESULTS

Body Weight Changes

Body weight changes followed very closely the pattern described in the first study.[16] Placebo rats lost about 2% of their body weight within the first two days following implantation. However, on day three they started regaining this loss. COR-implanted rats lost up to 8% of their body weight during the first eight days following implantation. Later, young rats regained weight at a rate similar to that of placebo rats, but their weight remained 6–8% lower until 95 days following implantation. The study in young rats was carried out in two consecutive identical experiments (12 rats in each experiment), and FIGURE 1 presents the weight data of the first experiment. Statistical analysis by ANOVA showed a significant difference between the groups $[F(1,20) = 38.98; p < 0.001]$. The second experiment displayed comparable data. Similar weight loss following each implantation was found in the middle-aged group, resembling the pattern described in the previous study.[16]

Plasma Corticosterone Levels

It was shown previously[16] that following COR pellet implantation, plasma concentrations of corticosterone were stable throughout the day, with no diurnal variation. COR plasma levels were within the range associated with mild stress. FIGURE 2 presents morning values of plasma COR concentrations for the two young experimental groups, at seven time intervals throughout the experiment. Plasma levels of COR-implanted rats were significantly elevated during the whole period, with a gradual decrease in COR values observed throughout the experiment. COR plasma concentrations were always above 150 ng/ml, a level that is characteristic for rats under mild stress.

An additional blood analysis was performed on day 95, to ensure the return to normal values before starting the behavioral tests (see FIGURE 2). As expected, plasma COR concentrations of the two groups were in the normal range of low morning values, and there was no difference between the groups.

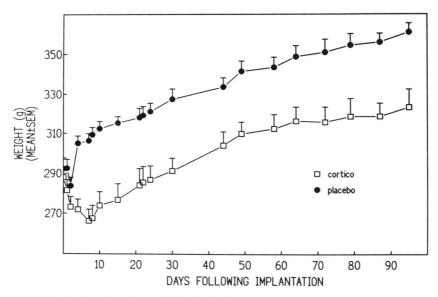

FIGURE 1. Body weight changes following implantation of corticosterone versus placebo SR pellets in young rats ($n = 6$ in each group).

In the older experimental groups, plasma concentrations following the repeated implantation procedure were similar to those found in the previous study, carried out in young rats.[16] COR levels were significantly different during the morning (9 AM) between placebo and COR-implanted rats [$F(1,10) = 380, p < 0.001$ by ANOVA; see TABLE 1]. No difference was found between evening (5 PM) values.

Young Rats—RAM Results

Prolongation of COR treatment from 63 to 90 days did not result in a pronounced cognitive impairment in young rats. The differences between the cognitive performance of placebo and drug-treated rats were not statistically significant. Quite a few rats did not complete the RAM test within the time allowed for the test each day (15

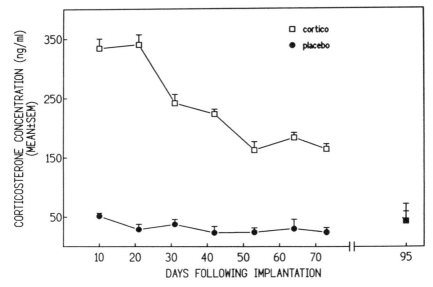

FIGURE 2. Plasma corticosterone concentrations following implantation of corticosterone versus placebo SR pellets in young rats (*n* = 12 in each group).

min). This fact made it difficult to analyze the parameter of daily errors. The number of rats that completed the task versus those that did not was analyzed instead (see FIGURE 3). Using χ^2 test for two independent variables, an overall significant difference [χ^2 (1) = 8.47; $p < 0.005$] between COR and placebo implanted rats was found. Significantly more COR implanted rats did not complete the task compared to placebo implanted rats. However none of the clearly cognitive parameters were statistically significant.

Middle-Aged Rats—MWM Results

Before starting the COR treatment, all rats were screened for their cognitive performance in the MWM, and divided between cognitively impaired and nonimpaired.

Compared to a group of young rats, all of which learned the maze easily, some of the middle-aged rats were as fast in learning the maze, while others had considerable difficulties. We used the combined escape latency data of the last two training days (3

TABLE 1. Plasma Corticosterone (COR) Concentrations 10 Days following Each Implantation, in Placebo versus Drug-Treated Groups[a]

Implantation	Placebo Group	COR Group
I	34.8 ± 5.3	127.8 ± 5.0
II	8.8 ± 2.3	144.9 ± 8.4
III	37.1 ± 7.7	176.4 ± 15.8

[a]Morning mean values ± standard error of the mean in ng/ml; *n* = 6.

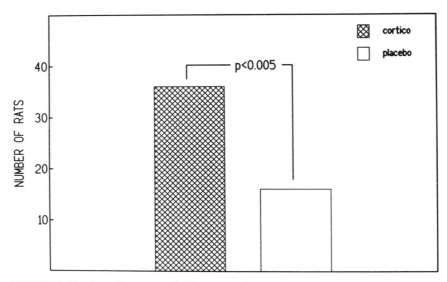

FIGURE 3. Number of young rats failing to complete the RAM test during maze acquisition ($n = 12$ rats × 12 days).

and 4) in order to rank the rats' performance. FIGURE 4 presents the wide range of escape latencies that were found in these middle-aged rats. It is obvious that the distribution of escape latencies does not resemble a normal homogenous distribution, but rather indicates two distinct subpopulations. We defined all rats with escape latency of 50 sec and below as "nonimpaired" and all those with escape latency of 80 and above as "impaired." Since the "impaired" group exhibited cognitive deficits due to normal aging, the effects of corticosterone will be discussed hereafter for the "nonimpaired" group only.

Middle-Aged Rats—RAM Results

All the cognitive parameters measured in the RAM exhibited significant differences between drug and placebo treated rats. As an example, the parameter of first error entry is shown in FIGURE 5. Two-way ANOVA with repeated measures showed a significant statistical difference between the groups [$F(2,19) = 41.97$; $p < 0.001$], with a day by group interaction [$F(28,266) = 1.88$; $p = 0.006$]. The number of rats that completed the task, versus those that did not, was also analyzed using the chi-square test for two independent variables. Similarly to the young rat group, an overall significant difference [$\chi^2 (1) = 52.5$; $p < 0.001$] between COR and placebo implanted rats was found (see FIGURE 6).

DISCUSSION

An animal model that simulates the high levels of corticosterone under stress was developed in Fischer 344 rats, in order to study the relationship between stress, aging, and the deterioration of cognitive functions. Middle-aged rats showed higher vulnerability to COR treatment compared to young ones. This conclusion is based on the severe cognitive impairment found in the present study in middle-aged rats, compared to the subtle learning deficit measured in an identical previous study in young rats.[16] Even the present prolongation of COR treatment in young rats from 63 to 90 days, with COR plasma levels somewhat higher, did not compensate for the difference in age.

In a recent *in vitro* study, carried out in hippocampal astrocyte cultures, Tombaugh and Sapolsky[22] investigated the temporal features and steroid specificity of the synergism between hypoxia and hypoglycemia and COR treatment. They concluded that at least 24 hours pretreatment of COR is needed for the toxic effect to emerge, and suggested that the effects that follow prolonged COR exposure are receptor mediated steroid specific. Our results demonstrated a synergism between COR treatment and aging, which in this case was analogous to "metabolic insult." It seems that young rats are more resistant to high levels of COR, as much as older animals are more sensitive and less adaptive to stress.[23] The exact age at which rats become more sensitive to high COR might be strain dependent. This hypothesis might explain the discrepancies between results obtained in various studies, in which rats of different strains and different age groups were used.[24–26] Furthermore, in studies in which rats were not prescreened as in the present study,[25] some of the placebo-treated rats might have exhibited normal age-related cognitive impairment. Such cognitive deficits, overlapping with COR effects, might obliterate the clear difference between the treatment groups.

The newly developed animal model ("nonimpaired" middle-aged rats, treated continuously with COR) can be used for testing the central protective effects of

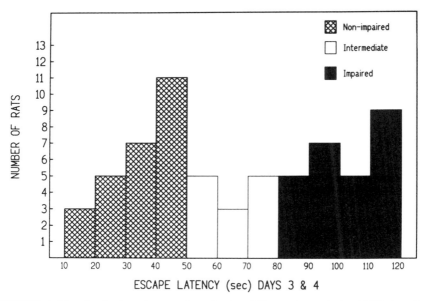

FIGURE 4. The distribution of escape latencies in middle-aged rats during MWM learning (number of rats for the combined latencies of training days 3 and 4).

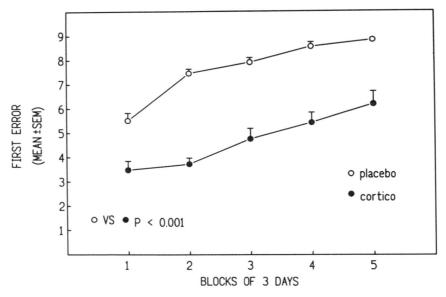

FIGURE 5. First error entry during acquisition of the RAM in corticosterone versus placebo-treated middle-aged rats (all rats in this study were classified before treatment as "nonimpaired" in an initial MWM screening).

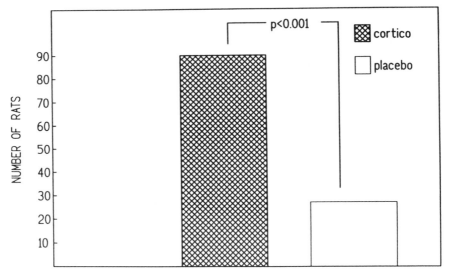

FIGURE 6. Number of middle-aged rats failing to complete the RAM test during maze acquisition ($n = 11$ rats $\times$ 15 days).

various drugs during either pathological or normal aging. Further careful histological and histochemical studies, in which the brain damage inflicted by the high COR treatment will be studied and compared to the damage caused by normal aging, are still required. Our preliminary observations suggest that while in normal aging the damage to hippocampal CA3 is more severe, under COR treatment the damage to CA1 and CA4 is more prominent. It is interesting to note that damage to the CA1 region of the hippocampus is the predominating pathological process in the brain of Alzheimer's disease patients.[27] Therefore, the exact applicability of the new model awaits further clarification.

SUMMARY

Stress was implied as involved in "enhanced aging," and prolonged administration of corticosterone was claimed to lead to central neuronal lesions. This study describes an animal model that simulates the steroid elevation associated with stress by a continuous slow-release administration of corticosterone, in young (3 months old) and middle-aged (12 months old) Fischer 344 rats. Plasma concentrations of corticosterone were stable throughout the day, with no diurnal variation, within the range associated with mild stress. Corticosterone prolonged treatment resulted in morphological changes mainly in the CA1, CA4, and dentate gyrus areas of the hippocampus.

Middle-aged rats showed higher vulnerability to the long-term COR treatment than young ones, even when COR treatment was prolonged in young rats from 63 to 90 days. Middle-aged rats were screened before the corticosterone treatment, using the Morris water maze, and divided between cognitively "impaired" and "nonimpaired" subpopulations. Severe cognitive damage during acquisition of the eight-arm radial maze was shown, after the continuous hormonal treatment, in rats initially defined as "nonimpaired" in the Morris water maze.

This animal model might be useful for testing the protective effects of drugs against brain changes and cognitive damage, during either pathological or normal aging.

REFERENCES

1. LANDFIELD, P. W., J. C. WAYMIRE & G. LYNCH. 1978. Hippocampal aging and adrenocorticoids: quantitative correlations. Science **202**: 1098–1102.
2. LANDFIELD, P. W. & J. C. ELDRIDGE. 1991. The glucocorticoid hypothesis of brain aging and neurodegeneration: recent modifications. Acta Endocrinol. **125**(S1): 54–64.
3. SAPOLSKY, R. M., D. R. PACKAN & W. W. VALE. 1988. Glucocorticoid toxicity in the hippocampus: in vitro demonstration. Brain Res. **453**: 367–371.
4. SAPOLSKY, R. M., L. C. KREY & B. S. McEWEN. 1985. Prolonged glucocorticoid exposure reduces hippocampal neuron number: implication for aging. J. Neurosci. **5**: 1222–1227.
5. UNO, H., R. TARARA, J. G. ELSE, M. A. SULEMAN & R. M. SAPOLSKY. 1989. Hippocampal damage associated with prolonged and fatal stress in primates. J. Neurosci. **9**: 1705–1711.
6. SAPOLSKY, R. M., L. C. KREY & B. S. McEWEN. 1986. The neuroendocrinology of stress and aging: the glucocorticoid cascade hypothesis. Endocrine Rev. **7**: 284–301.
7. SAPOLSKY, R. M. 1985. A mechanism for glucocorticoid toxicity in the hippocampus: increased neuronal vulnerability to metabolic insults. J. Neurosci. **5**: 1228–1232.
8. OLTON, D. S., J. A. WALKER & F. H. GAGE. 1978. Hippocampal connections and spatial discrimination. Brain Res. **139**: 295–308.

9. EICHENBAUM, H. & T. OTTO. 1992. The hippocampus—what does it do? Behav. Neural Biol. **57:** 2–36.
10. JACOBSON, L. & R. M. SAPOLSKY. 1991. The role of the hippocampus in the feedback regulation of the hypothalamic-pituitary-adrenocortical axis. Endocrine Rev. **12:** 118–134.
11. RANSMAYR, G., P. CERVERA, E. C. HIRSCH, W. BERGER, W. FISCHER & Y. AGID. 1992. Alzheimer's disease: is the decrease of the cholinergic innervation of the hippocampus related to intrinsic hippocampal pathology? Neuroscience **47:** 843–851.
12. SCHUURMAN, T., E. HORVATH, D. G. SPENCER & J. TRABER. 1986. Old rats: an animal model for senile dementia. *In* Senile Dementias: Early Detection. A. Bes, *et al.,* Eds.: 624–630. John Libbey Eurotext. London, England.
13. WIEGERSMA, S. & K. MEERTSE. 1990. Subjective ordering, working memory, and aging. Exp. Aging Res. **16:** 73–77.
14. THOMPSON, L. T., R. A. DEYO & J. F. DISTERHOFT. 1990. Nimodipine enhances spontaneous activity of hippocampal pyramidal neurons in aging rabbits at a dose that facilitates associative learning. Brain Res. **535:** 119–130.
15. KADAR, T., M. SILBERMANN, R. BRANDEIS & A. LEVY. 1990. Age-related structural changes in the hippocampus: correlation with working memory deficiency. Brain Res. **512:** 113–120.
16. DACHIR, S., T. KADAR, B. ROBINZON & A. LEVY. 1993. Cognitive deficits induced in young rats by long-term corticosterone administration. Behav. Neural Biol. **60:** 103–109.
17. LEVY A., T. KADAR & S. DACHIR. 1992. Nimodipine counteracts behavioral effects of long term corticosterone treatment. Soc. Neurosci. Abstr. **18**(1): 350.
18. GALLAGHER, M. & M. A. PELLEYMOUNTER. 1988. An age-related spatial learning deficit: choline uptake distinguishes impaired and unimpaired rats. Neurobiol. Aging **9:** 363–369.
19. TOLEDO-MORRELL, L., Y. GEINISMAN & F. MORRELL. 1988. Age-dependent alterations in hippocampal synaptic plasticity: relation to memory disorders. Neurobiol. Aging **9:** 581–590.
20. FISCHER, W., K. S. CHEN, F. H. GAGE & A. BJOERKLUND. 1991. Progressive decline in spatial learning and integrity of forebrain cholinergic neurons in rats during aging. Neurobiol. Aging **13:** 9–23.
21. HENRIKSSON, B. G., S. SODERSTORM, A. J. GOWER, T. EBENDAL, B. WINBALD & A. H. MOHAMMED. 1992. Hippocampal nerve growth factor levels are related to spatial learning ability in aged rats. Behav. Brain Res. **48:** 15–20.
22. TOMBAUGH, G. C. & R. M. SAPOLSKY. 1993. Endocrine features of glucocorticoid endangerment in hippocampal astrocytes. Neuroendocrinology **57:** 7–13.
23. MEIER-RUGE, W. 1975. Mini-review: experimental pathology and pharmacology in brain research and aging. Life Sci. **17:** 1627–1636.
24. BODNOFF, S. R., A. HUMPHREYS, G. M. ROSE & M. J. MEANEY. 1992. Effects of corticosterone and stress on spatial learning, hippocampal plasticity and neuron loss. Soc. Neurosci. Abstr. **18**(1): 534.
25. LUINE, V., R. L. SPENCER & B. S. MCEWEN. 1992. Effects of corticosterone on hippocampal 5HT and spatial memory. Soc. Neurosci. Abstr. **18**(1): 670.
26. AHLERS, S. T., D. SHURTLEFF, J. R. THOMAS & F. PAUL-EMILE. 1992. Glucose administration attenuates cold-induced impairment of matching-to-sample performance in rats. Soc. Neurosci. Abstr. **18**(1): 866.
27. HANKS, S. D. & D. G. FLOOD. 1991. Region-specific stability of dendritic extent in normal human aging and regression in Alzheimer's disease. I. CA1 of hippocampus. Brain Res. **540:** 63–82.

Early Postnatal Diazepam Treatment of Rats and Neuroimmunocompetence in Adulthood and Senescence[a]

OLGA BENEŠOVÁ, HANA TEJKALOVÁ,
ZDENA KRIŠTOFIKOVÁ, JAN KLASCHKA,
AND MIROSLAV DOSTÁL[b]

Psychiatric Center Prague
Ústavní 91
181 03 Prague 8, Czech Republic

[b]*Institute of Experimental Medicine*
Czech Academy of Science
Vídeňská 1083
14220 Prague 4, Czech Republic

Drugs administered in perinatal treatment of risk pregnancies and risk newborns may disturb the development of the fetal/neonatal brain and immune system, which pass through a highly vulnerable phase of intensive cytodifferentiation. Even fine deviations in the programmed developmental processes induced by drugs may initiate disorders in the formation of neural network and cytoarchitectonics as well as in the receptor-transmitter communication system. These alterations are not evident at birth but form the basis for various functional defects (functional teratogenicity) appearing gradually during further maturation or even in adulthood as various neuropsychic deviations (e.g., hyperkinetic syndrome in children, sensorimotor deficits, mental retardation, altered psychoemotional reactivity) or disorders of immunocompetence.[1,2] The functional teratogenic risk is especially high in drugs with receptor-mediated effects (psychotropics, hormones) since the majority of receptors necessary for their action are developing in the perinatal period.[2]

Diazepam, one of the most frequently used tranquilizers, belongs to this class of drugs. Detailed studies concerning late consequences of prenatal exposure to diazepam in rats (for review see References 3 and 4) reported various behavioral disturbances in the offspring (decreased adaptation and learning ability) associated with brain biochemical alterations (deficits of benzodiazepine receptors, altered transmitter turnover). Some recent papers indicated even impairment of immunoreactivity in the progeny of rats administered diazepam during pregnancy.[5,6]

In spite of these warning reports, diazepam is still widely prescribed in perinatal risk situations, e.g., in cases of imminent preterm labor or in resuscitated newborns when intubated—in both conditions for its tranquilizing and myorelaxing action. For the evaluation of a potential developmental hazard of perinatal diazepam treatment on the human level, all experiments with diazepam exposure during rat pregnancy mentioned above are not fully consistent due to the low ontogenic phase that was influenced by diazepam. In addition, there are species differences between rat and man in the ontogenetic maturity at birth, and the vulnerable period of intensive brain

[a]This study was supported by the grant IGA MZČR No. 0294-3.

cytodifferentiation and cell receptor formation that takes place perinatally in man is shifted to the first postnatal decade in rat.

Therefore, we decided to investigate the functional teratogenic potential of diazepam in animal model experiments using early postnatal diazepam administration in rats and long-term follow-up until the age of 18 months with the registration of behavior, reproductive functions, brain neurobiochemical parameters, and immunoreactivity.

MATERIALS AND METHODS

The experiments were performed in rats, strain Wistar, bred under controlled conditions. The standard pellet diet and water was given *ad libitum*. On the first day after delivery, the litter size was adjusted to 10 pups. The young were weaned on the 28th day, selected according to gender, and housed in plastic cages in groups of 4 animals per cage till the age of 6–7 months and in groups of 2 animals per cage after this age.

Diazepam was administered on the 7th postnatal day in the dose 10 mg/kg subcutaneously (sc). One-half of the litter was treated with diazepam, the other half with the same volume of the solvent (3 microl/g body weight, triethylenglycol + saline, aa) and served as controls. All animals were followed up during development, adulthood, and senescence until the age of 18 months with regard to behavior, reproduction, brain neurobiochemical parameters, and immunocompetence, including registration of weight, morbidity, and mortality. The tests for behavior and immunocompetence as well as brain biochemical analysis were carried out at the age of 6, 12, and 18 months in groups of male rats (at least 10 controls + 10 treated animals) which included siblings of 4–5 litters. Reproduction ability was assessed in females aged 8, 12, and 15 months, in males aged 13 months, selected on the basis of litters.

During the first two months of life, *developmental landmarks* (pinna and eye opening, incisor eruption, motor skill) and the onset of *sexual maturation* were registered.

Behavioral Tests

Spontaneous exploration of the "open field" (four 5-min sessions with 24-h intervals in the box 60 × 46 cm, height 35 cm). Videotaped recordings of the sessions were analyzed by the investigator blinded to the animal history. Frequency and duration of various behavioral elements (rearing, locomotion, immobility, freezing, grooming, air and floor sniffing, defecation, etc.) were registered and evaluated using computer and special programs.

Memory test—discrimination between a familiar and a new object,[7] using fine exploratory and approach elements of behavior (day 1: presentation of 2 identical objects in two 4-min sessions with 10 min pause; day 2: presentation of the same 2 objects in the first 4-min session, in the second 4-min session after 10 min, one of them is substituted by a new one of different form). Recording and evaluation as in open field.

Motor performance—balancing and running on the rotating cylinder (dia 17 cm, speed 270 cm/min) in two 2-min sessions with 24-h interval.

Reproductive Ability

In females: assessment of estrous cycles in the course of 21 days, ability to conceive in a 7-day mating test with a young male and to give birth to live pups.

In males: spermiogram in standard epididymis extract, ability to fertilize a young female in a 7-day mating test.

Biochemical Analysis of the Brain

After decapitation, the brain was quickly removed and—while on an ice-cooled plate—dissected in 4 regions (cortex, hippocampus, hypothalamus, striatum) for various neurobiochemical analyses.

Markers for central monoaminergic neurotransmission:
a. Concentration of noradrenaline (NA), dopamine (DA), and serotonin (5-HT) and their metabolites homovanilic acid (HVA), vanilmandelic acid (VMA), and 5-hydroxyindolacetic acid (5-HIAA) in the hypothalamus, using high-performance liquid chromatography (HPLC) assay;
b. Concentration of DA and HVA in the striatum, using the modification of the spectrophotometric method of Earley and Leonard.[8]

Marker for cholinergic neuronal activity:
High-affinity choline uptake in the hippocampus, using the combination of the methods of Collier et al.[9] and Pugsley *et al.*[10] as described in our previous paper.[11]

Markers for free radical induced membrane damage:
a. Lipid peroxidation in the cortex, using the method of Ohkawa *et al.*[12]
b. Protein insolubilization in the cortex, using the method of Zs.-Nagy *et al.*[13] as described in our previous paper.[14]

Immunological Tests

The rats were sequentially immunized by bovine serum albumin (BSA, day 0, dose 100 micrograms emulsified in an equal volume of Freund complete adjuvans, injected at the base of the tail) and sheep red blood cells [SRBC, dose 2. 10^2 injected intraperitoneally (ip) on day 3]. The immune response was assayed on day 8. Alternatively, the rats were immunized by ovalbumin (OVA, day 0) and SRBC (day 8) injected in the same way and doses as in the combination BSA + SRBC, and the immune response was assayed on day 15.

The delayed-type hypersensitivity (DHT) reaction to BSA was assayed 24 h after challenging the rats with the heat-aggregated BSA into the left hind foot. The swelling of the foot was measured using a calliper and expressed in percent of the thickness of the foot before the challenge.

The serum hemagglutinating antibodies against SRBC were determined by microtitration and expressed as the $-\log_2$ of the highest degree of dilution, where agglutination could still be observed. The titer of immunoglobulin G (IgG) was determined after mixing the serum with an equal volume of 0.2 M 2-mercaptoethanol. The titer of IgM was determined as the difference between total Ig (TIg) and IgG.

The amount of anti-SRBC class IgM antibodies secreted by immune spleen cells was measured using a spectrophotometric determination of lymphocyte-mediated SRBC hemolysis. Serum titers of IgG and IgM antibodies to ovalbumin were determined using the enzyme-linked immunosorbent assay.[15]

Proliferative response of spleen lymphocytes to concanavalin A (Pharmacia, Uppsala, Sweden) was assayed in the usual way.[16]

Statistical Evaluation of the Results

The results of behavioral tests were evaluated by analysis of variance, using the statistical program package BMDP (program 2V, 7D and 3D) and Student's t-test.

The statistical evaluation of biochemical results was performed using ANOVA and Bonferoni t-test (BMDP-7D).

In immunological results, the significance of the differences between reactions of control and experimental rats in individual litters was determined by the nonparametric analysis of variance Kruskal-Vallis.[17] The Mann-Whitney U test was used for statistical evaluation of the differences between the means of pooled results of experimental and control groups.

RESULTS

The administration of diazepam in the dose of 10 mg/kg sc to 7-day-old rat pups induced a significant growth retardation lasting for 1–2 days when compared with control littermates, injected by the solvent. However, the body weight of treated rats normalized rapidly and beginning from the weaning (PD 28) until the end of the life, there were no weight differences between treated and control animals. No significant alterations were found in registered developmental landmarks and onset of sexual maturation either in males or in females.

The main results of testing exploratory activity in the "open field" at the age of 6, 12, and 18 months are presented in FIGURE 1. When considering the items of gross motor exploratory behaviour—rearing (FIGURE 1a) and locomotion (FIGURE 1b)—in the first minute of the first session, i.e., the first reaction in the new environment, it is evident that this reaction is characterized in diazepam-treated rats by significantly higher rearing and running, especially when younger. On the other hand, they reveal a lower rate of fine exploratory activity (FIGURE 1c—air and floor sniffing) as well as immobile postures (FIGURE 1d). The rate of defecation in the "open field" which is considered as a marker of emotional reactivity was evaluated either as the latency to lay the first bolus in the first session (FIGURE 2a), or as the sum of boluses defecated in the whole session (FIGURE 2b). It is evident that at the age of 6 and 12 months, the time interval to the appearance of the first defecated bolus is shorter in diazepam-treated rats—i.e., their reaction was characterized by a prompt defecation—and, in addition, the total defecation rate was higher. These findings indicate an increased emotional reactivity in diazepam-treated animals.

No differences between control and diazepam-treated rats were found in applied tests of memory—discrimination of the familiar and new object—at any age category.

Assessment of motor coordination on a rotating cylinder indicated some differences only in senescent rats at the age of 18 months in terms of inferior performance in diazepam-treated animals: the criterion was achieved in 9 of 10 control rats (90%) and only in 5 of 13 treated rats (39%), $p < 0.05$.

The outcome of testing reproductive ability is summarized in TABLE 1. A higher

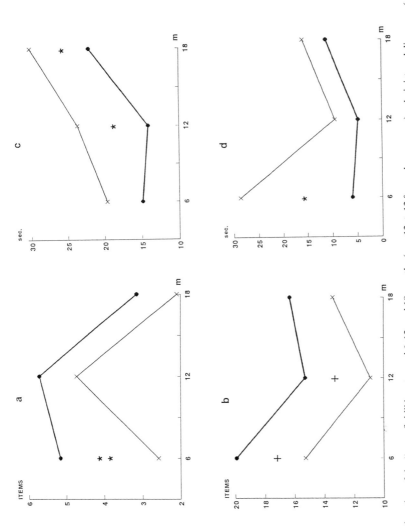

FIGURE 1. Exploration of the "open field" in rats aged 6, 12, and 18 months ($n = 12 + 12$ for each age group), administered diazepam (solid circles) or vehicle (crosses) on the 7th postnatal day. Rearing (a), locomotion (b), air and floor sniffing (c), and immobility (d) in the first minute of the first session. Statistical difference between treated and control rats: $^{**}p < 0.01$, $^{*}p < 0.05$, $^{+}p < 0.06$.

number of female diazepam-treated rats with irregular estrous cycles at the age of 8 and 12 months may be considered as a sign of some deficits of reproductive function, but the ability of conception was not inferior in comparison with age-matched controls. This fact is probably due to a long mating period (7 days) used in our experiments which allowed the animals to compensate some estrous cycle irregulari-

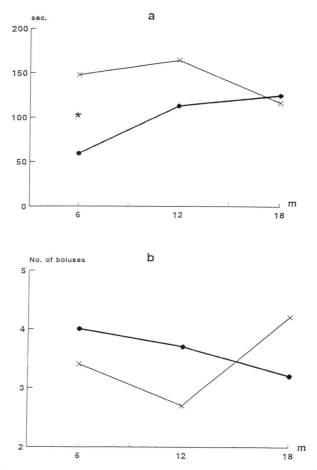

FIGURE 2. Defecation in the "open field" test. **a:** Latency to the first defecated bolus. **b:** Total of defecated boluses in the first session. For further description, see FIGURE 1.

ties, e.g., prolongation of interestrus intervals. No differences from age-matched controls were found in further criteria of fertility (pregnancy failure, live birth, litter size). At the age of 15 months, i.e., in the period of physiological extinction of reproductive functions, even the incidence of estrous cycle irregularity did not differ in both groups.

TABLE 1. Reproductive Ability in Adult Rats (Females and Males) Administered Diazepam or Vehicle on the 7th Postnatal Day

Age	Group	Percent of Rats with Irregular Estrus Cycles		Conception	
Females					
8 months	Control	31%	$n = 19$		
	Diazepam	71%[a]	$n = 14$		
12 months	Control	28%	$n = 14$	50%	$n = 14$
	Diazepam	67%[a]	$n = 15$	47%	$n = 15$
15 months	Control	53%	$n = 19$	0%	$n = 19$
	Diazepam	77%	$n = 13$	0%	$n = 13$

Age	Group	Spermiogram (% path. sperm cells)	Ability to Fertilize Normal Female	
Males				
13 months	Control	5.9%	27%	$n = 11$
	Diazepam	10.0%	0%	$n = 11$

[a] $p < 0.05$.

Male reproduction was examined in 13-month-old male rats, i.e., at the age of beginning senescence. At this age, the ability of fertilizing a young female is substantially decreased even in control animals and the minor inferiority of diazepam treated male rats registered in our experiment could not reach statistical significance.

Biochemical analysis of the brain revealed some deviations in the monoamine transmission in the striatum and the hypothalamus as demonstrated in TABLE 2. The differences between control and diazepam-treated rats seem to concern the turnover of dopamine in the striatum and probably also in the hypothalamus (significant alterations of DA and its metabolite HVA at the age of 6 and 18 months). More convincing, however, was the finding of significantly decreased concentration of both serotonin (5-HT) and its metabolite 5-HIAA in the hypothalamus of diazepam-treated rats aged 12 months. The same result was achieved in another series of 12-month-old animals ($n = 15$) using the spectrophotometric assay (5-HT in the hypothalamus of diazepam-treated rats = -55% of the control values, $p < 0.05$).

No deviations were found in other brain neurobiochemical markers tested in our experiments (HACU, lipid peroxidation, protein insolubilization).

TABLE 2. Concentration of Brain Monoamines and Their Metabolites in Adult Rats Administered Diazepam or Vehicle on the 7th Postnatal Day[a]

Age	n	a. Striatum		n	b. Hypothalamus					
		DA	HVA		5-HT	5-HIAA	NA	DA	HVA	VMA
6 months	17	+11	-53^c	12	-3	+21	-2	-4	$+88^c$	-1
12 months	14	+3	-26	15	-39^c	-37^c	+18	+9	+14	-30
18 months	23	$+13^b$	-4	23	+1	+8	-3	+20	-51	+53

[a] The results are presented as differences (+ or −) from control group values expressed in percents. (a) Spectrophotometric assay. (b) HPLC assay. For further abbreviations, see Methods.
[b] $p < 0.05$.
[c] $p < 0.01$.

The list of immunological assays performed in groups of 20 rats at the age of 6, 12, and 18 months is presented in TABLE 3. Statistically significant differences in the immune response of diazepam-treated and control rats are denoted by footnote symbols. A significantly decreased delayed-type hypersensitivity and lower proliferative response of spleen lymphocytes to concanavalin A of 6-month-old diazepam-treated rats in comparison with their untreated sibs indicated a depression of cell-mediated immunity. In 12-month-old animals, administered postnatally with diazepam, the delayed-type hypersensitivity did not differ from the controls. The significantly lower serum titers of anti-SRBC antibodies, however, suggested a depression of humoral immune response. The group of diazepam-treated female rats, aged 18 months, exhibited significant decrease of anti-SRBC IgM class antibodies secreted by spleen lymphocytes.

Regarding the differences in the assay spectrum, immunization scheme, and sex of rats in particular age groups, this pilot study does not allow analysis of the potential age-related variability of diazepam-induced depression of immunoreactivity in adult and senescent rats.

TABLE 3. The Synopsis of Immunological Assays Performed (+) and Statistically Significant Differences of the Results in Adult Rats Administered Diazepam or Vehicle on the 7th Postnatal Day[a]

Diazepam	10 mg/kg sc on postnatal day 7		
Sex	M	M	F
Age in months	6	12	18
Immunization	BSA	BSA	OVA
	SRBC	SRBC	SRBC
DTH	+[c]	+	−
Spleen − CON	+[c]	−	−
Spleen IgM (SRBC)	+	+	+[b]
Serum Ab (SRBC)	+	+[c]	+
Serum Ab (OVA)	−	−	+

[a]DTH = delayed-type hypersensitivity; BSA = bovine serum albumin; OVA = ovalbumin; SRBC = sheep red blood cells; CON = concanavallin A.
[b]$p < 0.05$.
[c]$p < 0.01$.

DISCUSSION

The present experiments have shown that diazepam administered in a single dose of 10 mg/kg sc to 7-day-old rats induced significant deviations of behavior, immune reactivity, and brain neurotransmission in adult life.

The behavior of diazepam-treated rats in the "open field" was characterized by altered strategy of exploring a new environment. While control rats begin with careful sniffing and fine exploratory movements followed gradually by locomotor activity and rearing, diazepam-treated animals react with high rate of rearing and running suggesting sometimes attempts of escape. This motor reaction was joined with increased emotional response as was indicated by intensified defecation rate. It may be assumed that diazepam-treated rats reveal higher emotionality as well as deviations in exploratory activity and adaptation that might compromise an individual's chance of survival. This behavioral difference between diazepam-treated and control rats was more evident in younger rats (age 6 months) and declined with aging, especially in elements of gross exploratory movements and immobility due probably to gradual physiological decrease of total gross motor activity in old animals. The character of behavioral changes described by various authors as late consequence of developmental exposure to diazepam was essentially very similar although the drug treatment was long term and applied prenatally. Kellogg[3] found alterations of adaptability and novelty reaction in adolescent rats (age 60 days) after prenatal diazepam administration (1–10 mg/kg over gestational days 13–20). The pattern of behavioral deviations in 6-month-old offspring of dams treated with diazepam (5.6 mg/kg between gestational days 15–20) reported by Marczynski and Urbancic[18] resembled surprisingly our findings: inability of habituation to novel environment, defective exploratory activity with sudden escape reactions, increased urination/ defecation scores. This behavioral profile was qualified as increased emotional tension, and the authors even proposed to use such animals as "models of chronic anxiety."

There are also references concerning late behavioral and endocrine changes following long-term postnatal administration of diazepam (10 mg/kg ip from the 2nd till 12th day of life).[19,20] This massive diazepam impact on early postnatal development induced lifelong body weight deficit and endocrine organ changes (higher hypophysis and thymus weight, lower relative weight of seminal vesicals). At the age of 65 days, diazepam-treated rats when exposed to new environment revealed hyperactivity with chaotic movements and an increased excitability, sometimes even aggressive acts against objects.

As is evident, the pattern of late behavioral deviations induced by diazepam administration during early ontogenic development is analogous in the reports of various authors and does not differ substantially from our findings. What is of interest in our experiments is the fact that a single injection of the drug in 7-day-old pups was sufficient for initiating the development of these behavioral abnormalities.

Similar reasoning may apply to another serious risk of early diazepam treatment, i.e., alteration of immune reactivity. Livezey *et al.*[5] administered diazepam (6 mg/kg per day sc) in female Sprague-Dawley rats during the last 5 days of pregnancy (days 15–20) and found lower titers of plasma IgG, a higher number of white blood cells, and lower hematocrit values in diazepam progenies aged 6 months. Some of these animals were followed up until the age of 20 months, and a higher incidence of medium to severe uterine, lung, and skin infections as well as tumors was found in the diazepam-treated group. Schlumpf *et al.*[6] observed a reduction of T-lymphocyte reactivity in 2–3 month old offspring of Long Evans dams treated with diazepam (1.25 mg/kg per day) from 14 to 20 days of gestation. Experiments with divided shorter periods of drug treatment indicated the dependence of this risk on the ontogenic stage of development in the time of drug administration. The mentioned immune deficit was found in the progeny of rats treated with diazepam during gestation days 16–20, but the same treatment applied earlier during gestation days 12–16 was ineffective. In our experiments (for more detailed description and discussion, see Reference 21), a single dose of diazepam administered postnatally to 7-day-old young had similar late consequences for adult immunocompetence as administration of diazepam to pregnant rats on several successive days at the end of pregnancy. These facts indicate an increased sensitivity to the deleterious action of diazepam at higher developmental stages. Apparently, the risk of adverse effects of this drug on the developing immune system is increasing along with advancing ontogenic development and expression of benzodiazepine receptors in differentiating cell population of the immune system.

It is possible to assume that in diazepam-treated rats, behavioral and immunological deviations might have some relations to brain neurobiochemical alterations reported in our and other authors experiments. This point of view is based firstly on the fact that benzodiazepine receptors, which are mediators of diazepam effects, are present both in the brain and in immune system cells (lymphocytes); secondly that diazepam is benzodiazepine with an equal affinity to both central (brain) and peripheral (lymphocytes) types of benzodiazepine receptors,[22] and thirdly that a decrease of benzodiazepine receptors was assessed in the brain of rats exposed to diazepam *in utero:* in the forebrain of 3-month-old[23] and in the thalamus of 12-month-old[24] animals.

Our findings of various deviations in striatal dopamine turnover appearing in diazepam-treated rats in the course of their lives fit in the scope of different reported brain dopamine alterations: increase of striatal dopamine in 60-day-old offspring of dams treated with diazepam (1 mg/kg per day sc) between gestational days 7–20[25] or decreased dopamine turnover in the mesolimbic system in 90-day-old rats that were subjected to the action of diazepam (5 mg/kg per day released from pellets implanted to dams) from prenatal day 8 through the first postnatal week.[26] On the other hand, Simmons *et al.*[27] found no changes of dopamine in the hypothalamus of 90-day-old rats exposed *in utero* to diazepam (1–10 mg/kg per day) over gestational days 13–20, but reported a dose-related decrease of noradrenaline turnover in this region. The important finding of these authors that the late gestation (days 17–20) is the period most sensitive to diazepam-induced alterations of hypothalamic noradrenaline turnover brought further evidence for increasing risk of functional teratogenicity of diazepam when it is applied at a higher stage of ontogenic development and receptor formation.

The variability of results concerning delayed effects of early diazepam treatment on brain catecholamine transmission both in our experiments and in above-mentioned references, which cannot be explained by the dosage and timing of diazepam administration or by the age of experimental rats when tested, does not allow us to draw satisfactory conclusions. In this context, it is worth mentioning our finding of another neurotransmission deficit, namely, the significant decrease of serotonin and its metabolite 5-HIAA in the hypothalamus of diazepam-treated rats, which was not reported so far. We have found it only at the age of 12 months and the result was confirmed in two different samples of rats using two different biochemical assays. No changes of brain serotonergic transmission were assessed either at the age of 6 months (mature adulthood) or at the age of 18 months (old age); the deficit was limited only on the age category of 12 months which represents in the rat life gradual onset of aging process. This age of 1 year appeared to be also a certain turning point in our experiments concerning behavior and reproduction (perhaps even immuno-competence).

These facts suggest that the manifestation of functional teratogenic defect may vary during the lifespan of the rat.[3,28] On the one hand, the developmental deviation may be masked by compensatory mechanisms that are most effective during adulthood, in the period of peak efficiency of the organism; thus the defect may become apparent when homeostatic balance breaks down at the age of aging process onset. On the other hand, along with progressing senescence, the functional deviation from normal values may gradually disappear due to physiological degeneration of functions in age-matched controls. Consequently, several functional abnormities and alterations may be apparent and detected only in certain periods of life. It is therefore very important to evaluate functional teratogenic potential of drugs in long-term animal studies covering the mentioned critical periods of life.

CONCLUSIONS

This long-term experimental study has shown that diazepam, injected as a single dose of 10 mg/kg sc to 7-day-old rats, induced in adult animals significant deviations of behavior (increased emotionality, defects in novelty reaction) and of immunocompetence (depression of immune response) as well as some transitional neurobiochemical alterations in the hypothalamus (5-HT) and striatum (DA). The fact that the manifestations of some functional abnormities vary during the life span and may not be detectable in certain periods of life emphasizes the necessity of lifelong follow-up of functional teratogenic sequellae.

The experimental data, indicating an increasing risk of functional teratogenic effects of diazepam when applied at higher ontogenic stages, have important clinical implications with regard to the still prevalent opinion that the risk of drug teratogenicity is limited to the first trimester of gravidity. This point of view arises from the traditional concept of teratogenicity as structural malformations. However, drugs with receptor-mediated effects may be of much higher risk at the end of gravidity or even in the neonatal period when relevant receptors necessary for their action are being formed. Preterm or inadequate activation of the developing receptors by the drug—as, e.g., by diazepam in our experiments—may initiate disorders in the receptor-transmitter communication systems that form the basis for persisting functional defects. The high risk of functional teratogenicity of diazepam, especially its immunoteratogenic effects, observed in our animal model experiments simulating clinical use of the drug in the perinatal period, should be a challenge for obstetricians and neonatologists using diazepam in risk pregnancies and risk neonates.

SUMMARY

Functional teratogenic risk of perinatal diazepam (D) treatment was studied in animal model experiments using early postnatal D administration in rats (single dose of 10 mg/kg sc in 7-day-old pups) and long-term follow-up till the age of 18 months with monitoring of behavior, reproductive functions, brain biochemical variables, and immune system reactivity. Behavioral tests carried out at the age of 6, 12, and 18 months indicated higher emotionality and deviations of novelty reaction in D rats in comparison with controls, and these differences decreased with aging. However, no deficits were found in memory testing. D rats revealed some transitional alterations of monoamine neurotransmission in the hypothalamus (5-HT) and striatum (DA) and minor defects in reproductive functions (irregular estrous cycles in females). Significant depression of immune response in D rats persisting for the whole life may be considered as a serious risk of neonatal D treatment.

REFERENCES

1. BENEŠOVÁ, O., J. PĚTOVÁ & A. PAVLÍK. 1984. Brain Maldevelopment and Drugs. Avicenum. Praha, Czechoslovakia.
2. BENEŠOVÁ, O. 1989. Perinatal pharmacotherapy and brain development. J. Prenatal Perinatal Studies **1:** 417–424.
3. KELLOG, C. K. 1988. Benzodiazepines: influence on the developing brain. *In* Biochemical Basis of Functional Neuroteratology. Permanent Effects of Chemicals on the Developing Brain. G. J. Boer, M. G. P. Feenstra, M. Mirmiran, D. F. Swaab & F. Van Haaren, Eds.: 207–228. Elsevier Publ. Amsterdam, the Netherlands.

4. TUCKER, J. C. 1985. Benzodiazepines and the developing rat: a critical review. Neurosci. Biobehav. Rev. **9:** 101–111.
5. LIVEZEY, G. T., T. J. MARZYNSKI, E. A. MCGREW & F. Z. BELUHAN. 1986. Prenatal exposure to diazepam: late postnatal teratogenic effect. Neurobehav. Toxicol. Teratol. **8:** 433–440.
6. SCHLUMPF, M., H. RAMSEIER, H. ABRIEL, M. YOUMBI, J. B. BAUMANN & W. LICHTENSTEIGER. 1989. Diazepam effects on the fetus. Neurotoxicol. **10:** 501–516.
7. ENNACEUR, A., A. CAVOY & J. DELACOUR. 1989. A new one-trial test for neurobiological studies of memory in rats. II. Effects of piracetam and pramiracetam. Behav. Brain Res. **33:** 197–207.
8. EARLEY, C. J. & B. E. LEONARD. 1978. Isolation and assay of noradrenaline, dopamine, 5-hydroxytryptamine and several metabolites from brain tissue using disposable Bio-Rad columns packed with Sephadex G-10. J. Pharmacol. Methods **1:** 67–70.
9. COLLIER, B., S. LOVAT, D. ILSON, L. A. BARKER & T. W. MITTAG. 1977. The uptake metabolism and release of homocholine: studies with rat brain synaptosomes and cat superior cervical ganglion. J. Neurochem. **28:** 331–339.
10. PUGSLEY, T. A., B. P. H. POSCHEL, D. A. DOWNS, Y. H. SHIH & M. I. GLUCKMAN. 1983. Some pharmacological and neurochemical properties of a new cognition activator agent, pramiracetam (Cl 879). Psychopharmacol. Bull. **19:** 721–726.
11. KRIŠTOFIKOVÁ, Z., J. KLASCHKA, H. TEJKALOVÁ & O. BENEŠOVÁ. 1992. High-affinity choline uptake and muscarinic receptors in rat brain during aging. Arch. Gerontol. Geriatr. **15:** 87–97.
12. OHKAWA, H., N. OHISHI & K. YAGI. 1979. Assay for lipid peroxides in animal tissues by thiobarbituric acid reaction. Anal. Biochem. **95:** 351–358.
13. ZS.-NAGY, I., K. NAGY, V. ZS.-NAGY, A. KALMAR & E. NAGY. 1981. Alteration of total content and solubility characteristics of proteins in rat brain and liver during aging and centrophenoxine treatment. Exp. Gerontol. **16:** 229–240.
14. KRIŠTOFIKOVÁ, Z., O. BENEŠOVÁ & H. TEJKALOVÁ. 1991. Changes in water solubility of proteins in aging rat brain. Arch. Gerontol. Geriatr. **12:** 41–48.
15. VOS, J. G., J. BOERKAMP, J. BUYS & P. A. STEERENBERG. 1970. Ovalbumin immunity in the rat: simultaneous testing of IgM, IgG and IgE response measured by ELISA and delayed-type hypersensitivity. Scand. J. Immunol. **12:** 289–295.
16. KRUISBECK, A. M. & E. SHEVACH. 1992. Proliferative assays for T cell function. *In* Current Protocols in Immunology. A. M. Kruisbeck, D. M. Margulies, E. M. Shevach & W. Strober, Eds. Green Publishing Assoc. & Wiley Interscience.
17. THEODORSSON-NORHEIM, E. 1986. Kruskal-Wallis test: basic computer program to perform nonparametric one-way analysis of variance and multiple comparisons on rank of several independent samples. Computer Methods Programs Biomed. Sci. **23:** 57–69.
18. MARCZYNSKI, T. J. & M. URBANCIC. 1988. Animal models of chronic anxiety and "fearlessness." Brain Res. Bull. **21:** 483–490.
19. FRAŇKOVÁ, S. & B. JAKOUBEK. 1974. Long-term behavioural effects of diazepam and ACTH, administered early in life. Activ. Nerv. Sup. (Praha) **16:** 247–249.
20. JAKOUBEK, B., M. KRAUS, R. ERDÖSOVÁ, J. LÁT & A. DĚDIČOVÁ. 1974. The effect of ACTH and diazepam, administered to infant rats on the body growth curve and some endocrine parameters measured in adult age. Activ. Nerv. Sup. (Praha) **16:** 246–247.
21. DOSTÁL, M., O. BENEŠOVÁ, H. TEJKALOVÁ & D. SOUKUPOVÁ. Immune response of adult rats is altered by administration of diazepam in the first postnatal week. Reprod. Toxicol. **8.** (In press.).
22. SCHLUMPF, M., R. PARMAR, H. R. RAMSIER & V. LICHTENSTEIGER. 1990. Prenatal benzodiazepine immunosuppression: possible involvement of peripheral benzodiazepine site. Dev. Pharmacol. Ther. **15:** 178–185.
23. KELLOGG, C. K., J. CHISHOLM, R. D. SIMMONS, J. R. ISON & R. K. MILLER. 1983. Neural and behavioral consequences of prenatal exposure to diazepam. Monogr. Neural Sci. **9:** 119–129.
24. LIVEZEY, G. T., M. RADULOVACKI, L. ISAAC & T. J. MARCZYNSKI. 1985. Prenatal exposure to diazepam results in enduring reactions in brain receptors and deep slow wave sleep. Brain Res. **334:** 361–365.

25. HOMFELD, B., E. DALITZ, H. MIDDLETON-PRICE & D. BIESOLD. 1987. Diazepam induced alterations in postnatal development. *In* Ontogenesis of the Brain. S. Trojan & F. Šťastný, Eds. **4:** 363–369. Universitas Carolina. Praha.
26. GRUEN, R. J., A. Y. DEUTCH & R. H. ROTH. 1990. Perinatal diazepam exposure: alterations in exploratory behavior and mesolimbic dopamine turnover. Pharmacol. Biochem. Behav. **36:** 169–175.
27. SIMMONS, R. D., C. K. KELLOGG & R. K. MILLER. 1984. Prenatal diazepam exposure in rats: long-lasting, receptor-mediated effects on hypothalamic norepinephrine-containing neurons. Brain Res. **293:** 73–83.
28. BENEŠOVÁ, O., H. TEJKALOVÁ & M. BUREŠOVÁ. 1992. Accelerated aging in rats as a consequence of disturbed perinatal development induced by drugs. *In* Ontogenesis of the Brain. S. Trojan & M. Langmeier, Eds. **5:** 135–139. Universitas Carolina Pragensis. Praha.

A Survey of the Available Data on a New Nootropic Drug, BCE-001

IMRE ZS.-NAGY

Fritz Verzár International Laboratory for
Experimental Gerontology (VILEG)
Hungarian Section
University Medical School
Debrecen, H-4012, Hungary

INTRODUCTION

The nootropic molecule coded BCE-001 (US Patent No. 4661618, 1985)[1] was born from a scientific research collaboration between BIOGAL Pharmaceutical Works Ltd. (Debrecen, Hungary) and the Hungarian Section of VILEG, University Medical School (Debrecen, Hungary).

The theoretical basis for the design of this new molecule was the membrane hypothesis of aging (MHA). MHA explains cell maturation and aging on the basis of the intrinsic biochemical and physicochemical interactions between the cell plasma membrane and basic oxidative processes of living systems. This working hypothesis has been elaborated since the late seventies;[2] it was based on the main achievements of previous experimental gerontological research, such as the cross-linking theory,[3-5] the free radical theory of aging,[6,7] and on available knowledge in cell physiology. The MHA has continuously been developed by checking experimentally various points of it in different biological models.[8-18] MHA was compared to the dysdifferentiation hypothesis of aging and cancer (DHAC), resulting in the conclusion that the two hypotheses are largely complementary to each other.[19] MHA is explained in detail in a recent monograph;[18] here we have space only for a short outline of MHA.

AN OUTLINE OF MHA

The main starting point of MHA is that the deterioration of the molecular components of living systems is mainly due to the biochemical effects of the oxygen free radicals (termed also active oxygen species). The most harmful active oxygen species is the OH· free radical causing a continuous alteration of molecular conformation through a forced rearrangement of the electron distribution on the external shells. The result of this type of rearrangement is either a simple oxidation or the formation of intra- or intermolecular cross-linking of proteins with any kind of other organic molecules (lipids, sugars, etc). Since the OH· free radicals react extremely fast, the only possible natural defense against them is the frequently repeated replacement of the damaged molecules by newly synthesized ones.

MHA takes into consideration that the OH· free radical reactions are by nature density dependent. This involves that the nearer the molecules are to each other, the more intermolecular cross-links are formed even at identical frequency of free radical events. The most compact cellular structures are the membranes; among them is the cell plasma membrane which is exposed also to so-called residual heat-induced damage (see References 8 and 18 for references). Therefore, the highest rate of damage is encountered in the cell membrane. As a consequence, the leading point of cell maturation and aging is a gradual loss of permeability of the cell membrane for monovalent ions (potassium and chloride) and most probably also for water. This trend results in a gradual increase of the intracellular density. It was predicted theoretically and has been proven experimentally that all enzyme activities decrease with the increasing density of their molecular environment. The increase of the intracellular density up to a certain level is required by cell maturation and differentiation. However, because of the ever ongoing character of this process, the increase of intracellular density becomes rate limiting for the replacement of the damaged components. The result of this situation is a dehydration of the intracellular mass, an accumulation of cross-linked proteins as well as of waste products (lipofuscin) in the cells, accompanied by a slowing down of the RNA synthesis rate (and protein turnover). Therefore, even if the rate of OH· radical formation decreases with the drop of oxygen consumption at later ages, the rate of direct damage may increase considerably. MHA is valid especially for postmitotic cells; however, with some modifications, it involves all types of cells.

PHARMACOLOGICAL TESTING OF MHA

MHA has been tested among others pharmacologically. The effects of centrophenoxine (CPH) have been summarized in detail before.[13] CPH is an ester of *p*-chlorophenoxyacetic acid (PCPA) and dimethylaminoethanol (DMAE) (FIGURE 1). It was classified formerly in human therapy as a brain metabolic stimulant (and the ill-defined term "neuroenergeticum" was applied to it), since it stimulates glucose uptake, oxygen consumption, and carbon dioxide production of the brain *in vivo* and also *in vitro* in brain slices. Early publications on the effects of CPH described a number of beneficial effects of CPH in cases like cerebral atrophy, brain injury, postapoplectic disorders, chronic alcoholism, barbiturate intoxications, etc. It has also been observed that prolonged administration of CPH to healthy old animals reduced significantly the accumulation of lipofuscin in the brain cells and myocardium. Furthermore, the medium life span of CPH-treated old animals increased significantly, and the learning ability of old, treated mice improved as compared to their age-matched controls (see Reference 13 for references). On the basis of these results, CPH could be considered as a potential antiaging drug.

CPH is classified nowadays as a nootropicum.[20] It is one of the most frequently used representative of nootropics in various countries. According to the most recent statistical data (MIDAS Data Base), its yearly sale amounts to about 20 tons; most of it is used in Japan.

Regarding the mechanism of action of CPH on the age-dependent decline of mental performance, the early suggestion was that the DMAE moiety of CPH enters the choline synthesis cycle (i.e., improves the acetylcholine supply of the brain).[21,22] However, this explanation has been contested by others.[23–25] It has been shown that a fraction of DMAE from CPH becomes indeed trimethylated in the liver resulting in an increase of free choline availability.[26–28] Considering that only a very small fraction of choline level is able to keep acetylcholine synthesis saturated, while the rest is necessary for phospholipid production,[23,29–32] an increased availability of choline caused by CPH or DMAE cannot be the only explanation of the effect of this drug. As a matter of fact, in this case, a choline-rich diet alone should have the same effect as CPH has, which is not observed.[24,25]

A step forward was the discovery of the strong OH· radical scavenger ability of DMAE. It has been shown both in chemical systems[33] and also by ESR–spin trapping techniques[34] that the effect of OH· free radicals generated by the Fenton reaction decreases to a considerable extent on both proteins and spin traps in the presence of DMAE.

Pharmacokinetic studies of CPH revealed that after intravenous administration of equimolar doses of ^{14}C-labeled DMAE or CPH, much higher levels of DMAE were found in the brain after CPH treatment, as compared to DMAE alone, since apparently the esterified form of DMAE with PCPA penetrates much easier the blood-brain barrier. CPH is hydrolyzed on both sides of the barrier *in vivo*. However, the DMAE moiety becomes phosphorylated in the brain and yields phosphoryl-DMAE, which is in turn converted to phosphatidyl-DMAE, seemingly the end-metabolite of DMAE in the brain.[35] Phosphatidyl-DMAE is incorporated in nerve

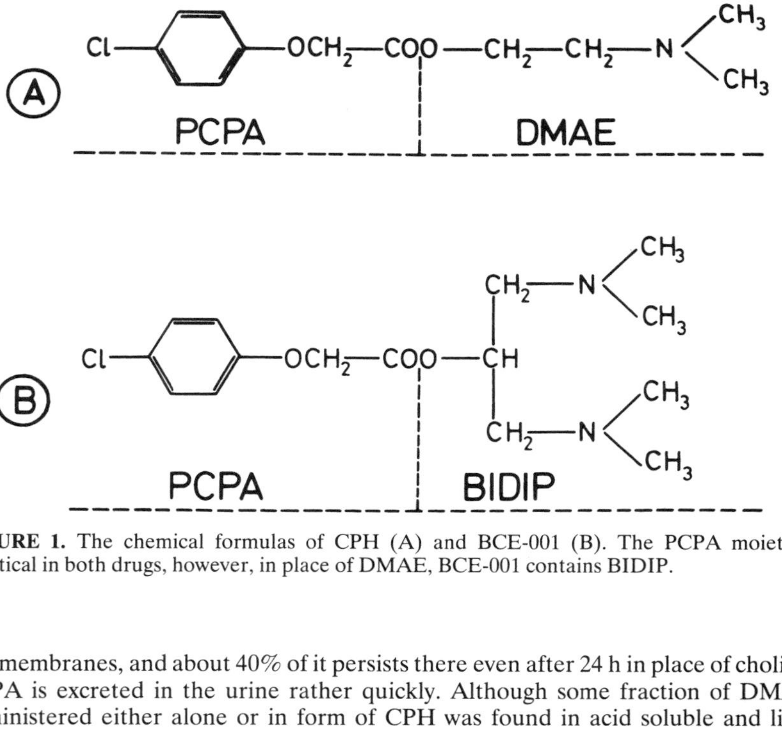

FIGURE 1. The chemical formulas of CPH (A) and BCE-001 (B). The PCPA moiety is identical in both drugs, however, in place of DMAE, BCE-001 contains BIDIP.

cell membranes, and about 40% of it persists there even after 24 h in place of choline. PCPA is excreted in the urine rather quickly. Although some fraction of DMAE administered either alone or in form of CPH was found in acid soluble and lipid cholines in the brain, evidence is available that trimethylation of DMAE does not take place in the brain but in the liver.[35] This fact suggested that its OH· radical scavenger ability shown *in vitro* may really be of significance also *in vivo*. The effects of CPH were studied in detail since 1976 parallel with the development of MHA. The conclusion was reached that the effects of CPH on the brain can be interpreted as an OH· free radical scavenging action of the DMAE moiety in the neuronal membranes.[13]

THE DESIGN OF BCE-001

It should be stressed that because of the extremely short lifetime of OH· free radicals, protection of neuronal membrane components against OH· radical damage can be imagined only if the following criteria are fulfilled.

1. The scavenger molecule should have a reaction rate with OH· radicals comparable to that of the target molecule to be protected.
2. The scavenger should get sufficiently close to the target and remain there as a component part for a sufficiently long time.
3. The scavenger must not exert any deleterious side effect (toxicity) for the organism in general or in the immediate vicinity of the target molecule.

The above-listed criteria imply that it is most probably a hopeless effort to start testing of various scavengers without having any particular knowledge about their molecular biology, binding sites, etc. It should be stressed that, unfortunately, most of the studies on dietary antioxidants were performed without having such special information. For example, Weber and Miquel[36] reviewed the available data on the effects of various radical scavenger compounds like butylated hydroxytoluene (BHT), 2-mercaptoethylamine (2-MEA), cysteine, 2,2'-diaminodiethyldisulfide, santoquine, vitamin E, ascorbic acid, D,L-methionine, Na-selenite, quercetin, thiazolidine-4-carboxylic acid, tocopheryl-*p*-chlorophenoxyacetate, nordihydroguaiaretic acid (NDGA), folcysteine, propyl gallate, diludine, and α-tocopherolchinone. The most striking observation was that although some antioxidant supplements are indeed capable of extending the life span of experimental animals, the observed effects are not consistent when studying the same drug in various species.

Considering all these data and the results obtained with CPH, a new drug was designed coded BCE-001, with the intention to increase the OH· radical scavenging ability of CPH in the cell membrane. BCE-001 is basically similar to CPH; the difference is that the PCPA moiety is esterified with 1,3-bis(dimethylamino)-2-propanol (BIDIP) instead of DMAE (FIGURE 1). The complete chemical name is 4-chloro-phenoxy-acetic acid-1,3-bis(dimethylamino)-2-propyl ester (PCPA-BI-DIP). It is a white, powderlike substance, displaying a melting point of 202–205°C. Its overall composition is $C_{15}H_{23}ClN_2O_3 \times 2HCl$, with a molecular mass of 387.7. BCE-001 is freely soluble in methanol, and in water (however, it rapidly hydrolyzes at neutral pH); moderately soluble in ethanol and acetonitrile; poorly soluble in acetone, dichlor-methane, and ethyl-acetate.

As regards the stability of BCE-001, tests were performed for 12 weeks at 4, 24, and 40°C. Extrapolating the results for 3 years, decomposition rates of 1.5, 4, and 10% were obtained in samples stored at the given temperatures, respectively. Therefore, the dry substance maintains its stability sufficiently for 3 years even at room temperature.

In solution, the molecule displays a pH dependence of stability: at pH 2.5 in aqueous solution about 50% of it is hydrolyzed during the first hour. At pH 7.0, the hydrolysis is immediate and 100%. Considering that the gastric pH is around 2.0, and assuming an absorption time of 20–30 min, one can accept that mostly the intact ester molecules are absorbed from the stomach. At the physiological pH 7.2–7.4, the ester molecule is most probably hydrolyzed, unless some yet unknown carrier molecules are not protecting it against the hydrolytic effect of this pH.

It is important to stress that BIDIP contains 2 dimethylamino groups, suggesting that twice as much loosely bound electrons are available in this moiety for the neutralization of OH· radicals. As will be demonstrated below, this property of the molecule proved to be biologically meaningful, since it resulted in a doubling of the rate constant of the reaction with OH· free radicals. BCE-001 proved to be a nootropic agent of low toxicity *in vivo*, which can be administered orally or even parenterally.

Acute toxicity studies in rodents revealed the LD_{50} values shown in TABLE 1. Details about the toxicity studies are available in unpublished documentation in possession of BIOGAL Pharmaceutical Works, Ltd. (Debrecen, Hungary). The acute toxicity tests repeatedly confirmed the values shown in TABLE 1 for both types of administration. Therefore, it can be concluded that BCE-001 is really of low toxicity, and it is somewhat better tolerated than CPH itself in mice. The latter displayed intravenous (iv) and peroral (po) LD_{50} toxicity values 385 and 2270 mg/kg body weight, respectively.[13] It is noteworthy that biologically effective doses applied po in rodents are in the range of 60–100 mg/kg body weight, i.e., far below the LD_{50} doses.

TABLE 1. LD_{50} Values of BCE-001 (mg/kg Body Weight) in CFY Rats and CFLP Mice of Both Sexes

	Males	Females
Per os		
	In rats	
	2719.1	2329.1
Range	(2573.8–2872.7)	(2231.8–2430.7)
	In mice	
	3904.1	3195.8
Range	(3852.7–3956.1)	(3107.4–3286.6)
Ip		
	In rats	
	872.08	827.03
Range	(846.62–898.31)	(802.43–852.38)
	In mice	
	957.7	890.9
Range	(917.56–999.6)	(864.89–917.73)

OH· FREE RADICAL SCAVENGING ABILITY OF CPH AND BCE-001

Protein Cross-Linking Model

In this model,[33] OH· free radicals are generated by Fenton reaction, attacking and cross-linking the proteins (e.g., bovine serum albumin = BSA) added to the reaction mixture. As a consequence, the water solubility of the protein (originally 100%) gradually decreases. Therefore, it is sufficient to measure the protein content and the molecular weight distribution of the still soluble fraction of BSA in the supernatant in order to reveal the effect of the OH· radicals and the influence of radical scavengers like DMAE or BIDIP on this reaction. These studies revealed that DMAE efficiently inhibits the polymerization of BSA induced by the OH· radicals, i.e., DMAE is a potent OH· radical scavenger under the given conditions. The polymerization of BSA could be detected not only as a precipitation of an insoluble, gluelike mass, but also in the still soluble rest of BSA in form of di-, tri-, and tetramerized molecules. The covalent character of the newly formed intermolecular bonds has been proven by chemical tests like treatment with concentrated (6 M) urea, etc.[33]

BCE-001 behaved similarly to DMAE with the only difference that equimolar amounts of it displayed a roughly twofold protective effect against the polymerization of BSA (unpublished results).

ESR–Spin Trapping Experiments

This technique applies specially designed compounds (spin traps) the reactions of which with various types of free radicals are well known. They form usually some relatively long-lived radicals (spin adducts). The concentration of spin adducts can be quantitatively measured under controlled conditions by means of their paramagnetic properties by ESR spectroscopy.[37-39] Using this technique, one can obtain data regarding the competition for the given type of radical generated in the reaction mixture, and in some cases also the rate constants of the radical scavenging process can be estimated.

The spin trapping experiments demonstrated that the CPH molecule and both components of it display a strong affinity toward OH· radicals.[34] In the case of DMAE, the reaction rate can be estimated at about 0.8×10^9 $M^{-1}s^{-1}$. This figure is quite comparable with that of the spin trap (DMPO) used.[39] Since most bioorganic compounds react with OH· radicals at rates[40] ranging from 10^7 to 10^{10} $M^{-1}s^{-1}$, DMAE really may exert a significant protection for numerous cell membrane components against OH· free radicals. It is noteworthy that BIDIP displayed a reaction rate constant with OH· free radicals of about 1.7×10^9 $M^{-1}s^{-1}$ in identical test conditions (unpublished results), which is quite near to the theoretically expected twofold increase, as compared to DMAE.

The OH· scavenger ability of DMAE[34] and BIDIP (unpublished results) has also been tested in some other spin trapping models using PBN and 4-POBN. In addition, proline and hydroxyproline were also tested as special spin traps.[34,41] All these investigations supported the OH· scavenger ability of DMAE and BIDIP. Therefore, these compounds, if incorporated into the plasma membrane of nerve cells, can really be considered as site-specific OH· free radical scavengers, i.e., their observed effects should be interpreted on this basis.

Although these experiments revealed also an OH· radical scavenger capability of the PCPA moiety present in both the CPH and BCE-001 molecules, PCPA cannot be responsible for the nootropic effects of either of them, since no binding of this compound is known in the brain. It cannot be excluded, however, that PCPA may have some physiologically meaningful effect in the blood or in some other tissues (e.g., kidney or liver) during its excretion.

The early data regarding OH· radical scavenger ability of DMAE and BIDIP have recently been confirmed in a completely different system, applying a gamma radiation source for generation of OH· free radicals as well as the measurement of the carbonyl group formation on the BSA (see Reference 42, in this volume). The quantitatively better properties of BIDIP could well be established also by these recent experiments.

IN VIVO BIOLOGICAL EFFECTS OF CPH AND BCE-001

Since the effects of BCE-001 were compared to those of CPH, we list below the main findings obtained in animal experiments with both drugs. Such a comparison may facilitate judgment on improvement of the effects with the new compound.

Obviously, neither the presence of DMAE in the brain nerve cell membranes[35] nor the *in vitro* OH· radical scavenging ability of this compound[34] proves directly that it acts as an OH· radical scavenger also *in vivo*. However, numerous experimental results, listed below, demonstrate indirectly that the presence of DMAE or BIDIP in the cell membrane is of physiological significance that can be attributed to their OH· radical scavenger properties.

Effects on Lipid Fluidity in Synaptosomal Membranes

The microviscosity of the membrane lipids was measured by means of a fluorescence polarization method after diphenyl-hexatriene (DPH) labeling of brain cortical synaptosomal membranes.[43]

Aging causes an increase of microsviscosity in the synaptosomal membranes (TABLE 2). If old rats had been treated with CPH for 60 days,[43] or with BCE-001 for 20 days (unpublished results), the membrane microviscosity decreased again significantly (about the same extent) as revealed by fluorescence anisotropy measurements

TABLE 2. Age-Dependent Alterations of the Microviscosity of the Lipid Layer of Synaptosomal Membranes in Rat Brain Cortex and the Effects of CPH and BCE-001 on This Parameter in Old Rats[a]

	Young	Adult	Old	Old + CPH	Old + BCE-001
Microviscosity (poise)	2.338	2.370	2.632[b]	2.466[c]	2.450[c]
±SD	0.016	0.022	0.035	0.018	0.010
n	61	51	71	44	45
Duration of treatment (days)				60	20

[a]Notes: n = number of measured points. SD = standard deviation. Significance: [b]old versus young and adult; [c]treated groups versus old; for both cases $p < 0.001$.

after DPH labeling (TABLE 2). These results imply that BCE-001 treatment improved the neuronal membrane lipid fluidity about three times faster than did CPH. Spin labeling ESR techniques[44] confirmed the validity of the results obtained by DPH labeling for both drugs (unpublished results). These results show indirectly that BIDIP reaches the brain synaptosomal membranes. Synaptosomal membranes were protected considerably by CPH pretreatment against the toxic effect of *in vivo* acute Fe^{2+} overload in the cerebrospinal fluid of young rats;[45] therefore, similar effects can be expected also from BCE-001.

Effects on Protein Molecular Weights in Synaptosomal Membranes

The molecular weight distribution of the proteins displays a considerable age-dependent shift toward higher values in the synaptosomes of the rat brain cortex. This is a clear sign of an increased cross-linking of the membrane proteins. A treatment of 60 days with CPH[46] or of 20 days with BCE-001 (unpublished results) reversed this tendency to a considerable extent in old rats.

Effects on the Lateral Mobility of Proteins in Hepatocyte Membrane

The lateral mobility of hepatocyte membrane proteins can be measured by means of the fluorescence recovery after photobleaching (FRAP) technique. The lateral diffusion constant (D) displays a characteristic, negative age correlation in Fischer 344 and Wistar rats, in C57BL black mice, as well as in wild mouse strains of considerably different longevity (*Peromyscus leucopus, Mus musculus*).[47-52] The striking fact is that the rate of decay of protein mobility in hepatocyte membranes is inversely proportional to the life span of the given strain. In the case of the wild mouse strains mentioned above, there exists a 2.6-fold difference in longevity in favor of *P. leucopus,* and the age-related decline of D is about 2.5 times slower in the longer-living species.[52]

FRAP experiments on 2-year-old Fischer 344 rats pretreated per os through gastric tube with aqueous solutions of 80 mg/kg CPH or BCE-001 for 5 weeks revealed a significantly higher value of D than in the controls. BCE-001 produced a quantitatively larger increase of the protein diffusion constant under identical dosage and time of treatment than did CPH.[51]

A further important observation was that the well-known, almost linear body weight loss of the Fischer 344 male rats above the age of 2 years was only slightly inhibited by CPH from the end of the 3rd week of treatment, whereas in the BCE-001-treated group, this loss of body weight was almost completely stopped after 1 week of treatment.[51] This observation indicates that the observed increase in D under the effect of CPH or BCE-001 is not only an improvement of a cellular parameter, but it is also meaningful from a general physiological point of view. An inhibition of the body weight loss in these animals is very convincing evidence for the overall improvement of the status of the animals, and is in agreement with the observed life-prolonging effect of BCE-001.

Effects on the Passive Potassium Permeability of Nerve Cell Membranes

The age-dependent decline of passive potassium permeability in the nerve cells is an important, key issue in brain aging, as explained by the MHA. CPH treatment of 60 days (80–100 mg/kg) in old rats reincreases the passive potassium permeability of the neuronal cell membrane, i.e., it decreases the intracellular potassium content and rehydrates the cytoplasm of brain neurons considerably.[53,54] BCE-001 was of the same effect. However, a lower dose (60 mg/kg) and shorter time (3–4 weeks) of treatment were sufficient to reach the same level of these improvements (unpublished observations).

These findings indicate that CPH and BCE-001 may be useful in the prevention or therapy of age-dependent brain disorders.

Effects on the Rates of Total and mRNA Synthesis in the Brain Cortex

The rate of synthesis of total as well as mRNA synthesis was measured by means of radioisotope methods *in vivo* in rats. An age-dependent decrease of the rates of total and mRNA synthesis was observed in the brain cortex of rats between 1 and 2 years of age (to 40–50% of the young-adult value).[55] The significance of this phenomenon in the age-dependent decrease of protein turnover rates has clearly been explained by MHA, as the main reason of the loss of physiological abilities of all cells and organs.

In vivo treatments with both CPH and BCE-001 reversed this tendency. CPH treatment of 60 days reincreased these rates to 80–90%,[56] whereas BCE-001 resulted in similar increases already during 40 days, and values up to 113% were obtained when the drug was applied for 60 days (unpublished results). Therefore, BCE-001 is not only a better OH· radical scavenger than CPH, but it is able to stimulate more efficiently the *in vivo* rates of brain RNA synthesis. This fact may have great significance in the prevention or therapy of human brain disorders like dementias, where the decreased RNA and protein synthesis is an obvious reason for the dysfunctions.

Survival Experiments

It has been observed by various authors that CPH treatment is capable of prolonging the medium life span of laboratory animals, especially if the treatment starts at relatively young ages (6 months). It improves also the learning ability of several species (see References 54 and 57 for references). In some cases an increase of the medium life span up to 30% was described in mice, but only if CPH treatment started at the age of 6 months.

The effect of BCE-001 on the medium life span was studied in one experiment when female CFY rats were treated from the age of 18 months intraperitoneally. The untreated controls displayed a medium life span of 23.6 months which is a quite usual value for this strain. The BCE-001 treatment increased the medium life span of these rats to 29 months (unpublished results). These experiments will be repeated by po treatment in the future.

Some Further Animal Experiments

BCE-001 in comparison with CPH was tested in further behavioral and other animal models on the basis of commissions from BIOGAL Pharmaceutical Works, Ltd. (Debrecen, Hungary), in various laboratories in Japan and Hungary. Although the results have not been published, we can mention here briefly the following results. Doses of 60–100 mg/kg of BCE-001 administered ip for 7–30 days in rats improves brain functions. It displays an effect on the neurotransmitters, particularly increases 5-HT content in the septum, and improves memory functions through a novel mechanism of action. It is particularly active in the hippocampus and modifies its dopaminergic system. It increases glucose utilization in the brain regions involved in memory and awakening such as the frontal cortex, nucleus basalis, nucleus lateralis thalami, hippocampus, and reticular formation. BCE-001 exerts a protective action against experimentally induced hypoxia, manifesting itself in a longer survival period. It also inhibits the formation of strokes in spontaneously hypertensive rats. Therefore, it can be considered as a cerebrovascular protective agent acting without any prolonged modification of the systemic circulation. Various tests on memory consolidation and retrieval demonstrated that BCE-001 has beneficial effects comparable to those of CPH. Therefore, the possibility of developing a useful nootropic drug for human use seems to be realistic. It is important to stress here that BCE-001 displayed a more advantageous effect in each of the listed experiments as compared to CPH.

Human Experiments with CPH

In order to create a basis of comparison for eventual future human application of BCE-001, specially designed human experiments were performed, and their results are summarized here. In a double-blind, randomized, human clinical trial, CPH treatment of 8 weeks improved psychometric and behavioral performance in about 50% of patients with medium level dementia (DSM III, Cat. 1; ICD No. 299); the placebo group displayed improvement only in 27%.[57] A considerable rehydration of the intracellular mass was observed in the verum group at the expense of the extracellular liquid; meanwhile, the body weight remained unchanged.[58] These data are mentioned here to demonstrate that nootropica like CPH (and most probably also BCE-001) behave also in humans as predictable on the basis of MHA. Similar human trials will be performed with BCE-001 as soon as the drug arrives at the human phase II of testing.

CONCLUSIONS

Experimental biological research is approaching a synthesis on the basis of which the understanding of the physicochemical reasons for the limited existence of living systems may become possible. The widest frame of this understanding actually is represented by the MHA, suggesting that an interdisciplinary approach to cell aging is necessary, possible, and hopeful at the same time. It describes a cellular mechanism explaining the effects of the oxygen free radicals with general validity and offers good chances for experimental testing. The hopes for an eventual possibility of slowing down the age-dependent decline of brain functions (and perhaps of prolonging human life span) are strengthened by the fact that according to the MHA, the rate-limiting process in cellular aging is the structural and functional deterioration of the cell membrane, which can be reached much more easily with properly designed pharmacological interventions than any other internal compartment of brain cells.

The experimental facts observed by applying special OH· radical scavengers like CPH and BCE-001 are consistent with the assumptions and predictions of the MHA. It has been demonstrated that alterations of the cell parameters through a reversal of the age-dependent deterioration of the membrane structure and function are really meaningful in physiological terms not only at the cellular level but also for the whole organism. The significance of these experimental results may be either in an immediate geriatric application of preventive character, or in the possible therapeutic use of BCE-001. Apart from that, the most important message of the results seems to be that a properly designed improvement of the defense against OH· free radical attacks in the brain cell membrane is beneficial. Following this route, a number of further new drugs can be designed, which may be helpful in the achievement of a real breakthrough in geriatric care.

One can predict that future life-span-influencing strategies can be based on the free-radical theory of aging. However, the old, simplistic approach according to which practically any kind of compound displaying radical scavenger ability *in vitro* was expected to exert a life-prolonging effect should be revised. Due to the known properties of OH· radical reactions, only a site-specific, nontoxic and physicochemically feasible radical protection offers the hope of success. It should also be stressed that in highly evolved living systems where natural radical protection is a priori much more efficient than in rodents, most probably only a multifactorial radical protection can be successful, if one intends to improve the natural defense system.

REFERENCES

1. 1985. USA Patent No. 4661618.
2. Zs.-NAGY, I. 1978. A membrane hypothesis of aging. J. Theor. Biol. **75:** 189–195.
3. BJORKSTEN, J. 1942. Chemistry of duplication. Chem. Industr. **49:** 2.
4. KING, A. L. 1946. Pressure volume relation for cylindrical tubes with elastometric walls: the human aorta. Appl. Phys. **17:** 501–505.
5. VERZÁR, F. 1955. Veränderungen der thermoelastischen Kontraktion der Sehnenfasern im Alter. Helv. Physiol. Pharmacol. Acta **13:** C64–C67.
6. HARMAN, D. 1956. Aging: a theory based on free radical and radiation chemistry. J. Gerontol. **11:** 298–300.
7. HARMAN, D. 1961. Mutation, cancer and aging. Lancet **1:** 200–201.
8. Zs.-NAGY, I. 1979. The role of membrane structure and function in cellular aging: a review. Mech. Ageing Dev. **9:** 237–246.
9. Zs.-NAGY, I. 1986. Common mechanisms of cellular aging in brain and liver in the light of the membrane hypothesis of aging. *In* Liver and Aging—1986, Liver and Brain. K. Kitani, Ed.: 373–387. Elsevier Science Publishers. Amsterdam, New York & Oxford.
10. Zs.-NAGY, I. 1987. An attempt to answer the questions of theoretical gerontology on the basis of the membrane hypothesis of aging. Adv. Biosci. **64:** 393–413. (Pergamon. London, England.)
11. Zs.-NAGY, I. 1988. The theoretical background and cellular autoregulation of biological waste product formation. *In* Lipofuscin—1987: State of the Art. I. Zs.-Nagy, Ed.: 23–50, Akadémiai Kiadó, Budapest. Elsevier Science Publishers, Amsterdam.
12. Zs.-NAGY, I. 1989. Functional consequences of free radical damage to cell membranes. *In* CRC Handbook of Free Radicals and Antioxidants in Biomedicine. J. Miquel, A. T. Quintanilha & H. Weber, Eds. **1:** 199–207. CRC Press, Inc. Boca Raton, Florida.
13. Zs.-NAGY, I. 1989. Centrophenoxine as OH· free radical scavenger. *In* CRC Handbook of Free Radicals and Antioxidants in Biomedicine. J. Miquel, A. T. Quintanilha & H. Weber, Eds. **2:** 87–94. CRC Press, Inc. Boca Raton, Florida.
14. Zs.-NAGY, I. 1989. On the role of intracellular physicochemistry in the quantitative gene expression during aging and the effect of centrophenoxine. A review. Arch. Gerontol. Geriatr. **9:** 215–229.
15. Zs.-NAGY, I. 1991. A review on the recent advances in the membrane hypothesis of aging. *In* Liver and Aging—1990. K. Kitani, Ed.: 321–334. Elsevier Science Publishers. Amsterdam, The Netherlands.
16. Zs.-NAGY, I. 1991. The horizons of an interdisciplinary synthesis in experimental gerontology. Arch. Gerontol. Geriatr. **12:** 329–349.
17. Zs.-NAGY, I. 1991. Dietary antioxidants and brain aging: hopes and facts. *In* The Potential for Nutritional Modulation of Aging Processes. D. K. Ingram, G. Baker & N. Shock, Eds.: 379–399. Food and Nutrition Press, Inc. Trumbull, Connecticut.
18. Zs.-NAGY, I. 1994. The Membrane Hypothesis of Aging. CRC Monoscience Series. CRC Press, Inc. Boca Raton, Florida. (In press.)
19. Zs.-NAGY, I., R. G. CUTLER & I. SEMSEI. 1988. Dysdifferentiation hypothesis of aging and cancer: a comparison with the membrane hypothesis of aging. Ann. N.Y. Acad. Sci. **521:** 215–225.
20. GIURGEA, C. & S. J. SARA. 1978. Nootropic drugs and memory. *In* Practical Aspects of Memory. M. M. Gruneberg, P. E. Morris & R. N. Sykes, Eds.: 754–763. Academic Press. London, New York & Oxford.
21. HOCHSCHILD, R. 1973. Effect of dimethylaminoethyl-*p*-chlorophenoxyacetate on the life span of male Swiss Webster albino mice. Exp. Gerontol. **8:** 177–183.
22. LONDON, E. D. & J. T. COYLE. 1978. Pharmacological augmentation of acetylcholine levels in kainate lesioned rat striatum. Biochem. Pharmacol. **27:** 2962–2965.
23. HAUBRICH, D. R., P. F. WANG, D. E. CLODY & P. W. WEDEKING. 1975. Increase in rat brain acetylcholine induced by choline or Deanol. Life Sci. **17:** 975–980.
24. ZANISER, N. R., D. CHOU & I. HANIN. 1977. Is 2-dimethylaminoethanol (Deanol) indeed a precursor of brain acetylcholine? A gas chromatographic evaluation. J. Pharmacol. Exp. Ther. **200:** 545–559.

25. JOPE, R. S. & D. J. JENDEN. 1979. Dimethylaminoethanol (Deanol) metabolism in rat brain and its effect on acetylcholine synthesis. J. Pharmacol. Exp. Ther. **211:** 472–479.
26. HAUBRICH, D. R., P. F. WANG & P. W. WEDEKING. 1975. Distribution of intravenously administered choline methyl-^{3}H and synthesis in vivo of acetylcholine in various tissues of guinea pigs. J. Pharmacol. Exp. Ther. **193:** 246–255.
27. HAUBRICH, D. R., N. H. GERBER & A. B. PFLUEGER. 1981. Deanol affects choline metabolism in peripheral tissues of mice. J. Neurochem. **37:** 476–482.
28. CEDER, G., L. DAHLBERG & J. SCHUBERTH. 1978. Effects of 2-dimethylaminoethanol (Deanol) on the metabolism of choline in plasma. J. Neurochem. **30:** 1293–1296.
29. FREEMAN, J. J. & D. J. JENDEN. 1976. The source of choline for actylcholine synthesis in brain. Life Sci. **19:** 949–962.
30. ANSELL, B. G. & S. SPANNER. 1977. Functional metabolism of brain phospholipids. Int. Rev. Neurobiol. **20:** 1–29.
31. HAUBRICH, D. R. & T. J. CHIPPENDALE. 1977. Regulation of acetylcholine synthesis in the nervous system. Life Sci. **20:** 1465–1478.
32. BARTUS, R. T., R. L. DEAN, J. A. GOAS & A. S. LIPPA. 1980. Age-related changes in passive avoidance retention: modulation with dietary choline. Science **209:** 301–303.
33. ZS.-NAGY, I. & K. NAGY. 1980. On the role of cross-linking of cellular proteins in aging. Mech. Ageing Dev. **14:** 245–251.
34. ZS.-NAGY, I. & R. A. FLOYD. 1984. Electron spin resonance spectroscopic demonstration of the hydroxyl free radical scavenger properties of dimethylaminoethanol in spin trapping experiments confirming the molecular basis for the biological effects of centrophenoxine. Arch. Gerontol. Geriatr. **3:** 297–310.
35. MIYAZAKI, M., K. NAMBU, A. Y. MINAKI, M. HASHIMOTO & K. NAKAMURA. 1976. Comparative studies on the metabolism of beta-dimethylaminoethanol in the mouse brain and liver following administration of beta-dimethylaminoethanol and its *p*-chlorophenoxyacetate, Meclofenoxate. Chem. Pharm. Bull. **24:** 763–769.
36. WEBER, H. U. & J. MIQUEL. 1986. Antioxidant supplementation and longevity. *In* Nutritional Aspects of Aging, L. H. Chen, **1:** 42–49. CRC Press, Inc. Boca Raton, Florida.
37. FLOYD, R. A. 1981. DNA–ferrous iron catalyzed free radical formation from hydrogen peroxide. Biochem. Biophys. Res. Commun. **99:** 1209–1215.
38. FLOYD, R. A. 1982. Observations on nitroxyl free radicals in arylamine carcinogenesis and on spin-trapping hydroxyl free radicals. Can. J. Chem. **60:** 1577–1586.
39. FLOYD, R. A. & C. A. LEWIS. 1983. Hydroxyl free radical formation from hydrogen peroxide by ferrous iron–nucleotide complexes. Biochemistry **22:** 2645–2649.
40. WALLING, C. 1975. Fenton's reagent revisited. Acc. Chem. Res. **8:** 125–131.
41. FLOYD, R. A. & I. ZS.-NAGY. 1984. Formation of long-lived hydroxyl free radical adducts of proline and hydroxyproline in a Fenton reaction. Biochim. Biophys. Acta **790:** 94–97.
42. NAGY, K., G. DAJKÓ, I. URAY & I. ZS.-NAGY. Comparative studies on the free radical scavenger properties of two nootropic drugs, CPH and BCE-001. Ann. N.Y. Acad. Sci. (This volume.)
43. NAGY, K., V. ZS.-NAGY, C. BERTONI-FREDDARI & I. ZS.-NAGY. 1983. Alterations of the synaptosomal membrane microviscosity in the brain cortex of rats during aging and centrophenoxine treatment. Arch. Gerontol. Geriatr. **2:** 23–39.
44. NAGY, K., P. SIMON & I. ZS.-NAGY. 1983. Spin label studies on synaptosomal membranes of rat brain cortex during aging. Biochem. Biophys. Res. Commun. **117:** 688–694.
45. NAGY, K., R. A. FLOYD, P. SIMON & I. ZS.-NAGY. 1985. Studies on the effect of iron overload on rat cortex synaptosomal membranes. Biochim. Biophys. Acta **820:** 216–222.
46. NAGY, K. & I. ZS.-NAGY. 1984. Alterations in the molecular weight distribution of proteins in rat brain synaptosomes during aging and centrophenoxine treatment. Mech. Ageing Dev. **28:** 171–176.
47. ZS.-NAGY, I., K. KITANI, M. OHTA, V. ZS.-NAGY & K. IMAHORI. 1986. Age-dependent decrease of the lateral diffusion constant of proteins in the plasma membrane of hepatocytes as revealed by fluorescence recovery after photobleaching in tissue smears. Arch. Gerontol. Geriatr. **5:** 131–146.
48. ZS.-NAGY, I., K. KITANI, M. OHTA, V. ZS.-NAGY & K. IMAHORI. 1986. Age-estimations of

rats based on the average lateral diffusion constant of hepatocyte membrane proteins as revealed by fluorescence recovery after photobleaching. Exp. Gerontol. **21:** 555–563.

49. KITANI, K., I. ZS.-NAGY, S. KANAI, Y. SATO & M. OHTA. 1988. Correlation between the biliary excretion of ouabain and the lateral mobility of hepatocyte plasma membrane proteins in the rat. The effects of age and spironolactone pretreatment. Hepatology **8:** 125–131.

50. ZS.-NAGY, I., K. KITANI & M. OHTA. 1989. Age dependence of the lateral mobility of proteins in the plasma membrane of hepatocytes in C57BL/6 mice: FRAP studies on liver smears. J. Gerontol. Biol. Sci. **44:** B83–B87.

51. ZS.-NAGY, I., M. OHTA & K. KITANI. 1989. Effect of centrophenoxine and BCE-001 treatment on the lateral diffusion constant of proteins in the hepatocyte membrane as revealed by fluorescence recovery after photobleaching in rat liver smears. Exp. Gerontol. **24:** 317–330.

52. ZS.-NAGY, I., R. G. CUTLER, K. KITANI & M. OHTA. 1993. Comparison of the lateral diffusion constant of hepatocyte membrane proteins in two wild mouse strains of considerably different longevity: FRAP studies on liver smears. J. Gerontol. Biol. Sci. **48:** B86–B92.

53. ZS.-NAGY, I., C. PIERI, C. GIULI & M. DEL MORO. 1979. Effects of centrophenoxine on the monovalent electrolyte contents of the large brain cortical cells of old rats. Gerontology **25:** 94–102.

54. LUSTYIK, GY. & I. ZS.-NAGY. 1985. Alterations of the intracellular water and ion concentrations in brain and liver cells during aging as revealed by energy dispersive X-ray microanalysis of bulk specimens. Scanning Electron Microsc. 1985/I: 323–337.

55. SEMSEI, I., F. SZESZÁK & I. ZS.-NAGY. 1982. In vivo studies on the age-dependent decrease of the rates of total and mRNA synthesis in the brain cortex of rats. Arch. Gerontol. Geriatr. **1:** 29–42.

56. ZS.-NAGY, I. & I. SEMSEI. 1984. Centrophenoxine increases the rates of total and mRNA synthesis in the brain cortex of old rats: an explanation of its action in terms of the membrane hypothesis of aging. Exp. Gerontol. **19:** 171–178.

57. PÉK, GY., T. FÜLÖP & I. ZS.-NAGY. 1989. Gerontopsychological studies using NAI ("Nürnberger Alters-Inventar") on patients with organic psychosyndrome (DSM III, Category 1) treated with centrophenoxine in a double blind, comparative, randomized clinical trial. Arch. Gerontol. Geriatr. **9:** 17–30.

58. FÜLÖP, T., JR., I. WÓRUM, J. CSONGOR, A. LEÖVEY, T. SZABÓ, GY. PÉK & I. ZS.-NAGY. 1990. Effects of centrophenoxine on body composition and some biochemical parameters of demented elderly people as revealed in a double blind clinical trial. Arch. Gerontol. Geriatr. **10:** 239–251.

Comparative Studies on the Free Radical Scavenger Properties of Two Nootropic Drugs, CPH and BCE-001

KATALIN NAGY, GÁBOR DAJKÓ,[a] ISTVÁN URAY,[a] AND
IMRE ZS.-NAGY

F. Verzár International Laboratory for
Experimental Gerontology (VILEG)
Hungarian Section
University Medical School
Debrecen, H-4012, Hungary

[a]*Institute of Nuclear Research of the Hungarian Academy of Sciences*
Debrecen, H-4001, Hungary

INTRODUCTION

Centrophenoxine has been found to slow down certain phenomena associated with aging.[1] Its effective portion is dimethylaminoethanol (DMAE), which is incorporated into nerve cell membranes of experimental animals in the form of phosphatidyl-DMAE.[2] DMAE has proven to be an efficient free radical scavenger *in vitro* as shown indirectly.[3] It has been established by ESR spectroscopy using spin trapping techniques that both CPH and DMAE were OH· free radical scavengers.[4] Centrophenoxine treatment of old animals reduced the lipofuscin content in neurons, myocardium, etc.[5] Chronic treatment of old rats with CPH exerted a protective effect on proteins against oxygen free radical induced cross-linking.[6]

These results suggested the synthesis of a new molecule, coded as BCE-001, which has recently been developed by the Hungarian Section of VILEG and BIOGAL Pharmaceutical Works Ltd, Debrecen (US Patent number 4661618, 1985). The new molecule contains bis-dimethylaminoisopropanol (BIDIP) in the place of DMAE (FIGURE 1). The present studies were aimed at testing the OH· free radical scavenging efficiency of BCE-001 and BIDIP in comparison to that of CPH and DMAE, respectively.

METHODS

Exposure of Bovine Serum Albumin to Oxygen Radicals

Bovine serum albumin (BSA) was exposed to oxygen free radicals using $^{60}Co\gamma$ radiation source under oxygen atmosphere, at room temperature.[7] The BSA solution (0.33 mg/ml) was prepared in double distilled and deionized water. Irradiation time was 3 hours, and the distance of samples from radiation source was varied in order to achieve oxygen radical exposures of approximately 1–100 nmol of radicals/nmol of BSA; total doses of irradiation were 1–80 kilorads.[8] The protein carbonyl content was determined spectrophotometrically using the 2,4-dinitrophenylhydrazine (DNPH) reaction.[9] Results were calculated from an extinction coefficient of 21.0 mM^{-1} cm^{-1}

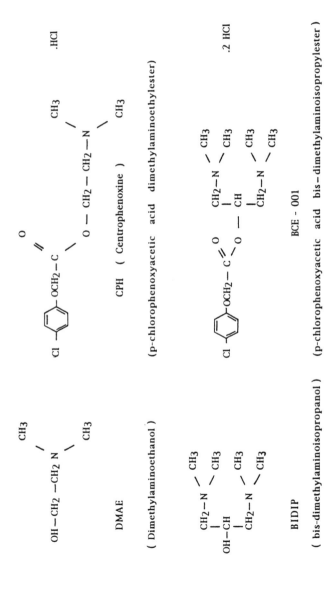

FIGURE 1. The molecular structure of the tested compounds.

for aliphatic hydrazones.[9] The protection displayed by nootropic drugs against free radical induced protein oxidation was tested. The applied concentrations of DMAE and BIDIP were 1 and 10 mM, respectively.

Spin Trapping with DMPO

The experimental method of Floyd and Levis[10] as described by Zs.-Nagy and Floyd[11] was followed. OH· free radicals were generated by the ADP–Fe(II)–H_2O_2 system and trapped by 5,5-dimethyl-1-pyrroline-*N*-oxide (DMPO). The concentration of DMPO was 20 mM. The ESR spectra were recorded with a JEOL JES-RE1X spectrometer. Typical instrumental parameters were as follows: modulation frequency 100 kHz, modulation amplitude 0.2 mT, time constant 1 s, receiver gain 5 × 10^2 at 4 mW power level. All the recordings were carried out at room temperature. The ESR signal intensity of DMPO-OH spin adduct was characterized by the height of the second peak.

The free radical scavenging ability of DMAE and BIDIP, or CPH and BCE-001, was tested and compared respectively in 1 and 10 mM concentrations. Stock solutions of DMAE and BIDIP were prepared in bicarbonate buffer and neutralized by adding concentrated HCI. CPH and BCE-001 were dissolved in polyvinylpyrrolidon (PVP), which is a known solvent of CPH for intravenous (iv) and intramuscular (im) administrations.

CHEMICALS AND DRUGS

BSA, DMAE, and DMPO were products of Sigma Chem. Co. CPH was used as a lyophylized powder from HELFERGIN 500 ampoules provided as a gift from PROMONTA Chemische Fabrik GmbH (Hamburg, Germany). BIDIP and BCE-001 were from BIOGAL Pharmaceutical Works Ltd. (Debrecen, Hungary). All other reagents were from Reanal Budapest (Hungary).

RESULTS

Protection against Protein Oxidation

The level of protein carbonyl groups can be used as a measure of oxygen radical mediated protein damage under various physiological conditions. Measurements of carbonyl content of BSA following exposure to increasing amount of oxygen radicals revealed a large and linear increase, as the control curve shows in FIGURE 2. In the presence of 1 mM BIDIP, irradiation induced a much smaller, by about 55% less, carbonyl content than in the control experiment. The protective effect of 1 mM DMAE against free radical attack of BSA was less effective by 15% than that of 1 mM BIDIP. In 10 mM concentration, both molecules protected the protein solutions very efficiently from oxidative damage, but BIDIP was again 15% more effective than DMAE.

Because the whole ester molecules CPH and BCE-001 disintegrated during irradiation, the system used by us is not suitable to compare the whole ester molecules.

Spin Trapping Experiments with DMPO

Electron spin resonance spectroscopy was applied using the spin trapping method for a semiquantitative comparison of the OH· radical scavenger properties of the compounds. FIGURE 3 shows the control spectrum of the DMPO-OH spin adduct. The amount of DMPO-OH spin adduct decreased considerably, if BIDIP or DMAE was present in the reaction mixture. Both BIDIP and DMAE decreased significantly the ESR signal intensity, in 10 mM concentration. But in equimolar concentrations, BIDIP was about twofold more efficient; the signal height of the

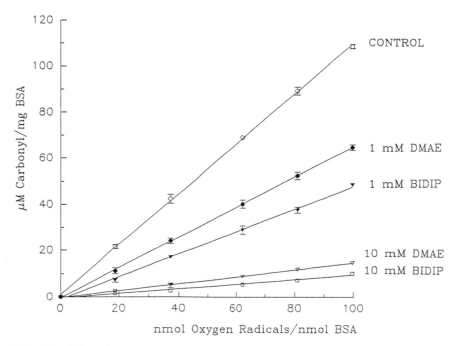

FIGURE 2. Effect of BIDIP and DMAE on the carbonyl content of BSA following exposure to OH· + O$_2^{\bar{}}$ (+O$_2$) at the radical/BSA molar ratios indicated. Values are means (± standard error of the mean) of three independent experiments.

second peak of BIDIP was about the half that of DMAE. In 1 mM concentration, the free radical scavenging effect of both molecules decreased very much, but BIDIP was still more effective than DMAE even in this low concentration.

Since BCE-001 and CPH were dissolved in PVP, a control curve was also taken in the presence of the same amount of PVP (FIGURE 4). Both BCE-001 and CPH reduced significantly the ESR signal intensity in 10 mM concentration, but BCE-001 was about twofold more efficient than CPH. In 1 mM concentration, we had the same result as in the case of alcoholic molecules—BCE-001 had still more OH· radical scavenging ability than CPH.

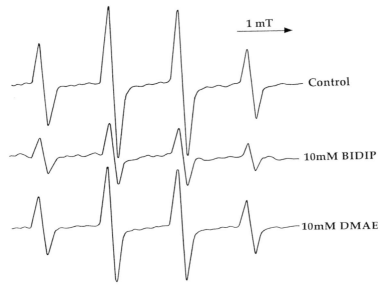

FIGURE 3. Effect of BIDIP and DMAE on the ESR spectra of DMPO-OH spin adduct, obtained in the ADP-Fe(II)-H_2O_2 mixture. The concentration of DMPO was 20 mM in each experiment.

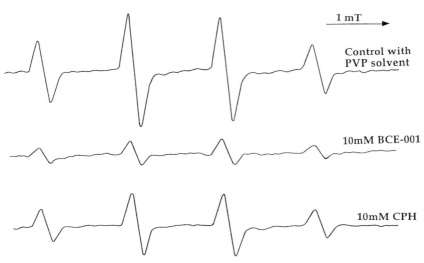

FIGURE 4. ESR spectra of the DMPO-OH spin adduct, in the presence of BCE-001 and CPH. The concentration of DMPO was 20 mM in each experiment.

DISCUSSION

As reported by Davies,[7] BSA exposed to $OH \cdot + O_2^{\bar{}} + O_2$ undergoes spontaneous fragmentation. Fragmentation of BSA produces new carbonyl groups with no apparent increase in free amino groups. In our experiments, we measured a significantly lower carbonyl content in the presence of both alcoholic molecules, compared to the control value. It means that both BIDIP and DMAE protected proteins against free radical attack and oxidative damage, but the protective effect of BIDIP was more efficient. This agrees well with the theoretical expectations based on the molecular structures of these compounds. On the basis of the experimental results, the free radical scavenger property of BIDIP and BCE-001 proved to be much more effective as compared to that of DMAE and CPH, respectively. (1) BIDIP protected proteins more efficiently against free radical attack and degradation than DMAE. (2) DMPO spin-trapping experiments also confirmed the much better $OH \cdot$ radical scavenging ability of BIDIP and BCE-001 relative to that of DMAE and CPH, respectively.

In vivo comparative experiments with CPH and BCE-001 on various parameters of old rats revealed not only a series of beneficial effects of both drugs, but also confirmed the increased efficacy of BCE-001 against equivalent doses of CPH. The free radical scavenger activities of these drugs were tested on the lateral diffusion constant of membrane proteins in hepatocytes.[12] The age-dependent decrease of the lateral diffusion constant of membrane proteins reincreased again in hepatocytes of old rats following a 5-week period of treatment with these drugs, but BCE-001 caused a significantly larger increase, and animals survived longer with better overall physiological parameters, as compared to the CPH-treated ones. Treatment of old rats with CPH resulted in significant rehydration of brain cell cytoplasm,[13] a considerable increase in the total and mRNA synthesis rate in the brain cortex of old rats,[14] and a beneficial influence on many other cellular and *in vivo* aging parameters.[15,16] BCE-001 showed effects similar to those of CPH, but to an even greater extent, that is, lower doses or shorter treatment periods gave similar results as compared to CPH (our unpublished results). Therefore, both drugs can be regarded as free radical scavengers and potential antiaging drugs.

REFERENCES

1. ZS.-NAGY, I., C. PIERI, C. GIULI & M. DEL MORO. 1979. Effects of centrophenoxine on the monovalent electrolyte contents of the large brain cortical cells of old rats. Gerontology **25:** 94–102.
2. MIYAZAKI, H., K. NAMBU, Y. MINAKI, M. HASHIMOTO & K. NAKAMURA. 1976. Comparative studies on the metabolism of beta-dimethylaminoethanol in the mouse brain and liver following administration of beta-dimethylaminoethanol and its *p*-chlorophenoxyacetate, Meclofenoxate. Chem. Pharm. Bull. **24:** 763–769.
3. ZS.-NAGY, I. & K. NAGY. 1980. On the role of cross-linking of cellular proteins in aging. Mech. Ageing Dev. **14:** 245–251.
4. ZS.-NAGY, I. & R. A. FLOYD. 1984. Electron spin resonance spectroscopic demonstration of the hydroxyl free radical scavenger properties of dimethylaminoethanol in spin trapping experiments confirming the molecular basis for the biological effects of centrophenoxine. Arch. Gerontol. Geriatr. **3:** 297–310.
5. ROY, D., D. N. PATHAK & R. SINGH. 1983. Effect of centrophenoxine on the antioxidative enzymes in various regions of the aging rat brain. Exp. Gerontol. **18:** 185–197.
6. NAGY, K. & I. ZS.-NAGY. 1984. Alterations in the molecular weight distribution of proteins in rat brain synaptosomes during aging and centrophenoxine treatment of old rats. Mech. Ageing Dev. **28:** 171–176.

7. DAVIES, K. J. A. & M. E. DELSIGNORE. 1987. Protein damage and degradation by oxygen radicals. III. Modification of secondery and tertiary structure. J. Biol. Chem. **262:** 9908–9913.
8. DAVIES, K. J. A. 1987. Protein damage and degradation by oxygen radicals. I. General aspects. J. Biol. Chem. **262:** 9895–9901.
9. LEVINE, R. L., D. GARLAND, C. N. OLIVER, A. AMICI, I. CLIMENT, A. G. LENZ, B. W. AHN, S. SHALTIEL & E. R. STADTMAN. 1990. Determination of carbonyl content in oxidatively modified proteins. Methods Enzymol. **186:** 464–478.
10. FLOYD, R. A. & C. A. LEWIS. 1983. Hydroxyl free radical formation from hydrogen peroxide by ferrous iron–nucleotide complexes. Biochemistry **22:** 2645–2649.
11. ZS.-NAGY, I. & R. A. FLOYD. 1984. Electron spin resonance spectroscopic demonstration of the hydroxyl free radical scavenger properties of dimethylaminoethanol in spin trapping experiments confirming the molecular basis for the biological effects of centrophenoxine. Arch. Gerontol. Geriatr. **3:** 297–310.
12. ZS.-NAGY, I., M. OHTA & K. KITANI. 1989. Effect of centrophenoxine and BCE-001 treatment on lateral diffusion of proteins in the hepatocyte plasma membrane as revealed by fluorescence recovery after photobleaching in rat liver smears. Exp. Gerontol. **24:** 317–330.
13. LUSTYIK, GY. & I. ZS.-NAGY. 1985. Alterations of the intracellular water and ion concentrations in brain and liver cells during aging as revealed by energy dispersive X-ray microanalysis of bulk specimens. Scan. Electron Microsc. 1985/I: 323–337.
14. ZS.-NAGY, I. & I. SEMSEI. 1984. Centrophenoxine increases the rates of total and mRNA synthesis in the brain cortex of old rats: an explanation of its action in terms of membrane hypothesis of aging. Exp. Gerontol. **19:** 171–178.
15. ZS.-NAGY, I. 1989. Centrophenoxine as OH· free radical scavenger. *In* CRC Handbook of Free Radicals and Antioxidants in Biomedicine. J. Miquel, H. Weber & A. Quintanilha, Eds. **2:** 87–94. CRC Press, Inc. Boca Raton, Florida.
16. ZS.-NAGY, I. A survey of the available data on a new nootropic drug, BCE-001. Annals N.Y. Acad. Sci. (This volume.)

The Potent Free Radical Scavenger α-Lipoic Acid Improves Cognition in Rodents

S. STOLL, A. ROSTOCK,[a] R. BARTSCH,[a] E. KORN,
A. MEICHELBÖCK, AND W. E. MÜLLER

Central Institute of Mental Health
Department of Psychopharmacology, J5
D-68072 Mannheim, Germany

[a] Arzneimittelwerk Dresden GmbH
a company of ASTA Medica
Meissner Strasse 191
D-01445 Radebeul, Germany

INTRODUCTION

α-Lipoic acid or thioctic acid is a coenzyme for the pyruvate dehydrogenase complex in the mitochondrial matrix. Presently it is mainly in theraputic use against diabetic polyneuropathy.[1,2] At least part of its therapeutic implications can be explained by the free radical scavenging properties of α-lipoic acid[3] and particularly of its reduced form dihydrolipoic acid.[4,5] Free radical damage may be an important cause of aging and age-related disease,[6] including Alzheimer's disease[6] and Parkinson's disease.[7] The membrane hypothesis of aging[8] argues that chronic damage by free radicals leads to changes in cell membrane properties that cause a deterioration of cellular function. Based on the membrane hypothesis of aging, we investigated whether a treatment with α-lipoic acid could improve memory function in young and aged mice. Because of the potential therapeutic importance of the results, we performed a parallel experiment in young rats using α-lipoic acid and the known cognition enhancer piracetam[9,10] to see whether the results in mice can be generalized.

MATERIALS AND METHODS

Animals

Female NMRI mice had been purchased from Interfauna, Tuttlingen, Germany. Young-adult ones (3–6 months) had been transferred to our animal facilities at least two weeks before the beginning of the tests. Old female NMRI mice were received at the age of 12 months as retired breeders and kept in our animal facilities from then on until they were 20 to 23 months old. Young (2 months) male CrI: (Wi)BR rats had been purchased at Charles River, Bad Sulzfeld, Germany. They were transferred to the testing facilities 4 days before the test.

Treatment

Orally treated mice received 100 mg/kg body weight α-lipoic acid in Methocel (1%) administered once per day for 15 days for the test of habituation in the open field. Controls received Methocel alone. Mice treated by intraperitoneal injection (ip treatment) got 100 mg/kg body weight α-lipoic acid as its trometamol salt (Thioctacid T solution for injection from Asta Medica, Frankfurt, Germany) for 15 days during the test in the Morris water maze. Controls were treated with saline. On days of behavioral testing, the treatments were given after the tests. Rats received 1 and 10 mg/kg α-lipoic acid in 5% dimethylaminoacetamide (DMA) or 100 mg/kg and 300 mg/kg piracetam in saline intraperitoneally one hour before the tests. Controls received the respective vehicle alone.

Behavioral Testing

Habituation in the Open Field

This test has been described in detail in Stoll *et al.*[11] In short, mice were placed in an open field (50 × 50 × 20 cm) the floor of which was divided in squares. Horizontal activities were measured as the number of squares entered with the forepaws. The animals were placed in the open field for 3 minutes, repeating this exposure after 15 minutes and after 24 hours. The test started on day 14 of oral treatment.

Morris Water Maze

The maze consisted of a black round pool (diameter 56 cm) that was filled with water of 27°C. The pool was divided into 4 quadrants. A black platform (diameter 4 cm) was placed about 1 cm below the waterline in the center of a quadrant. One test block included 4 trials on the first day and 1 trial on the second day. If a mouse did not find the platform within 60 seconds, it was guided to it. After finding the platform, the animal had to stay there for 30 seconds. Starting positions varied from trial to trial, platform positions from block to block. Six test blocks were performed: the first one began on day 4 before the start of ip treatment, the second to sixth ones on days 1, 4, 8, 11, and 14 of ip treatment. Swimming distances were measured with a Video Path Analyzer.

Active Avoidance Learning

The rats were placed in the active avoidance learning box (31 cm × 35 cm × 50 cm) where a tone signal (1.6 kHz, 8 s) (the conditioned stimulus) was followed by a foot shock (40 V, 12 s) (the unconditioned stimulus). Animals could avoid the shock by jumping to a suspended pole. During training and the retention test (24 hours after the training), each animal got 20 randomly distributed stimulus combinations. The test criterion for a conditioned response (CR) was that a rat jumped onto the pole in three succeeding stimulus combinations during the tone signal. Further, the latency from the start of the tone up to jumping onto the pole was registered.

Statistics

Statistical analyses apart from the Mann-Whitney rank sum test were performed with the SAS system for personal computers, release 6.03. In the Morris water maze task, swimming speeds of mice finding the platform are significantly higher than those of animals who do not, possibly distorting the distribution of the distances swum. To adjust for this difference as individually as possible and, therefore, with as little influence on variance as possible, the distance swum by a mouse that did not find the platform in a particular trial was adjusted. It was set to the maximum of the measured swimming distance and of the distance computed from the average swimming speed of the animal in the case of finding the platform in the block. That is, the computed swimming distance was the product of the individual blockwise swimming speed and the trial time of 60 seconds.

RESULTS

Habituation in the Open Field

A highly significant repetition of trials effect indicating learning was found in young (y), 3 months old, and aged (a), 20–23 months old, mice (see TABLE 1 for statistics). *Post hoc* comparisons of horizontal activities using the paired t-test revealed habituation in the 15 minute trial for both age groups in treated (tr) and control (co) animals (y-co: $p < 0.0001$, $t = 7.78$, $n = 15$; y-tr: $p < 0.0001$, $t = 6.87$, $n = 10$; a-co: $p < 0.0001$, $t = 7.40$, $n = 19$; a-tr: $p < 0.0001$, $t = 10.85$, $n = 10$). They also revealed no significant loss of habituation in the 24 hours trial as compared to the 15-minute trial for young mice either treated or controls. Aged control mice showed significant forgetting ($p < 0.003$, $t = 3.43$, $n = 19$). However, no significant forgetting between the 15-minute trial and the 24-hour trial could be found in aged treated mice.

Morris Water Maze

The time-course of swimming distances is shown in FIGURE 1. Both young (co: $n = 17$, tr: $n = 16$) and aged mice (co: $r = 14$, tr: $n = 14$) showed significant effects of block (y: $p < 0.0001$, $F = 7.35$, 5 DF; a: $p < 0.0001$, $F = 15.06$, 5 DF) and trial (y: $p < 0.0001$, $F = 15.77$; 4 DF; a: $p < 0.0001$, $F = 8.89$, 4 DF). The interaction of block and trial was significant in young animals ($p < 0.0069$, $F = 1.98$, 20 DF). A significant effect of treatment was found only in aged mice ($p < 0.0444$, $F = 4.43$, 1

TABLE 1. Habituation in the Open Field in Young and Aged Mice under Treatment with 100 mg/kg α-Lipoic Acid[a]

	Q0	Q15'	Q24h	n
Young control	98.07 ± 2.72	64.33 ± 5.27	75.53 ± 4.54	15
Young treated	88.70 ± 5.88	57.30 ± 6.37	68.30 ± 6.94	10
Aged control	61.79 ± 5.81	77.00 ± 5.51	77.00 ± 5.51	19
Aged treated	111.80 ± 13.17	64.90 ± 9.59	66.30 ± 7.76	10

[a]Q0 is the initial horizontal activity, Q15' the activity 15 minutes after the first trial, Q24h the activity 24 hours after the first trial. All means are given with SEMs. For statistics see text.

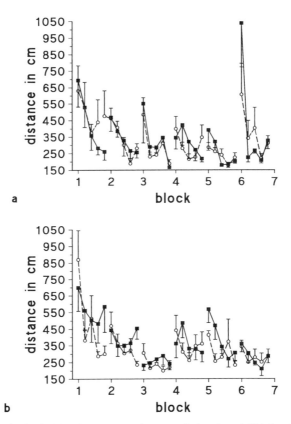

a   block

b   block

FIGURE 1. Learning in the Morris water maze in young (1a) and aged (1b) female NMRI mice under treatment with 100 mg/kg α-lipoic acid. Controls are indicated as open circles, treated animals as solid squares. A significant main effect of treatment could be found in aged mice. Values are means ± standard errors of the means (SEMs). For statistics see text.

DF). However, there were no significant interactions among treatment, block, and trial. For this reason, a separate analysis of the last three training blocks was performed. An interaction of treatment and trial close to significance could be found there ($p < 0.0611$, $F = 2.32$, 4 DF).

Active Avoidance Learning

Controls did not reach the criterion for a CR either during training or during the retention trial (FIGURE 2, FIGURE 3). However, both α-lipoic acid (FIGURE 2) and piracetam (FIGURE 3) improved performance during training and the retention trial in a dose-dependent way. Latencies decreased from training to the retention trial. This decrease was more pronounced in animals treated with either 1.0 or 10.0 mg/kg thioctic acid or 300 mg/kg piracetam (TABLE 2).

DISCUSSION

Age differences in habituation in the open field[11,12] and the Morris water maze task[13] have been described previously. The results presented in this paper give further support to the hypothesis that α-lipoic acid is able to improve cognitive function in rodents. The results of habituation in the open field and of the Morris water maze task support the notion that age-related deficits of cognition are attenuated: aged mice showed an improvement of memory in the habituation in the open field task as can be seen in the 24 hour activities (for a further discussion of this topic see Stoll *et al.*[11] A significant main effect of treatment for aged mice in the Morris water maze task hints at an age-specific effect of α-lipoic acid on learning or memory. Further, the interaction between treatment and trial during the last three water maze blocks that was close to significance in aged mice suggests a time-

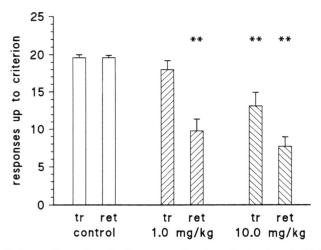

FIGURE 2. Active avoidance learning in young male rats under treatment with 1.0 and 10.0 mg/kg α-lipoic acid. Values are means ± SEMs. ** indicates $p < 0.01$ in the Mann-Whitney rank-sum test (1.0 mg, 24 hour retention: U = 3.5; 10.0 mg, training: U = 2.9; 10.0 mg, 24 hour retention: U = 3.5).

dependent effect of α-lipoic acid. This is in accordance with the hypothesis that increased oxidative stress with aging may be one cause of age-related cognitive decline. Since α-lipoic acid improves glucose utilization in a manner additive to insulin[14–17] and since glucose meabolism is impaired in patients with Alzheimer's disease,[18,19] a specific effect of α-lipoic acid may add to its radical scavenger function in aged individuals. This notion is supported by casuistic descriptions of a partial attenuation of behavioral deficits in Alzheimer's patients.[20] Improved active avoidance learning in young rats hint in a further direction: a nootropic component in the action of α-lipoic that is also found in piracetam cannot be excluded. Preliminary data for aged rats hint in the same direction.[21] Apart from improvements in cognition, α-lipoic acid may have additional effects on motor functions as may be suggested by the high initial activity of treated aged mice in the open field (TABLE 1) even though there was no significant difference to aged controls. Effects on motor

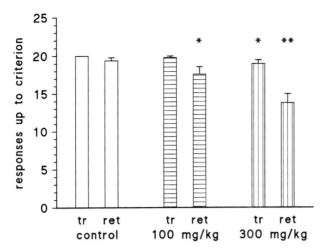

FIGURE 3. Active avoidance learning in young male rats under treatment with 100 and 300 mg/kg piracetam. Values are means ± SEMs. * indicates $p < 0.05$, ** indicates $p < 0.01$ in the Mann-Whitney rank-sum test (100 mg, 24 hour retention: U = 1.9; 300 mg, training: U = 2.2; 300 mg, 24 hour retention: U = 3.5).

functions may influence the results of the Morris water maze task and active avoidance learning as well. Our data hint at an action of α-lipoic acid on different areas of learning, as in the Morris water maze and active avoidance learning, and memory, as in habituation and the water maze. The effects seem to depend on species, model, and age. However, improved cognitive function is found in all models described here. Further experiments taking into account these possible differential effects of α-lipoic acid as well as possible effects on motor functions are necessary to elucidate the effects and the mechanisms of action of α-lipoic acid. The same is true regarding its biochemical mechanisms of action for the effects on learning and memory as suggested previously.[11] In summary, our data suggest that a treatment with free radical scavengers may be a useful treatment for age-related memory decline.

TABLE 2. Active Avoidance Learning in Young Male Rats under Treatment with α-Lipoic Acid or Piracetam[a]

Treatment	mg/kg	Training	U	Retention	U	n
Control	—	11.7 ± 0.3	—	8.0 ± 0.4	—	10
α-Lipoic acid	1.0	10.6 ± 0.3[c]	2.3	6.2 ± 0.2[c]	3.3	10
α-Lipoic acid	10.0	9.0 ± 0.3[c]	3.6	4.9 ± 0.5[c]	3.7	10
Control	—	10.8 ± 0.4	—	7.9 ± 0.3	—	10
Piracetam	100	10.8 ± 0.3	0.1	7.7 ± 0.3	0.6	10
Piracetam	300	9.9 ± 0.3[b]	1.9	7.0 ± 0.3[b]	2.3	10

[a]The mean latencies to jump to the pole after the tone signal started are given with SEMs. [b]Indicates $p < 0.05$, [c]$p < 0.01$ versus control in the Mann-Whitney rank sum test. U is the U-value of the Mann-Whitney Rank sum test.

REFERENCES

1. DIMPFEL, W., M. SPULER, F. K. PIERAU & H. ULRICH. 1990. Thioctic acid induces dose-dependent sprouting of neurites in cultured rat neuroblastoma cells. Dev. Pharmacol. Ther. **14**(3): 193–199.
2. SUZUKI, Y. J., M. TSUCHIYA & L. PACKER. 1992. Lipoate prevents glucose-induced protein modifications. Free Radical Res. Commun. **17**(3): 211–217.
3. EGAN, R. W., P. H. GALE, G. C. BEVERIDGE, G. B. PHILLIPS & L. J. MARNETT. 1978. Radical scavenging as the mechanism for stimulation of prostaglandin cyclooxygenase and depression of inflammation by lipoic acid and sodium iodine. Prostaglandins **16**: 861–869.
4. KAGAN, V. E., A. SHVEDOVA, E. SERBINOVA, S. KHAN, C. SWANSON, R. POWELL & L. PACKER. 1992. Dihydrolipoic acid—a universal antioxidant both in the membrane and in the aqueous phase. Reduction of peroxyl, ascorbyl and chromanoxyl radicals. Biochem. Pharmacol. **44**(8): 1637–1649.
5. SCHOLICH, H., M. E. MURPHY & H. SIES. 1989. Antioxidant activity of dihydrolipoate against microsomal lipid peroxidation and its dependence on α-tocopherol. Biochim. Biophys. Acta **1001**: 256–261.
6. HARMAN, D. 1986. Free radical theory of aging: role of free radicals in the origination and evolution of life, aging, and disease processes. *In* Free Radicals, Aging and Degenerative Diseases. Alan R. Liss, Inc. New York, N.Y.
7. KISH, S. J., K. SHANNAK, A. RAJPUT, J. H. N. DECK & O. HORNYKIEWICZ. 1992. Aging produces a specific pattern of striatal dopamine loss: implications for the etiology of idiopathic Parkinson's disease. J. Neurochem. **58**: 642–648.
8. SUN, A. Y. & G. Y. SUN. 1979. Neurochemical aspects of the membrane hypothesis of aging. Interdiscip. Top. Gerontol. **15**: 34–53.
9. GIURGEA, C. E. 1982. The nootropic concept and its prospective implications. Drug Dev. Res. **2**: 441–446.
10. STOLL, L., T. SCHUBERT & W. E. MÜLLER. 1991. Age-related deficits of central muscarinic cholinergic receptor function in the mouse: partial restoration by chronic piracetam treatment. Neurobiol. Aging **13**: 39–44.
11. STOLL, S., H. HARTMANN, S. A. COHEN & W. E. MÜLLER. The potent free radical scavenger α-lipoic acid improves memory in aged mice. Putative relationship to NMDA receptor deficits. Pharmacol. Biochem. Behav. **46**: 799–805.
12. STOLL, S. & W. E. MÜLLER. 1992. Habituierung in Open Field und Objektgedächtnis in Altersabhängigkeit bei der weiblichen NMRI-Maus. Z. Gerontologie **24**: 300–301.
13. STOLL, S., U. PASCHE, R. WEIGEL, U. HUBER & W. E. MÜLLER. A test battery of cognitive decline with aging in the mouse with partial retest capability. 1993. *In* Acta of the World Congress of Gerontology—XVth Congress of the International Association of Gerontology. Mon Editore. Bologna, Italy. (In press.)
14. HAUGAARD, N. & E. S. HAUGAARD. 1970. Stimulation of glucose utilization by thioctic acid in rat diaphragm incubated in vitro. Biochim. Biophys. Acta **222**: 583–586.
15. BASHAN, N., E. BURDETT & A. KLIP. 1993. Effect of thioctic acid on glucose transport. *In* The Role of Antioxidants in Diabetes Mellitus. PMI Verlag. Landsberg, Germany. (In press.)
16. WAGH, S. S., C. V. NATRAJ & K. K. G. MENON. 1987. Mode of action of lipoic acid in diabetes. J. Biosci. **11**: 59–74.
17. NATRAJ, C. V., V. M. GANDHI & K. K. G. MENON. 1984. Lipoic acid and diabetes: effect of dihydrolipoic acid administration in diabetic rats and rabbits. J. Biosci., **6**: 37–46.
18. HOYER, S. 1992. Abnormalities of glucose metabolism in Alzheimer's disease. Ann. N.Y. Acad. Sci. **527**: 53–58.
19. CRAFT, S., G. ZALLEN & L. D. BAKER. 1992. Glucose and memory in mild senile dementia of the Alzheimer type. J. Clin. Exp. Neuropsychol. **14**: 253–267.
20. BOYSEN, K.-H. 1967. Erfahrungen mit dem Präparat Thioctacid auf einer psychiatrischen Station. Med. Welt. **7**(1967): 395–400.
21. ROSTOCK, A. *et al.* Unpublished observations.

Age Dependence of the Glutamate Antagonistic Effect of GYKI 52466 in Snail Neurons[a]

I. TARNAWA,[b] S. TÓTH,[c] J. SÁRMÁNY,[c] AND I. PÉNZES[c]

[b]Institute for Drug Research
Post Office Box 82
H-1325 Budapest, Hungary

[c]Institute of Anesthesiology
Semmelweis Medical School
Diósárok st. 1
H-1122 Budapest, Hungary

INTRODUCTION

GYKI 52466 [1-(4'-aminophenyl)-4-methyl-7,8-methylenedioxy-5H-2,3-benzodiazepine] has recently been shown to specifically inhibit neuronal excitation mediated by the non-N-methyl-D-aspartate (non-NMDA) type glutamate receptors, in mammalian neurons[1,2] with a novel, noncompetitive mode of action.[3,4] The drug aroused a great scientific interest, as there are only few specific and potent antagonists of these receptors available. Moreover, the use of the other antagonists is rather limited in *in vivo* experiments, because they do not cross the blood-brain barrier easily. On the contrary, GYKI 52466 and some of its new analogues have good parenteral and oral effectiveness, which offers a good opportunity for a comparison of *in vivo* and *in vitro* experimental data. During the last couple of years, the role of non-NMDA receptors in neurodegenerative diseases has been extensively studied. Now, it is more or less generally accepted that they are significantly involved in several acute and chronic disorders of the central nervous system.[5–8] This suggests that the antagonists of this receptor may have a potential therapeutic value. It is very probable that similarly to several neurological diseases where the role of glutamate neurotoxicity is well established, the overexcitation of glutamate receptors is also involved in the development of certain neurological involution symptoms associated with normal and pathologically accelerated aging processes. Thus, GYKI 52466 is a potentially important research tool for investigating these phenomena and, theoretically, for controlling certain degenerative processes involved in aging. As non-NMDA antagonists will probably be introduced into the therapy as neuroprotective drugs in the not very far future, and because the acute and chronic conditions that need neuroprotective treatment are much more frequent among the elderly population, it is important to investigate the aging correlates of the action of such drugs.

Identified neurons of the pond snail (*Lymnaea stagnalis L.*) are suitable objects for studying age-related alterations in the neuronal membrane's functions.[9,10] Besides the methodological convenience that these giant cells offer for electrophysiologists, *Lymnaea* has a relatively short life span (similar to that of the rat), which makes this species preferable for comparative gerontological studies. Besides certain differ-

[a]This work was supported by OTKA 5424.

129

ences, there are also several similarities in the neurotransmitter mechanisms and in the basic transmembrane conductance mechanisms between molluscs and mammals; thus part of the electropharmacological results obtained in snails can be applied to higher animals as well.[11] In our present study, we used GYKI 52466 for studying age-related alterations in glutamate-evoked calcium currents in snail neurons and, further, to obtain preliminary experimental data concerning the possible geriatric use of a GYKI 52466-like compound.

METHODS AND MATERIALS

Experimental animals derived from an inbred strain of *Lymnaea stagnalis* and were kept under standardized laboratory conditions. Snails were allocated into "adult" (6–12 months) and "old" (more than 24 months) groups. For electrophysiological investigation, the central nervous system (suboesophageal ganglion ring) of the animal was removed and carefully freed from the covering connective tissue sheet to make the neurons visible under microscope and accessible for the glass microelectrodes. Some of the experiments were performed *in situ,* on identified neurons (mainly on VV 1–6 from the visceral and LPV 1–3 from the left parietal ganglia, according to the neuronal map of Benjamin)[12] of the isolated ganglion ring. The recording chamber (2 ml) was continuously perfused with an artificial medium (t = 20°C), the ionic composition of which was similar to the *Lymnaea* hemolympha (in mM: NaCl 44, KCl 2, CaCl$_2$ 4, MgCl$_2$ 1.5, TRIS 10); the pH was set to 7.4. For measuring calcium currents, sodium-free medium was used containing KCl 2, CaCl$_2$ 4, MgCl$_2$ 4, TRIS 10, TEA 50, and in some experiments part of CaCl$_2$ was replaced with BaCl$_2$. Drugs (AMPA.HBr, Research Biochemicals Inc.; L-glutamate, Sigma; GYKI 52466.HCl, synthesized at Institute for Drug Research) were dissolved in water and added to this medium. In other experiments, the same identified cells were dissociated[13] without any proteolytic treatment. For measuring electrophysiological parameters, standard current clamp and single electrode voltage clamp recordings were applied.

RESULTS AND DISCUSSION

The glutamate sensitivity of gastropoda neurons has long been known.[14] The majority of snail neurons are excited by glu, but it is not very well known if the receptors mediating its actions are the same as in higher animals. In the case of the neurons involved in this study, AMPA (a prototypic agonist compound at one of the non-NMDA receptor subtypes) was without any effect up to 20 μM; thus we used L-glutamate. Glutamate (100 μM) had a rather variable excitatory action, depending on the activity characteristics of the particular cell. The most prominent actions of glutamate on synaptically driven neurons were a substantial membrane potential decrease (depolarization), decrease of the spike amplitude, increase of the spontaneous spiking frequency, and an increase of the duration of the spike potential, which was mainly due to the slower repolarization. In intrinsically spiking (or pacemaker) cells, the decrease of the spike amplitude was the most apparent. It was frequently seen that spikes were sitting on the top of regularly occurring waves of membrane potential. Spikes could not follow the increase of the frequency of these pacemaker potentials. At first only some of the spikes failed to appear, later all of them disappeared. The onset of the action of glutamate was very fast, and a full recovery was seen if the duration of glu application was not longer than a few minutes. FIGURE 1 illustrates the rapidly developing actions of glutamate on the time course of the spike potential in a synaptically driven (A) and in a pacemaker neuron (B), respectively. Bottom traces show that GYKI 52466 (100 μM), applied shortly after

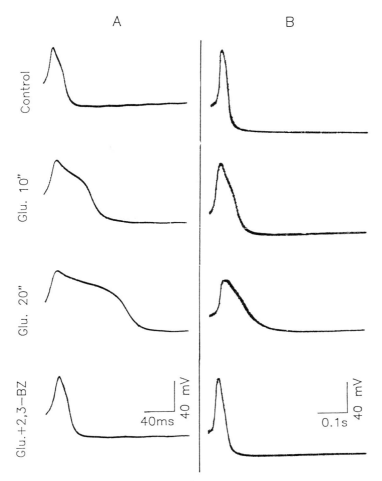

FIGURE 1. The rapidly developing actions of glutamate on the time course of the spike potential in a synaptically driven (A) and in a pacemacer neuron (B), respectively (both from the visceral ganglion). The spike amplitude was more affected in cell B. Bottom traces show that GYKI 52466 (100 μM) restored the parameters of the action potentials.

the start of the perfusion with glutamate, was able to completely restore the parameters of the action potentials. This is the first demonstration of the glutamate antagonistic action of this compound in invertebrates. When the perfusion of GYKI 52466 started with a delay, when the depolarizing and frequency elevating effect of glutamate had already fully developed, and the spike activity disappeared as a consequence of a depolarization block, GYKI 52466 gradually repolarized the cell to near the control value, but spontaneous activity did not come back again. However, when the cell was depolarized by intracellular current injection, the spike parameters were the same as in the control situation. The explanation of this apparent irreversible action on spontaneous spike activity can be that either some intracellular metabolic processes were triggered by glutamate influencing spiking or, more probably, that glutamate blocked the synaptic transmission at a site further from the surface of the ganglion, and the slowly acting GYKI 52466 did not have time to reach that region by diffusion to exert its blocking action. In the ganglia of the snail central nervous system, the somata of the neurons are localized at the surface, while the majority of the synaptic contacts are formed in the middle of the ganglion (i.e., in the neuropil), far from the cell bodies.

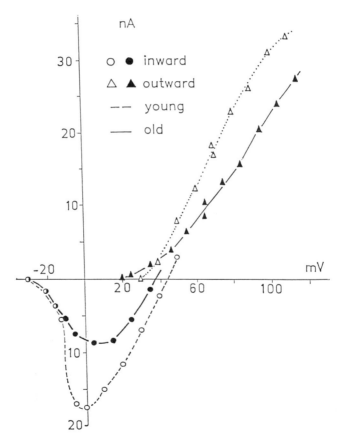

FIGURE 2. Current-voltage curves of an identified, isolated neuron of the visceral ganglion from control (adult) and old animals, in sodium-free medium. The high voltage activated calcium (inward) current was substantially smaller in the case of old neurons. The curve representing outward currents was shifted to the right.

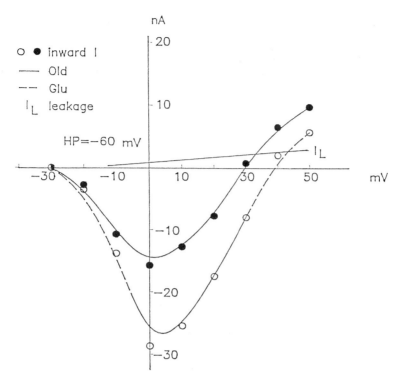

FIGURE 3. Effect of glutamate on the inward (calcium) currents in sodium-free medium, in a dissociated visceral ganglion cell of an old animal. A substantial potentiation of calcium currents is seen, especially at high membrane potentials.

GYKI 52466 alone sometimes caused as great as 10–20 mV hyperpolarization (not illustrated). As the effects of glutamate (e.g., increase of the spiking frequency, the longer repolarization time) can be partially due to its depolarizing effect, the antagonistic effect of GYKI 52466 could be explained simply with the hyperpolarization it caused. It was very important to investigate this interaction in voltage clamp experiments, when the membrane potential could be fixed at any desired level by intracellular current injection. These studies were performed on dissociated, isolated neurons. With this method, the exact measurements of transmembrane ionic currents at various clamped membrane potential values were performed. In FIGURE 2 the averaged current-voltage curves of an identified neuron of the visceral ganglion from control adult and old animals are compared, without any drug. Membrane potential was fixed at near the resting potential, and then depolarizing impulses of gradually increasing amplitude were applied. The evoked inward and outward currents are plotted against the voltage steps applied. The perfusion solution did not contain sodium (it was substituted with other cations), so that the inward current consisted of exclusively calcium currents. As it is seen in FIGURE 2, calcium currents, especially the high-voltage activated calcium current component, were substantially smaller in the case of old neurons. The curve representing outward currents was shifted to the right, but in the present paper only the calcium currents are discussed.

In old neurons, application of 100 μM glu resulted in a marked (from 12.5 to 27.5 nA), increase of the amplitude of calcium currents (FIGURE 3). The peak current was higher than the mean control current recorded from the neurons of young animals. Young animals also responded with an increased calcium current (from 21.5 to 40.0 nA), but the relative increase (86%) was smaller than in the case of old neurons (120%).

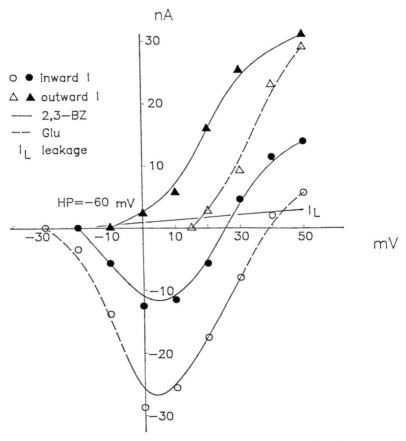

FIGURE 4. GYKI 52466 antagonizes the glutamate-induced increase of calcium currents in an old neuron (dissociated from the visceral ganglion). The activation of outward currents starts at lower potentials in the presence of GYKI 52466.

GYKI 552466 (100 μM) antagonized the calcium current enhancing effect of glutamate. To some extent, GYKI 52466 alone was able to inhibit calcium currents (not illustrated), but this effect was much less significant than its effect on the glutamate-potentiated currents. It is seen in FIGURE 4 that the activation threshold for inward currents shifted from 20 to 30 mV, suggesting that the low-threshold, rapidly inactivating calcium current component was also depressed. The glutamate antagonistic effect of GYKI 52466 did not differ in old and young neurons qualitatively; the inhibition was slightly stronger (53% v.s. 44%) in old neurons. The presently available data, however, do not make possible an exact quantitative analysis, as GYKI 52466 was studied only at one concentration level (at 100 μM, which is a relatively high concentration), and the comparison of dose-response curves to obtain proper quantitative data remains to be performed.

Considering that transmembrane calcium currents (especially glu-evoked Ca currents) are inhibited by GYKI 52446, the question may arise if the age-related impairment of the neuronal functions (reflected also in a smaller calcium current) will not be further weakened by the application of this compound. Indeed, one must be very careful when applying such drugs in geriatric population, where the applied doses can be markedly different from what is usually used. Most depressant drugs have more pronounced effects in elderly people than in adults, so it is important to find the optimal doses in every case.

By now, glutamate is generally accepted as one of the key factors involved in several neurodegenerative disorders.[5,6] Under certain conditions, sustained elevated extracellular concentration of glutamate can be measured and this high glutamate concentration can lead to cell toxicity in different ways.[15] Until recently, the activation of NMDA receptors has been regarded as the most important means of toxic calcium accumulation in the neuron, but during the last few years a large amount of evidence has accumulated suggesting a major role of non-NMDA receptors and voltage-dependent calcium channels in mediating excitotoxicity. Non-NMDA antagonists, among them GYKI 52466, have been proven to be neuroprotective in several animal models of neurotoxicity.[3,7,8] Our present results may supply further evidence about the potential use of such compounds in preventing glutamate and calcium induced neurotoxicity. It is now generally accepted that altered calcium homeostasis is one of the key features of aged neurons.[16] According to the membrane hypothesis of aging,[9,17] due to the changes in the colloidal state (dehydration, decreased ionic mobility) of the cell membrane and cytoplasm, the local concentration of calcium near the inner side of the neuronal membrane can reach extremely high values. Thus, the toxic effect of calcium currents caused by glutamate and the therapeutic potential of drugs influencing this process may be of special importance in aged people.

ACKNOWLEDGMENTS

We are grateful for the technical assistance of Terike Tóth.

REFERENCES

1. TARNAWA, I., I. ENGBERG & J. A. FLATMAN. 1989. *In* Amino Acids: Chemistry, Biology and Medicine. G. Lubec & G. A. Rosenthal, Eds.: 538–546. Escom Science Publishers. Leiden, The Netherlands.
2. ENGBERG, I., I. TARNAWA, J. DURAND & M. OUARDOUZ. 1993. Acta Physiol. Scand. **148:** 97–100.
3. ZORUMSKI, C. H., K. A. YAMADA, M. T. PRICE & J. W. OLNEY. 1993. Neuron **10:** 61–67.
4. DONEVAN, S. D. & M. A. ROGAWSKI. 1993. Neuron **10:** 51–59.
5. MELDRUM, B. S. & J. GARTHWAITE. 1990. Trends Pharmacol. Sci. **11:** 379–386.
6. KLOCKGETHER, T., L. TURSKI, T. HONORE, Z. ZHANG, D. M. GASH, R. KURLAN & J. T. GREENAMYRE. 1991. Ann. Neurol. **30:** 717–723.
7. LEPEILLET, E., B. ARVIN, C. MONCADA & B. S. MELDRUM. 1992. Brain Res. **571:** 115–120.

8. SMITH, S. E. & B. S. MELDRUM. 1992. Stroke **23:** 861–864.
9. ZS.-NAGY, I., S. TÓTH & G. LUSTYK. 1985. Arch. Gerontol. Geriatr. **4:** 53–66.
10. FROLKIS, V. V., A. S. STUPIA, O. A. MARTINENKO, S. TÓTH & A. I. TIMCHENKO. 1983. Mech. Ageing Dev. **25:** 91–102.
11. OSBORN, N. N. 1980. Trends Pharmacol. Sci. **1:** 290–291.
12. BENJAMIN, P. R. & C. T. INGS. 1972. Z. Zellforsch. **128:** 564–582.
13. CHAD, J. & H. WHEAL., EDS. 1991. Cellular Neurobiology, a Practical Approach. Oxford University Press. Oxford, England.
14. KERKUT, G. A., J. D. C. LAMBERT, R. J. GAYTON, J. E. LOKER & R. J. WALKER. 1975. Comp. Biochem. Physiol. **50A:** 1–25.
15. CHOI, D. W. 1988. Trends Neurosci. **11:** 465–469.
16. GIBSON, G. E. & C. PETERSON. 1989. Neurobiol. Aging **8:** 329–343.
17. ZS.-NAGY, I. 1989. Neurobiol. Aging **8:** 370–372.

Morphological Alterations of Synaptic Mitochondria during Aging

The Effect of Hydergine® Treatment

CARLO BERTONI-FREDDARI, PATRIZIA FATTORETTI,
TIZIANA CASOLI, CARLA SPAGNA,
AND WILLIAM MEIER-RUGE[a]

Center for Surgical Research (Neurobiology)
I.N.R.C.A. Research Department
60121 Ancona, Italy

[a] *Institute of Pathology*
University of Basel
CH-4003 Basel, Switzerland

Synaptic junctions, while being well-differentiated areas of the neuronal membrane, are reported to be very dynamic structures capable of consistent morphological rearrangements even in the fully developed adult system.[1] During aging, this plastic potential of the synaptic junctions appears to be considerably impaired. Quantitative studies on the morphology of the synaptic junctional areas in old laboratory animals and human beings have shown that the number of synapses decreases while the size of the single contact increases. As a final result of these opposite changes, the total synaptic contact area/μm^3 appears to be significantly reduced in the old central nervous system (CNS).[2–6]

Modulation of synaptic morphology is an ongoing physiological and multifactorial process,[1,7–9] thus it is not feasible to single out a unique factor to explain the age-dependent decay in synaptic structural dynamics. In spite of the reliability of this last assumption, a time-related decay of the neuronal metabolism in the old CNS has been proposed as an early deteriorative event that, in turn, may lead to a progressive deafferentiation of the synaptic circuitries.[10–16] Nerve cells and particularly their synaptic terminals need a high and constant energy supply: besides the restoration of the ionic concentration within the cell following the transmission of the nervous impulse, a steady part of the energy produced by the neurone is used to maintain the internal household of the cell including genesis and transportation of organelles to synaptic terminals. Conceivably, any impairment in the actual and proper energy supply at synaptic regions may play a crucial role in derangements of cell-to-cell information processing due to age.

With these concepts in mind, the aim of the present study was a computer-assisted morphometric study on the ultrastructural features of synaptic mitochondria of different ages and in old animals chronically treated with Hydergine, a pharmacon known to improve nerve cell metabolism[17,18] and reported to exert its action at nerve terminals.[19,20]

AGE-RELATED CHANGES IN THE MORPHOLOGY
OF SYNAPTIC MITOCHONDRIA

Young (3 months), adult (12 months), and old (24–26 months) rats were perfused with saline followed by a fixation solution (glutaraldehyde 2%, formalin 4%, 0.005 $CaCl_2$ in 0.1 M cacodylate buffer pH 7.4) through the left ventricle. Each group consisted of 5 animals; 5 tissue samples were taken from the cerebellar cortex of each animal and processed according to conventional electron microscopic procedures. Morphometry of mitochondria in the cerebellar glomeruli (FIGURE 1) was carried out in a semiautomatic mode by means of a computer-assisted image analyzer (FIGURE 2) as reported in detail in our previous paper.[21] The fraction of cytoplasmic volume occupied by mitochondria (volume density: Vv), the number of mitochondria/ μm^3 (numerical density: Nv), and their average size (skeleton: Sk) were the three parameters measured by us.

The choice of a proper anatomical model fulfilling the morphometric criteria currently adopted by scientists to perform quantitative morphological studies is a very difficult task when dealing with the nervous tissue. However, despite its anisotropic anatomy, even within the CNS, it is possible to sample very discrete areas and get reliable results correlated to specific performances. With the above caveats in mind, we chose the cerebellar glomerulus as anatomical model for our studies. Although the glomeruli do not show well-outlined borders, both under the optic and the electron microscope, they appear as easily identifiable large zones surrounded by the granule cell bodies in the cerebellar granular layer. The peculiar feature that has led us to investigate the glomeruli is that these areas of the cerebellar cortex are constituted of an enlargement of the mossy fiber intermingled with claw dendrites of the granular cells and with axons of Golgi cells. Thus, the mitochondria seen in cross-sectioned glomeruli are those organelles located at nerve terminals. This is not a mere anatomical consideration; on the contrary, it stresses the fact that within the regionally differentiated nerve cells, a mitochondrial heterogeneity has been clearly identified. Biochemical differences between the mitochondria located at the nerve cell body and those at axon terminals have led these organelles to be classified into two discrete populations: the "perikarial" and the "synaptic" mitochondria.[22-24] The pattern of metabolic activities carried out by these two populations of organelles is still under investigation; however, the peculiar functions of nerve terminals have been shown to require specific amounts of energy to cope with actual performances.[25-27] Taking into account this metabolic compartmentation of nerve cell mitochondria, in the present investigation, we intended to evaluate quantitatively the organelles directly subserving synaptic activities.

The results of our study in rats of different ages are summarized in FIGURE 3. We did not find any change due to age in the mitochondrial volume density (Vv) in the three groups analyzed. On the contrary, the number of mitochondria/μm^3 (Nv) appears to undergo significant changes both in adulthood and aging when compared with the data from the young group of rats, namely, Nv increases at 12 months of age whereas it decreases in 24–26 month old animals. The average skeleton (Sk) of the mitochondria shows an opposite trend as compared with Nv: in adulthood we found a decrease and in aging an increase, respectively, of the length of the organelles. To investigate the composition of the mitochondrial population present at synaptic regions with respect to their skeleton, we performed a percentage distribution of the single measurement regarding Sk (FIGURE 4). As better pointed out in the note on the right, it is clearly evident that in old animals 20.6% of the mitochondria exceed 5

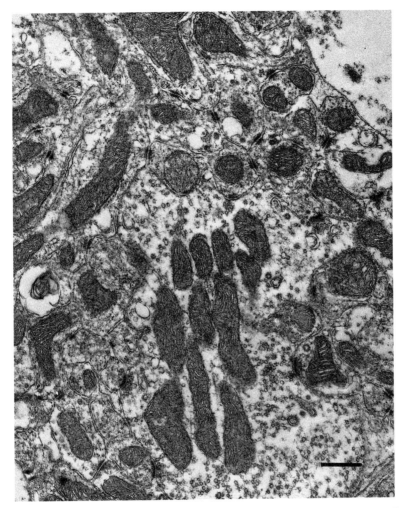

FIGURE 1. Electron microscopic picture of rat synaptic mitochondria from a cross-sectioned cerebellar glomerulus. The high numerical density of the organelles present in this area of the CNS lends further support to the reliability of the glomerulus as anatomical model for morphometric studies. Bar = 0.5 μm.

μm in length: a percentage that is consistently higher than in young (8.6%) and adult rats (5.3%).

Vv, Nv, and Sk, while reporting on specific morphological aspects of the mitochondria present at nerve endings, appear to be in a reciprocal relationship which can be supposed to have a true biological basis since these parameters are calculated independently using different morphometric formulas. Going into details, we would like to remark that the total volume of the mitochondria/μm^3 (Vv) seems to represent the final outcome of the inverse changes occurring in number (Nv) and size, or length (Sk), of these organelles. Thus, in addition to the widely documented plasticity of the synaptic contact zones,[2-8] we maintain that also the synaptic mitochondria are in a very dynamic condition that aims at rearrangements of their

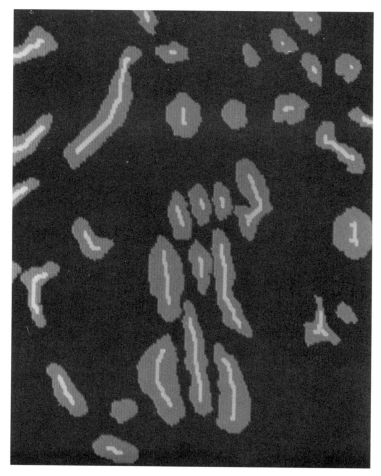

FIGURE 2. Video picture from our image analysis system of the same mitochondria shown in FIGURE 1. The whiter ribbon within each organelle provides information on mitochondrial skeleton (Sk) or length.

morphology to set up the proper "hardware" for the production of the energy needed to cope with specific demands of the synaptic network they subserve.[21] We are aware of the speculative character of the above assumption. Nevertheless, taking into account our previous studies on synaptic morphological changes at different

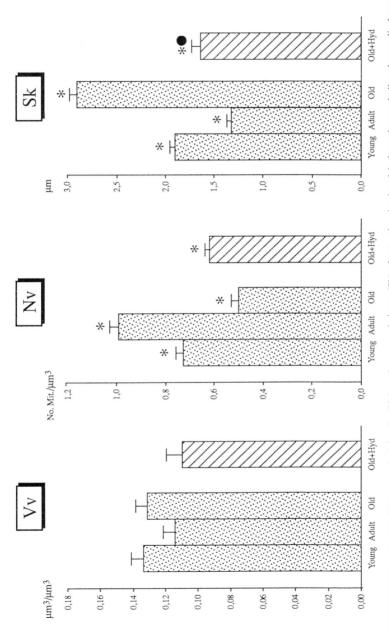

FIGURE 3. Volume density (Vv), numerical density (Nv), and average skeleton (Sk) of synaptic mitochondria from the cerebellar glomeruli of rats of different ages and in old, Hydergine-treated animals (mean ± standard error of the mean). Significance of intergroup differences (Student's *t*-test): *$p < 0.001$; •$p < 0.02$ vs. the adult group.

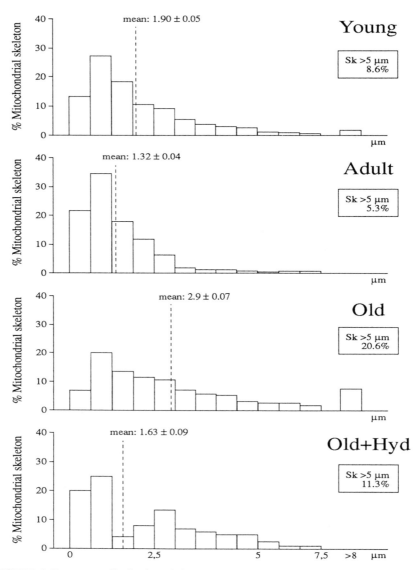

FIGURE 4. Percentage distribution of the skeleton (Sk) of synaptic mitochondria in rats of different ages and in old, Hydergine-treated animals. During aging, 20.6% of the mitochondrial population present at nerve endings is constituted by elongated organelles (>5 μm). Chronic Hydergine administration to old rats reduced this percentage to 11.3%.

ages[2-4,7,20] and the present data on synaptic mitochondria, parallel alterations in the ultrastructural features of the synaptic junctional areas and mitochondria can be clearly envisaged. In agreement with this rationale on mitochondrial morphological adaptability, our present finding reporting a life span constancy in the cytoplasmic volume fraction (Vv) occupied by the synaptic mitochondria shows that the potential for energy production seems to be unaffected by time. We have found age-related differences only in the composition of the mitochondrial population with reference to the percent of organelles of the same size or length (FIGURE 4). Thus, in adult animals, the energy needed at synaptic regions is provided by a high number of small mitochondria, whereas in old rats, synaptic performances depend on the energy supplied by a reduced number of elongated organelles. At synaptic regions, mitochondrial activities aim at providing in due time elevated amounts of ATP needed for the prompt reply to environmental stimuli: any delay in the supply of the proper energy may result in synaptic malfunction and lead to progressive disuse of the contact(s). Current biochemical results have clearly documented consistent decreases in the functionality of enzymes of the respiratory chain in old animals as a consequence of sustained stimulations.[10,19,24-26,28-31] The present results may represent the morphological aspect of these biochemical data: we maintain that the few enlarged organelles present at the synapses of old rats may be unable to accomplish their tasks especially when the demand is high.

On the basis of the wealth of reports on the impairment of cellular metabolism during aging, some authors support a "power failure hypothesis" as the causative mechanism leading to the progressive deterioration in cellular functions due to time.[13,14,32,33] At present, the still debated question is whether an impaired metabolism is the primary cause or the consequence of aging. With regard to synaptic terminal regions, it must be stressed that energy metabolism and functional activity are closely coupled,[15,32] a decline in synaptic performances results in a matched reduction of the metabolic demand which, in turn, depends on both the functional and morphological conditions of the tissue. Any change in mitochondrial ultrastructure may play a crucial role in these balanced relationships by contributing to the reinforcement and stabilization or to the weakening and deterioration of the synaptic circuits. During physiological aging, metabolic decay appears to be a subtle process actively counteracted by different cellular recovery strategies even in postmitotic cells like neurons. The identification of the many factors involved in the age-dependent impairment of the maintenance of a steady metabolism at synaptic endings represents an early step to program any type of intervention aimed at ameliorating synaptic capabilities.

CAUSATIVE EVENTS LEADING TO POSSIBLE MODIFICATIONS OF MITOCHONDRIAL MORPHOLOGY

In the present paper, we will discuss the many factors able to influence the activities of mitochondria and supposed to modify their morphology. At present, we cannot indicate a unique cause for the alterations found by us at the synaptic mitochondria of old rats. Conversely, the peculiar biogenesis of these organelles support that their morphology may be modulated by several facts and circumstances.

Mitochondria increase in mass and number by accretion and integration of newly synthesized material into preexisting organelles. The nuclear and the mitochondrial DNA (mitDNA) participate in the synthesis and subsequent assembling of these sets of structural proteins and lipids. Both genomes are coordinated through cellular signals to carry out this highly ordered sequence of events.[34,35] Derangements at any step in these processes may represent potential drawbacks both for mitochondrial activities and for their morphological features. First of all, it must be stressed that mitDNA is very sensitive to mutagens because of (1) its supercoiled structure; (2) the lack of protection from histone and/or nonhistone proteins; (3) the high frequency of point mutations associated with limited DNA repair mechanisms; (4) the presence of respiratory enzymes that can activate chemical carcinogens. An indirect threat to mitDNA integrity is also represented by the fact that it is attached to the inner membrane of the organelle. Thus, any alteration in the mitochondrial membrane structure may result in an impaired control of the respiratory chain with the consistent production of dangerous electrophiles (peroxides, epoxides, nitroxides, semiquinones) capable of prompt reactions with mitochondrial genes. As a support to this rationale, during aging it has been clearly documented that mitochondrial membranes undergo several deteriorative events, including a decrease in the unsaturation of the fatty acids of their phospholipids,[28] an increase in cholesterol content,[36] and an impairment in the Ca^{2+} uptake and release mechanisms.[33,37] Oxygen free radicals generated during cellular respiration are reported to be the main cause of mitochondrial membrane damage.[30] In turn, oxygen can attack other molecules and produce further reactive compounds. Because of the known short life of free radicals, this vicious circle appears to be particularly dangerous for mitochondrial structural molecules closely involved in the oxidative phosphorylation processes.

Different circumstances, including aging of insects and mammals, are reported to bring about an enlargement or elongation in mitochondria.[39–42] Only tentative explanations have been proposed so far for such a change in the morphology of these functional units of the cellular metabolism, and they claim a time-related progressive inability of mitochondria to divide or the fusion of small organelles into larger ones.[39–41] Taking into account the age-related alterations of the mitochondrial membrane structure and of its molecular composition together with the high vulnerability of mitDNA, we maintain that the elongated organelles are those unable to divide, with the consequence that in old individuals also the number of mitochondria is markedly reduced. Quantitative measurements on the morphology of muscle mitochondria in young and old human beings following physical training have shown that in both the groups analyzed, the mitochondrial volume fraction was augmented, but this was due to an increase in the number of organelles in younger subjects and to a significant enlargement of mitochondrial size in older individuals, respectively.[27] Thus, under stimulation, it seems that mitochondrial population is capable of functional adaptive rearrangement of its morphological features according to the age of the individual: with specific reference to the old organisms, our present data and those of Kiesling[27] support that the genesis of new mitochondria appears to stop at the intermediate step of accretion in size of the organelles, but it is not followed by their division.

Mitochondrial potential for function could be maintained through *de novo* formation of metabolically competent organelles. In agreement with their plastic condition, the turnover rate of the mitochondria is different from organ to organ. Neurons have been reported to renew their mitochondrial population at the slowest rate (24.4 days).[43] Conversely, these postmitotic cells utilize high levels of O_2 to support their specialized functions. Thus, in neurons the mitochondrial population is at a high risk of damage from free radicals and any delay in the renewal/substitution of irreversibly damaged organelles may result in potential impairments of synaptic structure and function. This last assumption is particularly true for synaptic mitochondria, which are not only transported from the nerve cell body to dendritic terminals and back via axonal flow,[44] but also depend on axonal transport for the biogenesis and eventual substitution of the majority of their constitutive molecules.[44,45]

THE EFFECT OF HYDERGINE® ON THE MORPHOLOGY OF SYNAPTIC MITOCHONDRIA OF OLD RATS

Hydergine (co–dergocrine mesylate: a fixed combination of four ergot alkaloids) is widely used in the treatment of the variety of symptoms underlying the typical impairment of cerebral functions known as age-related mental decline. In the early forties prescribed as a vasodilator, Hydergine is now currently administered as a metabolic enhancer able to improve several aspects of the neuronal metabolism and neurotransmitter activity.[46] It is widely documented that this pharmacon increases the stores of ATP,[19] stabilizes the cAMP content of the nerve cells,[48] improves brain glucose utilization[17,18] and, in turn, cerebral microcirculation.[49] In consideration of these effects and of the plastic condition of the mitochondria, we hypothesized that chronic Hydergine administration to old rats may be able to modify the ultrastructural features of the very discrete population of organelles directly supporting the metabolic needs of synaptic terminal regions.

The drug was dissolved in distilled water and administered to old rats (5 animals) by intubation into the stomach once a day for 4 weeks at a dose of 3 mg/kg of body weight.[20] Tissue processing for electron microscopy and morphometric measurements were carried out according to the procedure used for the untreated groups. The results of our investigation are reported in FIGURE 3. No significant difference was found with regard to Vv in the treated rats vs. the other groups taken into account. Nv significantly increased after Hydergine administration comparing old controls and treated animals, although in this latter group the number of organelles was still significantly lower than in young and adult animals. Sk is significantly decreased in the treated group as compared with young and old rats, but it is significantly higher vs. the adult animals. The percentage distribution of Sk reported in FIGURE 4 shows that, comparing the old Hydergine treated rats with the age-matched controls, the fraction of organelles longer than 5 μm is reduced from 20.6 to 11.3%.

These data support that chronic Hydergine treatment is able to reverse partially the age-related alterations in the morphology of synaptic mitochondria. Namely, in the old treated animals the steady value of Vv appears to be maintained through balanced changes of Nv and Sk opposite to those observed in the age-matched controls. The interesting finding of the reduction in the percentage of the elongated organelles in old rats (by about 45%) following Hydergine treatment further supports the idea that this drug is able to counteract the age-related impairment in the morphological structural dynamics of the population of synaptic mitochondria.

In looking for possible explanations of such an effect, both the mechanism of action of Hydergine and the morphological plasticity of synaptic mitochondria must be taken into account. Despite the fact that no molecular mechanism of action of Hydergine has been clearly identified, an extensive experimental and clinical research has yielded data supporting the idea that this drug exerts direct mixed agonistic and antagonistic effects on dopaminergic, serotoninergic, and alpha-adrenergic receptors. Namely, Hydergine is reported to be able to compensate for eventual deficit and, at the same time, to counteract the overactivity of monoaminergic systems in different areas of the brain, thus restoring the balance in the functional interplay among these molecules.[50–52] Besides these effects, receptor binding studies have shown that Hydergine facilitates evoked acetylcholine release[52] and increases the activity of cholineacetyltransferase (CAT)[53] in the hippocampus of old rats; therefore this drug has multiple actions on several neurotransmitter systems. In agreement with these data, studies on the localization of the labeled pharmacon in the CNS have shown that synaptic terminal regions are the major site of Hydergine action.[47]

As discussed above, the morphological features of synaptic mitochondria appear to be actively modulated by several cellular and environmental factors. The final outcome of these "stimulations" is an overall rearrangement of the mitochondrial population structural dynamics at synaptic terminals which aims at the assembling of the proper "hardware" able to cope with actual metabolic requests of ATP. These adaptive changes appear to be specific with regard to the synaptic connectivity where the mitochondria are located, e.g., the cerebellar glomeruli of young, adult, and old rats. In our previous studies, we found that chronic Hydergine administration to old rats resulted in a significant increase of the number of synaptic contacts both in the hippocampal dentate gyrus and in the cerebellar granular layer.[20,54] Our present data support that this positive effect of Hydergine on synaptic plasticity may be due to an improved efficiency in the metabolic machinery present at nerve endings. Although it cannot be claimed whether the early change due to Hydergine administration occurs at synaptic contact zones or mitochondria, it is widely reported that a constant and adequate use maintains the competence of any system/organ. Conceivably, good synaptic performances are well coupled with an efficient metabolism. A marked, significant increase in synaptic size has been reported by many authors both in old laboratory animals and human beings.[2-7] At present, it is not known whether this age-related change is due: (1) to an enlargement of the persisting contacts, (2) to the physiological elimination of the smaller, trophic-impaired junctions, or (3) to both these circumstances. As a matter of fact, the proper maintenance of a high number of synapses, typical of a finely tuned neuronal network, requires high amounts of ATP upon request. Conversely, any delay in the prompt supply of energy may result in deleterious effects for the scarcely used contacts. In addition to favoring a better synaptic functionality, the neuronal preservation of ATP stores brought about by Hydergine treatment[19] may support the activity of a high number of junctions including the smaller ones, thus postponing or possibly avoiding their elimination. We are aware that this assumption is speculative. Nevertheless, the improved metabolic economy in the nerve cells of Hydergine-treated animals is carried out also via the stabilization of neuronal cAMP content[9,51] and this fact may be relevant in view of the specific effect of cAMP on the formation and reinforcement of new synaptic contacts as reported in cultured neuroblastoma cells.[55]

Age-related mental decline has a multifactorial pathogenesis. Therefore any intervention aimed at the recovery of a single deteriorated aspect (e.g., cerebral blood flow or serotoninergic transmission) represents a weak theraupetic approach because of the several mechanisms involved. In consideration of these concepts, the pattern of information reporting the multiple modes of action of Hydergine has provided a rationale for the administration of this drug in the symptomatic treatment of the cerebral insufficiency of elderly people. Our present data further widen the biological range of action of Hydergine supporting that it has a favorable modulating effect on the dynamic morphology of the mitochondrial "hardware" present at synaptic terminals.

REFERENCES

1. COTMAN, C. W., N. NIETO-SAMPEDRO & E. W. HARRIS. 1981. Synapse replacement in the nervous system of adult vertebrates. Physiol. Rev. **61:** 684–784.
2. BERTONI-FREDDARI, C., C. GIULI, C. PIERI & D. PACI. 1986. Quantitative investigation of the morphological plasticity of synaptic junctions in rat dentate gyrus during aging. Brain Res. **366:** 187–192.

3. BERTONI-FREDDARI, C., W. MEIER-RUGE & J. ULRICH. 1988. Quantitative morphology of synaptic plasticity in the aging brain. Scann. Microsc. **2:** 1027–1034.

4. BERTONI-FREDDARI, C., P. FATTORETTI, T. CASOLI, W. MEIER-RUGE & J. ULRICH. 1990. Morphological adaptive response of the synaptic junctional zones in the human dentate gyrus during aging and Alzheimer's disease. Brain Res. **517:** 69–75.

5. DEKOSKY, S. T. & S. W. SCHEFF. 1990. Synapse loss in frontal cortex biopsies in Alzheimer's disease: correlation with cognitive severity. Ann. Neurol. **27:** 457–464.

6. SCHEFF, S. W., S. T. DEKOSKY & D. A. PRICE. 1990. Quantitative assessment of cortical synaptic density in Alzheimer's disease. Neurobiol. Aging **11:** 29–37.

7. BERTONI-FREDDARI, C. 1989. Synaptic plasticity in the cerebellar glomeruli of rats: effects of aging and vitamin E deficiency. *In* CRC Handbook of Free Radicals and Antioxidants in Biomedicine. J. Miquel, A. T. Quintanilha & H. Weber, Eds.: 255–267. CRC Press. Boca Raton, Florida.

8. CALVERLEY, R. K. S. & D. G. JONES. 1990. Contributions of dendritic spines and perforated synapses to synaptic plasticity. Brain Res. **15:** 215–249.

9. DESMOND, N. L. & W. LEVY. 1988. Anatomy of associative long-term synaptic modification. *In* Long-Term Potentiation: from Biophysics to Behavior. P. W. Landfield & S. A. Deadwyler, Eds.: 265–305. Alan R. Liss Inc. New York, N.Y.

10. HANSFORD, R. G. 1983. Bioenergetics in aging. Biochim. Biophys. Acta **726:** 41–80.

11. HOYER, S. 1985. The effect of age on glucose and energy metabolism in brain cortex of rats. Arch. Gerontol. Geriatr. **4:** 193–205.

12. MEIER-RUGE, W. 1985. Neurochemistry of the aging brain and senile dementia. *In* Aging 2000: Our Health Care Destiny. C. M. Gaitz & T. Samorajski, Eds. **1:** 101–112. Springer-Verlag. New York, N.Y.

13. MIQUEL, J., J. E. JOHNSON & J. CERVOS-NAVARRO. 1983. Comparison of CNS aging in humans and experimental animals. *In* Brain Aging: Neuropathology and Neuropharmacology, Aging. J. Cervos-Navarro & H. I. Sarkander, Eds. **21:** 231–258. Raven Press. New York, N.Y.

14. MIQUEL, J. & J. E. FLEMING. 1984. A two-step hypothesis on the mechanisms of in vitro cell aging: cell differentiation followed by intrinsic mitochondrial mutagenesis. Exp. Gerontol. **19:** 31–36.

15. SIESJO, B. K. & S. REHNCRONA. 1980. Adverse factors affecting neuronal metabolism: relevance to the dementias. *In* Biochemistry of Dementia. P. J. Roberts, Ed.: 91–120. J. Wiley & Sons Ltd. London, England.

16. SOKOLOFF, L. 1977. Relation between physiological function and energy metabolism in the central nervous system. J. Neurochem. **29:** 13–26.

17. KAWASHIMA, K., K. KOGURE & T. IDO. 1988. Increase in cerebral metabolic rate of glucose in multi-infarct dementia following intravenous administration of co-dergocrine mesylate (Hydergine). J. Neurol. **235** (Suppl. Abstr.): 10, 52.

18. NAGASAWA, H., K. KOGURE & T. KAWASHIMA. 1989. Influence of Hydergine on brain cell metabolism as demonstrated by PET. *In* Cerebral Insufficiency. Trends in Research and Treatment. A. Carlsson, S. Kanowski, H. Allain & R. Spiegel, Eds.: 169–178. Parthenon Publishing Group. Carnforth & Park Ridge.

19. MEIER-RUGE, W., A. ENZ & P. GYGAX. 1975. Experimental pathology in basic research of the aging brain. *In* Genesis and Treatment of Psychologic Disorders in the Elderly. S. Gershon & A. Raskin, Eds. **2:** 55–126. Raven Press. New York, N.Y.

20. BERTONI-FREDDARI, C., C. GIULI, C. PIERI & D. PACI. 1987. The effect of chronic Hydergine treatment on the plasticity of synaptic junctions in the dentate gyrus of aged rats. J. Gerontol. **42:** 482–486.

21. BERTONI-FREDDARI, C., P. FATTORETTI, T. CASOLI, C. SPAGNA, W. MEIER-RUGE & J. ULRICH. 1993. Morphological plasticity of synaptic mitochondria during aging. Brain Res. **628:** 193–200.

22. LAI, J. C. K., J. M. WALSH, S. C. DENNIS & J. B. CLARK. 1977. Synaptic and non-synaptic mitochondria from rat brain: isolation and characterization. J. Neurochem. **28:** 625–631.

23. VILLA, R. F., A. GORINI, D. GEROLDI, A. LO FARO & C. DELL'ORBO. 1989. Enzyme

activities in perikaryal and synaptic mitochondrial fractions from rat hippocampus during development. Mech. Age Dev. **49:** 211–225.

24. CURTI, D., M. C. GIANGARE, M. E. REDOLFI, I. FUGACCIA & G. BENZI. 1990. Age-related modifications of cytochrome c oxidase activity in discrete brain regions. Mech. Age Dev. **55:** 171–180.

25. DESHMUKH, D. R. & M. S. PATEL. 1982. Age-dependent changes in pyruvate uptake by nonsynaptic and synaptic mitochondria from rat brain. Mech. Age Dev. **20:** 343–351.

26. HARMON, H. J., S. NANK & R. A. FLOYD. 1987. Age-dependent changes in rat brain mitochondria of synaptic and nonsynaptic origins. Mech. Age Dev. **38:** 167–177.

27. KIESLING, K. H., I. PILSTROM, J. KARLSSON & K. PIEHL. 1973. Mitochondrial volume in skeletal muscle from young and old physically untrained and trained healthy men and from alcoholics. Clin. Sci. **44:** 547–554.

28. NOHL, H. & D. HEGNER. 1978. Do mitochondria produce oxygen radicals in vivo? Eur. J. Biochem. **82:** 563–567.

29. PATEL, M. S. 1977. Age-dependent changes in the oxidative metabolism in rat brain. J. Gerontol. **32:** 643–646.

30. SOHAL, R. S. & B. H. SOHAL. 1991. Hydrogen peroxide release by mitochondria increases during aging. Mech. Age Dev. **57:** 187–202.

31. SYLVIA, A. & M. ROSENTHAL. 1979. Effects of age on brain oxidative metabolism in vivo. Brain Res. **165:** 235–248.

32. SMITH, C. B. 1984. Aging and changes in cerebral energy metabolism. Trends Neurol. Sci. (June): 203–208.

33. LESLIE, S. W., L. J. CHANDLER, E. M. BARR & R. P. FARRAR. 1985. Reduced calcium uptake by rat brain mitochondria and synaptosomes in response to aging. Brain Res. **329:** 177–183.

34. ATTARDI, G. & G. SCHARTZ. 1988. Biogenesis of mitochondria. Annu. Rev. Cell Biol. **4:** 289–333.

35. WILKIE, D., I. H. EVANS, V. EGILSSON, E. S. DIALA & D. COLLIER. 1983. Mitochondria, cell surface, and carcinogenesis. Int. Rev. Cytol. **15:** 157–189.

36. GRINNA, L. S. 1977. Age related changes in the lipids of the microsomal and the mitochondrial membranes of rat liver and kidney. Mech. Age Dev. **6:** 197–205.

37. MARTINEZ, A., J. VITORICA, E. BOGONEZ & J. SATRUSTEGUI. 1987. Differential effects of age on the pathways of calcium influx into nerve terminals. Brain Res. **435:** 249–257.

38. GABEL, K. & B. I. ROOTS. 1989. Stereological analysis of mitochondria from brains of temperature acclimated goldfish, Carassius Aratus L. (5 and 30 C). J. Therm. Biol. **14:** 187–190.

39. SOHAL, R. S. & R. G. BRIDGES. 1978. Associated changes in the size and number of mitochondria present in the midgut of the larvae of the housefly., *Musca Domestica* and phospholipid composition of the larvae. J. Cell Sci. **34:** 65–79.

40. SOHAL, R. S. & R. G. BRIDGES. 1977. Effects of experimental alterations in phospholipid composition on the size and number of mitochondria in the flight muscles of the housefly, *Musca Domestica.* J. Cell Sci. **27:** 273–287.

41. TAUCHI, H. & T. SATO. 1985. Cellular change in senescence: possible factors influencing the process of cellular aging. *In* Thresholds in Aging. M. Bergener, M. Ermini & H. B. Stahelin, Eds.: 91–113. Academic Press Inc. London, England.

42. TAVARES, M. A. & M. M. PAULA-BARBOSA. 1983. Mitochondrial changes in rat Purkinje cells after prolonged alcohol consumption. J. Submicrosc. Cytol. **15:** 713–720.

43. MENZIES, R. A. & P. H. GOLD. 1971. The turnover of mitochondria in a variety of tissues of young, adult and aged rats. J. Biol. Chem. **246:** 2425–2429.

44. GRAFSTEIN, B. & D. S. FORMAN. 1980. Intracellular transport in neurons. Physiol. Rev. **60:** 1167–1283.

45. LASEK, R. J. & M. J. KATZ. 1987. Mechanisms at the axon tip regulate metabolic processes critical to axonal elongation. *In* Neural Regeneration, Progress in Brain Research. F. J. Seil, E. Herbert & B. M. Carlson, Eds. **71:** 49–60. Elsevier. Amsterdam, The Netherlands.

46. KRASSNER, M. B. 1984. Mechanism of action of Hydergine (ergoloid mesylates) in relation to organic brain disorders. Adv. Ther. **1:** 172–189.

47. Iwangoff, P., W. Meier-Ruge, C. Schieweck & A. Enz. 1976. The uptake of DH-ergotoxine by different parts of the cat brain. Pharmacology **14:** 27–38.

48. Markstein, R. & H. Wagner. 1978. Effect of dihydroergotoxine on cyclic AMP generating systems in rat cerebral cortex slices. Gerontology **24:** 94–105.

49. Sinzinger, H. 1985. Double-blind study of the influence of co-dergocrine on platelet parameters in healthy volunteers. Eur. J. Clin. Pharmacol. **28:** 713–716.

50. Ermini, M. 1985. The effects of Hydergine on neurotransmitters. Br. J. Clin. Prac. **39:** 11–14.

51. Markstein, R. 1985. Hydergine: interaction with neurotransmitter systems in the central nervous system. *In* Aging 2000: Our Health Care Destiny. C. M. Gaitz & T. Samorajski, Eds.: 361–375. Springer Verlag. New York, N.Y.

52. Ermini, M. & R. Markstein. 1982. Hydergine therapy: mechanism of action. Br. J. Clin. Prac. **16:** 27–32.

53. Dravid, A. R. 1983. Deficits in cholinergic enzymes and muscarinic receptors in the hippocampus and striatum of senescent rats. Effect of chronic Hydergine treatment. Arch. Int. Pharmacodyn. Ther. **264:** 195–202.

54. Bertoni-Freddari, C., P. Fattoretti, T. Casoli, M. Gambini & W. Meier-Ruge. The effect of Hydergine on synaptic terminals of the ageing cerebellum. *In* Individualized Hydergine Treatment in the Ageing Patient. (In press.)

55. Nirenberg, M., S. Wilson, H. Higashida, A. Rotter, K. Krueger, N. Busis, R. Ray, J. G. Kenimer & M. Adler. 1983. Modulation of synapse formation by cyclic adenosine monophosphate. Science **222:** 794–799.

Mitochondrial DNA Transcription and Translation in Aged Rat

Effect of Acetyl-L-carnitine[a]

M. N. GADALETA, V. PETRUZZELLA, L. DADDABBO,
C. OLIVIERI, F. FRACASSO, P. LOGUERCIO POLOSA,
AND P. CANTATORE

Department of Biochemistry and Molecular Biology
University of Bari
Bari, Italy

INTRODUCTION

Mitochondrial DNA (mtDNA) carries the information for 13 of the 60 polypeptides of mitochondrial respiratory complexes: therefore, it is responsible together with nuclear DNA (nDNA) for the biogenesis of this essential organelle. Aging is a complex phenomenon mainly associated with loss of mitochondrial bioenergetic capacity. Therefore, it has been hypothesized that the degenerative processes of senescence could be caused by defects of mtDNA.[1-5] In fact, mtDNA is localized near the cell's most active compartment for the production of oxygen free radicals, it is unprotected by hystonelike proteins, and it lacks efficient repair mechanisms. Furthermore, it is a highly compact molecule so that most mutational changes in mtDNA might have injurious effects. According to this hypothesis, damaged mtDNA molecules should accumulate with age, particularly in terminally differentiated tissues such as muscle and brain, altering the normal synthesis of mtDNA encoded polypeptides of respiratory complexes as well as ATP production.[2] Recently, sporadic and inherited mutations of mtDNA have been found in different human mitochondrial pathologies.[6] It has been suggested that aging could be the most widespread mitochondrial pathology.[7] We used the rat to study the role of the mitochondrial genetic system in aging. We found in aged rat brain and heart a reduced steady-state level of mt transcripts[8] due to reduced RNA synthesis,[9] an unchanged mitochondrial DNA copy number per cell,[10] a reduced number of mtDNA molecules harboring the triplex strand structure in the "D-loop region,"[11] and a low but increasing age-related content of mtDNA molecules harboring a 4.8 K base deletion.[12] We found, furthermore, that the reduced steady-state level of mt transcripts is reversible: 1 h acetyl-L-carnitine (AC) pretreatment of senescent rats is able to bring back the level of mt transcripts to the value of adult rat.[8]

In this paper, we report data showing that the effect of AC on the level of mt transcripts in aged rat heart is time and dose dependent. Furthermore, we report that the rate of both mtRNA and protein synthesis is activated by *in vivo* administration of AC.

[a]The financial support of Telethon-Italy to the project Decrease in Micocondrial Capacity and Changes of Mitochondrial DNA Structure and Expression in Muscle and Brain: a Comparative Study Using Rat as a Model is gratefully acknowledged. This work has been accomplished also with funds from CNR P.F. "INVECCHIAMENTO" Code No. 931345 and from Sigma-Tau Company.

MATERIAL AND METHODS

Animals

Fisher 344 male rats 7 months or 26–27 months old, fed *ad libitum*, were used. They were kept in an animal room under controlled conditions up to the moment of use.

Isolation of Heart Mitochondria and Nucleic Acid Extraction

Mitochondria from heart were isolated, and the steady-state mt transcript analysis was carried out as already reported.[8]

MtRNA Synthesis in Free (Nonsynaptic) Mitochondria

Free (nonsynaptic) mitochondria were isolated from cerebral hemispheres, and *in vitro* RNA synthesis was carried out as already reported.[9]

Isolation of Synaptosomes

All the following preparative steps were carried out at 4°C. The cerebral hemispheres were aseptically dissected out from three rats and minced in 10 volumes of 10% (w/v) sucrose in 0.005 M Tris-HCl (pH 6.7 at 25°C), 0.2 mM EDTA (medium ST). This suspension was hand processed with a Dounce homogenizer. The crude homogenate was centrifuged at $1300 \times g$ for 5 min, and the low speed supernatant was then recentrifuged at $12,000 \times g$ for 5 min to produce the $12,000 \times g$ membrane fraction. The pellet was resuspended in 1 ml of medium ST/g of original wet tissue. Synaptosomes were isolated according to the procedure by Nagy and Delgado-Escueta[13] with few modifications. Briefly, the $12,000 \times g$ membrane fraction was diluted with 4 volumes of 8.5% Percoll, 0.25 M sucrose medium (final concentration of Percoll, 6.8%), and the suspension (3 ml) was then layered onto a two-step Percoll density gradient (4 ml, 16%; 4 ml, 10%), and centrifuged at $15,000 \times g$ for 20 min in a Beckman Ty70 fixed angle rotor. Synaptosomes, which formed a diffuse band at the 10–16% Percoll interphase, were collected and used without further purification.

Protein Labeling

Protein labeling was essentially carried out as reported in Reference 14. Synaptosomal fraction (1.5 ml) recovered from the Percoll/sucrose gradient was mixed with 2 ml of methionine-free Dulbecco's modified Eagle's medium and incubated for 2 min at 37°C under continuous gentle shaking. After that, 100 µg/ml of the cytoplasmic protein synthesis inhibitor cycloheximide was added and incubated for 5 min. Finally, 1 mCi of [^{35}S]methionine (15 µCi/µl, 1100 Ci/mmol; Amersham Corp.) was added and protein labeling allowed to proceed for 20 min. Less than 1 h passed between killing the animals and beginning the protein-labeling experiment. In some experiments, the effect of the mitochondrial protein synthesis inhibitor, chloramphenicol, added to a final concentration of 100 µg/ml, was investigated. Incorporation was terminated by the addition of 5 volumes of ice-cold incubation medium. Synaptosomes were collected by centrifugation at 12,000 × g for 10 min, washed two times with 0.25 M sucrose in 5 mM Tris, 0.1 mM EDTA, pH 7.0 (medium A), and finally resuspended in a small volume (300 μl) of this medium in the presence of 5 mM phenylmethylsulfonyl fluoride. Protein concentration was determined by the Bradford method.[15]

Electrophoretic Analysis of In Vitro Translation Products

A sample of the synaptosomal suspension (150 μg of protein) was run on a sodium dodecyl sulfate (SDS)–15% polyacrylamide gel. The gel was prepared for fluorography by incubating it overnight at 4°C in 30% methanol–10% acetic acid, then at room temperature for 30 min in Amplify (Amersham). The intensity of the bands in the autoradiographs was determined by densitometry (LKB laser, scanning densitometer). Exposure times were chosen to fall in the linear response range.

Analysis of Synaptosomal mtDNA

In order to normalize the protein synthesis data from different experiments to a common internal marker, the mtDNA content of the synaptosomal fractions was determined. For this purpose, total nucleic acids extracted from a portion (0.7–0.8 mg of protein) of each synaptosomal suspension used in the [^{35}S]methionine-labeling experiments were digested for 3 h with Eco RI in the presence of RNase A (0.4 mg/ml). After incubation with 100 μg/ml proteinase K at 37°C for 20 min, portions of the samples were directly electrophoresed on a 1% agarose gel in 40 mM Tris acetate (pH 7.8), 1 mM EDTA. The gel was stained with ethidium bromide, destained, and then photographed under UV light. mtDNA fragments were quantitated by densitometry using, as a standard, known amounts of CsCl-purified rat liver mtDNA digested with Eco RI.[8]

RESULTS

Time and Dose Dependence of Acetyl-L-carnitine Effect In Vivo on the Steady-State Level of mt Transcripts

We already reported that the steady-state levels of 12S rRNA and Col mRNA, as representatives of the two transcription units of mtDNA,[8] in 27-month-old rats were differently affected by aging in the various organs examined. In cerebellum and cerebral hemispheres, the mt transcript level was reduced by about 70%, in the heart it was reduced by 30% whereas in liver it was not significantly reduced. However, the reduction was not irreversible: administration of AC (300 mg/kg bw, 1 h) to senescent rats enhanced the concentration of heart and brain 12S rRNA and Col mRNA to values similar to those, if not even higher, found in adult rats.

In FIGURE 1, the results obtained by measuring the effect of AC on the steady-state level of mtDNA transcripts in heart mitochondria of 27-month-old rat at different times after a single injection of 300 mg/g bw are reported. The maximum effect of a single dose of AC is obtained 3 h after injection; however, at 24 h the effect is similar to that shown at 1 h after treatment. These results confirm the data already obtained in brain.[17]

In FIGURE 2 the results obtained by measuring the effect of different doses of AC

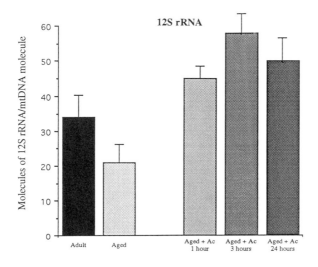

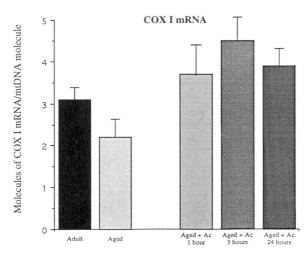

FIGURE 1. Time dependence of acetyl-L-carnitine effect on the 12S rRNA and COX I mRNA content in heart of aged rat. Data are obtained by hybridizing mtRNA isolated from heart with mt riboprobes. For details about the calculation of the number of molecules of mtRNA/ mtDNA molecule, see Reference 8. The values reported are the mean ± standard deviation (SD) of at least three different experiments.

on the steady-state level of mtDNA transcripts in heart mitochondria of aged rat 3 hours after injection are reported. As it is possible to see, the *in vivo* administration of 100 mg of AC to senescent rats does not affect the steady-state level of mt transcripts. However, the administration of 200 mg and of 300 mg of the drug increases mt transcript level.

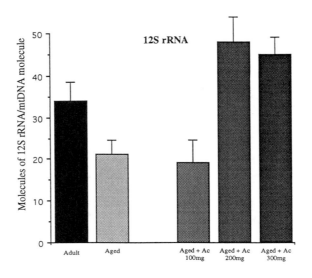

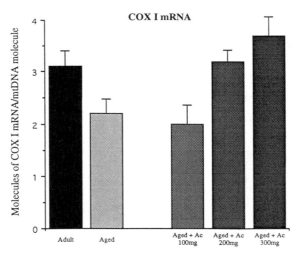

FIGURE 2. Dose dependence of acetyl-L-carnitine effect on the 12S rRNA and COX I mRNA content in the heart of aged rat. Data are obtained by hybridizing mtRNA isolated from heart with mt riboprobes. For details about the calculation of the number of molecules of mtRNA/mtDNA molecule, see Reference 8. The values reported are the mean ± SD of at least three different experiments.

RNA Synthesis in Free (Nonsynaptic) Mitochondria from Cerebral Hemispheres of 27-Month-Old Rat: Effect of Acetyl-L-carnitine

We already reported that the reduced steady-state level of mt transcripts in senescent rat depended, at least in part, on reduced synthesis of mtRNA.[9] To understand which step of the transcription process could be influenced by *in vivo* AC administration, we measured RNA synthesis in free (nonsynaptic) mitochondria isolated from cerebral hemispheres of senescent rats pretreated with AC.

In FIGURE 3, a representative electrophoretic pattern and densitometric analysis of the poly A$^-$ RNA fraction synthesized in free (nonsynaptic) mitochondria) isolated from cerebral hemispheres of adult, senescent, and senescent rats treated with AC (3 h, 300 mg/kg bw) are reported. *In vitro* RNA synthesis was measured as already reported.[9] The results confirmed by three different preparations show that *in vitro* mtRNA synthesis in old rats is activated by AC treatment.

Mitochondrial Protein Synthesis in Synaptosomes Isolated from Cerebral Hemispheres of 27-Month-Old Rat: Effect of Acetyl-L-carnitine

We already reported that mitochondrial protein synthesis was reduced by about 60% in 27-month-old rat in comparison with the 7-month-old rat.[18] In FIGURE 4, a representative electrophoretic pattern of the products obtained after 20 min incubation of synaptosomes with [^{35}S]methionine in the presence and in the absence of chloramphenicol is reported. The electrophoretic pattern of labeled products has been compared with that reported by Loguercio Polosa and Attardi.[14] All major bands corresponding to the more represented products of mitochondrial protein synthesis are evident. The labeling of all the bands in the synaptosome pattern, with the exception of the slower band, is found to be sensitive to 100 μg/ml chloramphenicol, as expected for mitochondrial translation products. The band resistant to chloramphenicol probably reflects some form of end-labeling phenomenon as suggested by Reference 14. In FIGURE 5, the 20 min [^{35}S]methionine labeling pattern of the synaptosome mitochondrial translation products from 26-month-old rats pretreated or not with AC (3 h, 300 mg/kg bw) is reported. An increase of about 40–50% has been calculated by densitometric scanning of the autoradiograph. The same result was obtained with three independent preparations.

DISCUSSION

Reduced efficiency of the mitochondrial respiratory chain activity with age in different tissues of human, primate, and rat has been reported.[19-24] Respiratory complex I and complex IV seem to be preferentially involved. Moreover, a focal deficit of cytochrome *c* oxidase (COX) activity in human muscle fibers has been detected: COX-deficient muscle fibers lie side by side with enzymatically active muscle fibers, and the number of COX-deficient fibers increases randomly with age.[25]

Since 1972, mitochondria have been suggested as a possible biological clock:[1] it was proposed that oxidative damage to mitochondrial structures and to mtDNA could be responsible for the functional energetic deficit associated with aging. Since then many studies have been performed to verify this possibility. An age-related increase of H_2O_2 production rate in mitochondria was reported in insects and in various rat

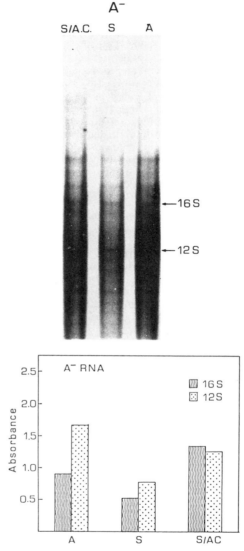

FIGURE 3. Electrophoretic pattern of the poly A⁻ mtRNA synthesized by isolated mitochondria from rat cerebral hemispheres (top panel). The densitometric analysis of the corresponding lanes in the autoradiograph of the gel is reported (bottom panel). S/A.C. = senescent rat pretreated with acetyl-L-carnitine (300 mg/kg bw, 3 h). S = senescent rat. A = adult rat.

tissues.[26] An extensive level of oxidative mtDNA damage was measured as 8-hydroxy-deoxyguanosine (8-OH-dG) in rat liver;[27] 8-OH dG increases exponentially with age in human and rat heart.[24] It has been suggested that the oxidative damage of mtDNA could cause deletions of different sizes:[24] an age-related increase of deleted mtDNA molecules has been reported in different tissues of aging human, mainly myocard and brain.[28,29] The deletions seem to accumulate in different organs with a time course that roughly parallels that of metabolic activity.[30] A kind of mosaicism was also reported in the distribution of the so-called common deletion among different human brain areas: its highest level was found in substantia nigra, caudate, and putamen and the lowest in cerebellar grey matter.[28,29] However, the highest percentage of the mtDNA molecules bearing this deletion was reported to be 0.46% in substantia nigra by Soong *et al.*[29] and 12% in putamen by Corral-Debrinski *et al.*[28] We identified a 4.8-kb mtDNA deletion in rat brain and liver[12] and, recently, two new deletions of 6.8 and 9.1 kb have been detected (unpublished results). Quantitative analysis of the mtDNA molecules carrying the 4.8 kb deletion in aged rat brain and liver showed that they were about 0.1% of total mtDNA molecules in both tissues. Although more than 10 deletions have been found in the same elderly subject,[31] due to their low absolute number, it is difficult to think that a linear quantitative correlation between damage to mtDNA and alteration in respiratory chain function exists.[32] Much higher levels of deleted molecules have been reported in mitochondrial pathologies[6] for obvious detrimental effects in oxidative phosphorylation and protein synthesis.

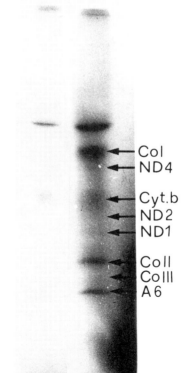

+CAP 27m

Col
ND4

Cyt.b
ND2
ND1

CoII
CoIII
A6

FIGURE 4. Electrophoretic pattern of protein synthesis products in synaptosomes from 27-month-old rat. CAP indicates protein synthesis performed in the presence of cloramphenicol (100 μg/ml): 150 μg of protein was loaded on each lane.

Here we report that both mtDNA transcription and translation are not irreversibly damaged in old rat; in fact, both processes can be restored by *in vivo* treatment
of senescent rat with AC. AC is a physiological molecule synthesized in mitochondria
by the reversible acetylation of L-carnitine by the enzyme carnitine acetyltransferase.
AC after injection reaches rapidly several tissues including muscles and brain, and
enters lipid biosynthetic pools in 10 min.[33] According to Siliprandi *et al.,*[34] AC may be
considered a reservoir of readily utilizable, activated, acetyl groups able to stimulate
the mitochondrial respiratory chain. Furthermore, AC affects energetic and choliner-

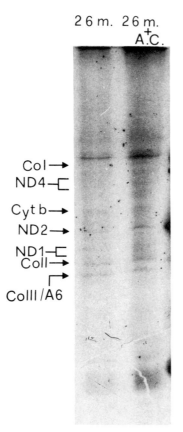

FIGURE 5. Electrophoretic pattern of protein synthe-
iss products in synaptosomes from 26-month-old rat
pretreated (AC) or not with acetyl-L-carnitine (300
mg/kg bw, 3h): 75 μg of protein was loaded on each
lane.

gic metabolism in rat brain;[35] it reduces lipofuscin accumulation in aged brain and
brings back to the adult value the reduced level of total carnitines in different tissues
of aged rat;[36] finally AC modulates the enzymes involved in the acylation-reacylation
process of membrane phospholipids.[37] Reduced mtDNA transcription and translation in aging rat could not depend on mtDNA mutation, both because the level of
mtDNA molecules affected is very low and because the machinery for RNA and
protein synthesis seems not to be irreversibly altered, nor might it be reduced
transcription responsible for reduced translation of mtDNA, according to Attardi.[38]

We propose here that less efficient mtDNA transcription and translation in aging rat could be mainly caused by oxidative damage to mitochondrial membranes, which also takes place in aging.[39] Oxidative damage to mt membranes might alter the optimal conditions of energy and cations for both processes.[8] Results already obtained by us on the effect of AC on the lipid composition of mt membranes and on the transport of some metabolites in aged rat seem to favor this hypothesis.[40,41]

ACKNOWLEDGMENTS

The authors are grateful to Miss R. Longo for word processing.

REFERENCES

1. HARMAN, D. 1972 J. A. Geriatr. Soc. **20:** 145–147.
2. MIQUEL, J. & J. E. FLEMING. 1986. *In* Free Radicals, Aging and Degenerative Diseases. J. E. Johnson, *et al.* Eds.: 51–74. Alan R. Liss. New York, NY.
3. LINNANE, A. W., S. MARZUKI, T. OZAWA & M. TANAKA. 1989. Lancet **i:** 642–645.
4. 1992. Mutation Research, DNAging 1992. Special Issue on Molecular Basis of Aging: Mitochondrial Degeneration and Oxidative Damage (L. Joeny, Ed.) **275:** 113–414.
5. 1993. Bulletin of Molecular Biology and Medicine 1993 Special Issue on Mitochondria and Aging **18:** 1–178.
6. WALLACE, D. C. 1992. Annu. Rev. Biochem. **61:** 1175–1212.
7. GROSSMAN, L. I. 1990. Am. J. Hum. Genet. **46:** 415–417.
8. GADALETA, M. N., V. PETRUZZELLA, M. RENIS, F. FRACASSO & P. CANTATORE. 1990. Eur. J. Biochem. **187:** 501–506.
9. FERNANDEZ-SILVA, P., V. PETRUZZELLA, F. FRACASSO, M. N. GADALETA & P. CANTATORE. 1991. Biochem. Biophys. Res. Commun. **176:** 645–653.
10. GADALETA, M. N., G. RAINALDI, A. M. S. LEZZA, F. MILELLA, F. FRACASSO & P. CANTATORE. 1992. Mutat. Res. **273:** 181–193.
11. PETRUZZELLA, V., F. FRACASSO, M. N. GADALETA & P. CANTATORE. 1992. Ann. N.Y. Acad. Sci. **673:** 194–199.
12. LEZZA, A. M. S., G. RAINALDI, P. CANTATORE & M. N. GADALETA. 1993. Bull. Mol. Biol. Med. **18:** 67–80.
13. NAGY, A. & A. V. DELGADO-ESCUETA. 1984. J. Neurochem. **43:** 1114–1123.
14. LOGUERCIO POLOSA, P. & G. ATTARDI. 1991. J. Biol. Chem. **266:** 1–7.
15. BRADFORD, M. 1976. Anal. Biochem. **72:** 248–254.
16. LAEMMLI, U. K. 1970. Nature **227:** 680–685.
17. GADALETA, M. N., V. PETRUZZELLA, M. RENIS, F. FRACASSO & P. CANTATORE. 1990. *In* Structure, Function and Biogenesis of Energy Transfer Systems. E. Quagliariello *et al.,* Eds.: 135–138. Elsevier. Amsterdam, the Netherlands.
18. DADDABBO, L., C. OLIVIERI, F. FRACASSO, P. LOGUERCIO POLOSA, P. CANTATORE & M. N. GADALETA. 1993. XX Nat. Congr. GIBB, Bari, Italy, Abstract book.
19. TROUNCE, I., E. BYRNE & S. MARZUKI. 1989. Lancet **i:** 637–639.
20. YEN, T.-C., Y. S. CHEN, K.-L. KRUG, S.-H. YEH & Y.-H. WEI. 1989. Biochem. Biophys. Res. Commun. **165:** 994–1003.
21. TORII, K., S. SUGIYAMA, K. TAKAGI, T. SATAKE & T. OZAWA. 1992. Am. J. Respir. Cell Mol. Biol. **6:** 88–92.
22. GUERRIERI, F., G. CAPOZZA, M. KALOUS, F. ZANOTTI, Z. DRAHOTA & S. PAPA. 1992. Arch. Gerontol. Geriatr. **14:** 299–308.
23. BOWLING, A. C., E. M. MUTISYA, L. C. WALKER, D. L. PRICE, L. C. CORK & M. FLINT BEAL. 1993. J. Neurochem. **60:** 1964–1967.
24. HAYAKAWA, M., S. SUGIYAMA, K. HATTORI, M. TAKASAWA, & T. OZAWA. 1993. Mol. Cell. Biochem. **119:** 95–103.
25. MÜLLER-HÖCKER, J. 1992. Brain Pathol **2:** 149–158.

26. SOHAL, R. S. & B. H. SOHAL. 1991. Mech. Ageing Dev. **57:** 187–202.
27. RICHTER, C., J.-W. PARK & B. N. AMES. 1988. Proc. Natl. Acad. Sci. USA **85:** 6465–6467.
28. CORRAL-DEBRINSKI, M., T. HORTON, M. T. LOTT, J. M. SHOFFNER, M. F. BEAL & D. C. WALLACE. 1992. Nature Genetics **2:** 324–329.
29. SOONG, N. W., D. R. HINTON, G. CORTOPASSI & N. ARNHEIM. 1992. Nature Genetics **2:** 318–323.
30. SOONG, N. W., D. R. HINTON, G. CORTOPASSI & N. ARNHEIM. 1993. Bull. Mol. Biol. Med. **18:** 41–55.
31. ZHANG, C. A., BAUMER, R. J. MAXUELL, A. W. LINNANE & P. NAGLEY. 1992. FEBS Lett. **297:** 34–38.
32. HARDING, A. E. 1992. Nature Genetics **2:** 251–252.
33. FARRELL, S., J. VOGEL & L. L. BIEBER. 1986. Biochim. Biophys. Acta **876:** 175–177.
34. SILIPRANDI, N., D. SILIPRANDI & M. CIMAN. 1965. Biochem. J. **96:** 777–789.
35. NAPOLEONE, P., F. FERRANTE, O. GHIRARDI, M. T. RAMACCI & F. AMENTA. 1990. Arch. Gerontol. Geriatr. **10:** 173–185.
36. MACCARI, F., A. ARSENI, P. CHIODI, M. T. RAMACCI & L. ANGELUCCI. 1990. Exp. Geront. **25:** 127–134.
37. AURELI, T., A. MICCHELI, R. RICCIOLINI, M. E. DI COCCO, M. T. RAMACCI, L. ANGELUCCI, O. GHIRARDI & F. CONTI. 1990. Brain Res. **526:** 108–112.
38. ATTARDI, G., A. CHOMYN, M. P. KING, B. KRUSE, P. LOGUERCIO POLOSA & N. NARASIMHAN MURDTER. 1990. Biochem. Soc. Trans. **18:** 509–513.
39. PARADIES, G., F. M. RUGGIERO & E. QUAGLIARIELLO. 1992. Ann. NY Acad. Sci. **673:** 160–164.
40. PARADIES, G., F. M. RUGGIERO, M. N. GADALETA & E. QUAGLIARIELLO. 1992. Biochim. Biophys. Acta **1103:** 324–326.
41. PARADIES, G., F. M. RUGGIERO, G. PETROSILLO, M. N. GADALETA & E. QUAGLIARIELLO. Ann. N.Y. Acad Sci. (This volume.)

Effect of Life Span Prolonging Drugs (Geroprotectors) on Spontaneous and Induced Carcinogenesis

VLADIMIR N. ANISIMOV

Laboratory of Experimental Tumors
N. N. Petrov Research Institute of Oncology
St. Petersburg 189646, Russia

DEMOGRAPHY AND DISEASES

Mankind is rapidly growing old. In 1975, 5.3% of 4.1 billion people were over 65 years old. In 2000, it is expected that 6–8% of humans will be older than 65. In economically developed countries, 10–14% of the population are elderly and their part in the 20s of the 21st century will double. Large cities are the homes of pensioners. It should be noted that aging of the population is not caused only by increasing life span, but by decreasing birth rate as well.[1] Advances in medicine, pharmacology, and health services have led to higher living standards and longevity within the past 100 years. If earlier only 1 of 10 people survived until 65, now about 80% of the population reach this level. The population of age 80 and older will be twice as large in 2000 as compared to 1970. The rapid growth of mean life span in many countries has changed the demographic situation significantly, and some experts predict that the expected life span will be about 85 years in the near future.[1] However, in the 1960s and 1970s, a sharp decrease in the increase of mean life span occurred mainly in developed countries.

In addition to this, and despite evident progress in the development of health services and welfare, there is a slowdown in the rise of expected life span. Only some countries, particularly Japan, demonstrate the most rapid development of modern technology and an increase in the expected life span in women (over 80 years) and in men, leaving behind many countries of Europe and North America.[1]

Human life span has had a tendency to increase throughout the world but at different rates. Despite some remarkable (and probably mythical) cases of longevity, it should be noted that the maximal life span of humans living about 2000 years ago in Ancient Rome, in Europe in the Middle Ages, and in the last third of the 20th century has not changed and has not exceeded 100 years. Gavrilov and Gavrilova[2] consider the age of 95 + 2 to be the maximum human life span on the basis of kinetic calculations of the dependance of biological components of mortality on human age in different countries. They have shown that the total increase in the average life span in this century depended on a decrease in mortality from stochastic, accidental causes unrelated to age (disasters, accidents, morbidity with high letality). The exponential parameter of the Gompertz-Makeham equation describes the dependence of mortality on age:

$$R = R_0(\exp t) + A,$$

where A is the mortality from causes not connected with age, R is the probability of human death at age (t), R_0 is mortalitry at the moment of birth $(t = 0)$, and is constant, which has not changed throughout the history of mankind.

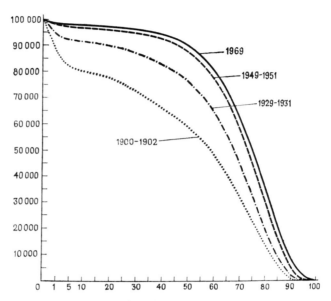

FIGURE 1. Trends in survival curves in United States. Ordinate: survivor number. Abscissa: age, years.

As seen from FIGURE 1, the human survival curve has become more rectangular in shape, i.e., more people live to maturity and old age whereas the maximum life span does not increase. According to Ludwig,[3] modern health services try to diminish the gap between average and maximal longevity; the interval left is filled with age-related diseases. Actually, the main causes of morbidity and mortality for many centuries have been natural disasters, plague epidemic, cholera, smallpox, and more recently tuberculosis, diphtheria, influenza, pneumonia, and childhood mortality. The increase in living standards, sanitation, medicine, and health services has significantly changed the character of morbidity. The main causes of death in the most developed countries appear to be cardiovascular diseases, cancer, diebetes mellitus, mental depression, and obesity. About 85 of 100 people die from these diseases. Unfortunately, the greater the increase in life span, the more years the population is living with bad health and in a state of dependence.[4]

Attempts to explain this burst in diseases of civilization are not clear. Contamination of the environment may account for only 5% of all cancers in humans.[5] Since the start of the industrial revolution, there is a parallel increase in mortality due to both cardiovascular disease and cancer.[6] This might provide a suggestion that environmental pollution by carcinogens does not reveal cancer morbidity as well as some carcinogenic factors of the external environment might cause cardiovascular diseases. It was shown that carcinogenic polycyclic aromatic hydrocarbons induce atherosclerotic patches in aorta.[7]

It is obvious that many factors in our life-style, such as inactivity, overeating, alcohol consumption, and tobacco smoking, do not help our medical and health services to decrease mortality. According to Doll and Peto,[5] alcohol drinking and diet can account for at least two-thirds of the cases of cancer in humans. However, the recent decrease in tobacco smoking in several countries has not resulted in the expected increase in the average life span. It should be noted that living conditions, habits, diet, and many other life-style factors are changing quickly, sometimes within one or two generations. It makes it difficult to analyze the biological changes occurring because all calculations of longevity cannot take into account all life-style changes even in the near future of people on our small and fragile planet.

Together with mathematic modeling as a method of studying the relationships between age, diseases, and mortality, experiments on animals are of great impor-tance. *Drosophila* and nematoda are important models to study the influence of genetic factors on aging and the effects of environmental factors on longevity. However, is often preferable to use mammalian models, such as mice and rats, in experiments since they have similar diseases to humans. For example, neoplasms are one of main causes of death in rats as well as in humans.

PARADOX OF GERONTOLOGY

To better understand the correlation between diseases and changes in average longevity, let us consider when the living conditions in a given population do not vary between generations but may vary between different populations of animals of the same species. It is seen in FIGURE 2 that the rate of mortality in three groups of animals with similar mean life spans is different: it is higher in the third group, but

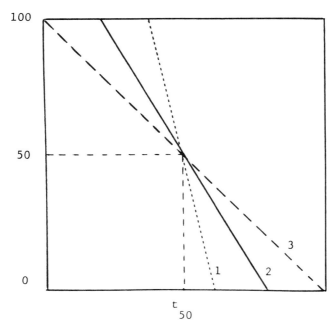

FIGURE 2. The relationship between survival and aging rate of a population. Ordinate: survival, %; abscissa: age.

lower in the first group as compared to the second group. The question is whether the cause of death will be similar in groups that have similar average, but different maximal, life span.

One of the inexplicable paradoxes of gerontology, especially involving the study of geroprotectors (drugs that increase life span) is that sometime after a 3–4 year long experiment, only one conclusion concerning the effect of a tested geroprotector on life span has been made. The survival curves of animals in experimental and control groups usually are presented in these reports. More information gives studies that include, together with the data on survival, the results of assay of the several parameters change under the influence of geroprotector tested (e.g., the level of enzymes in tissues, of hormones, mediators or immune response, number of receptors or their affinity, etc.). However, it is important to know the causes of death of animals in the control group and those groups where the life span of animals was prolonged. There are a lot of reports where these data are absent (for review, see Reference 8).

In some other papers, life span prolongation induced by these or those drugs is accomplished by some serious pathology. Thus, Cotzias et al.[9] have increased the life span of mice by 40% by feeding high dose of L-dihydroxyphenilalanine (DOPA), a precursor in the biosynthesis of catecholamines by nerve cells. Unfortunately, the authors did not report the causes of death of the long-living mice. They only stated that aged mice developed cataracts resulting in blindness. Administration of beta-aminopropionitrile to mice prolongs their mean life span, but serious pathology—lathirism—is a cost for life span prolongation.[10] The best approach to prolong life span of rodents is a caloric restricted diet.[11,12] At the same time, in caloric restricted animals, deceleration of body growth and maturity has been reported as well as inhibition of reproductive system function.[11]

GEROPROTECTORS AND CANCER

It is well known that the incidence of most neoplasms increases with age. Many researchers attribute this phenomenon to the simple accumulation of doses of carcinogen(s) with age, and some of them stressed that "there is no such thing as aging and cancer is not related to it."[13] Others suggest that the age-related increase in cancer rate is a result of changes developing in the internal milieu of the body in the process of ontogenesis, that is to say, metabolic, hormonal, and immunological shifts.[14,15] Obviously, both hypotheses explaining the mechanism of the age-related increasing of tumor incidence correspond to two main hypotheses of modern gerontology: the stochastic theory of aging (explaining aging as a result of accumulation of "errors" and damages leading to disturbance of functions and disregulation), or the theory of programmed aging, including genoregulatory, immunological, and neurohumoral theories.[16]

It should be noted that the relationship between age and mortality on the one hand, and between the incidence of the majority of cancers both in humans and animals and age as described by exponential equations and comparison of the parameters of these equations in the same population has great biological meaning.[8]

One of the most available methods to investigate the relationship between aging and cancer development is to examine the influence of some actions or substances that increase life span on tumor development.[8] It was shown that more than 20 chemicals could increase the life span of animals in experimental condition, and they were called "geroprotectors."[17] They belong to different chemical groups, have different mechanisms of action, and comparison of the data on the effect of these chemicals on life span and tumor development makes it possible to better understand the mechanisms of relationships between two fundamental biological processes—aging and carcinogenesis.

In 1978, Emanuel and Obukhova[17] proposed a classification of known geroprotectors based on the kinetic characteristics of delayed aging caused by gerorprotectors.

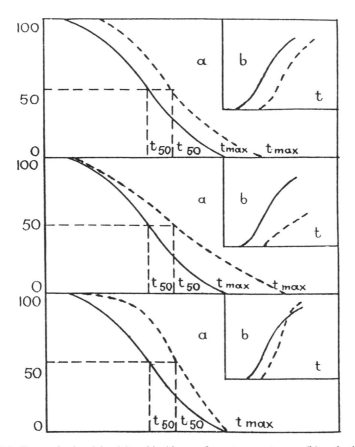

FIGURE 3. Types of aging delay (a) and incidence of spontaneous tumors (b) under influence of geroprotectors. Ordinate: (a) number of survival animals, %; (b) tumor rate, %. Abscissa: age; solid line = control, broken line = administration of geroprotector.

It is seen in FIGURE 3a (top) that there are geroprotectors that do not influence the rate of aging of treated population (slopes of survival curves in control and treated groups are equal)—they simply shift the survival curve to the right. Some other geroprotectors do not greatly change the survival of animals at young ages, but increase the maximal life span, delaying the aging rate of population (FIGURE 3b). Finally, there are geroprotectors that do not prolong maximal life span of animals, but the increase in their average life span is due to increased survival in childhood and young adult age (FIGURE 3c).

It should be noted that this classification scheme does not take into account the mechanisms of geroprotection but only the changes in the survival curves caused by geroprotectors. Besides, the cause of death in control and groups of animals treated with life span prolonging agent is not taken into consideration as well. It is a very important question.

It appears[8,18] that the incidence of tumor development in animals exposed to geroprotectors of the first type did not change but only the tumor latency was postponed. The geroprotectors that slow down aging according to the second type were highly effective—they increase tumor latent period and decrease the rate of its development. The least effective class was the increase in life span caused by geroprotectors of the third type where the frequency of tumor development was elevated even in comparison to the corresponding control (FIGURE 3b).

The results show a direct correlation between the rate of tumor development and the aging rate of the population. Taking all this into account, and the data on environment factors (overeating, exposure to constant light, chemical carcinogens, ionizing irradiation, etc.) that may cause premature aging,[8] the rate of aging is supposed to be the function of such influence.

When we compare FIGURE 1 with the last panel of FIGURE 3, we find that the method of increasing life span "used" by humans appeared to be the most ineffective and unfavorable. In fact, this approach increases cancer morbidity. Moreover, the higher the slope of the survival curve (e.g., "rectangularization" of the Gompertz curve), the higher the frequency of malignant and benign neoplasms. The epidemiological data support this conclusion for all developed countries. In fact, the prognosis of cancer morbidity is rather unfavorable up to the end of the 20th century. What can be done? The most favorable way to prolong life span and decrease tumor incidence is by the second type of geroprotector, though the first type was also successful.

THREE APPROACHES TO POSTPONEMENT OF AGING

Speaking about methods and perspectives of increasing active and healthy life, it is necessary to consider what compounds and factors may be assigned to one or other group of geroprotectors. The most typical representatives of the first type that slow down the onset of aging are antioxidants. Harman[19] suggests the use of drugs that decrease the number of free radicals in order to increase life span. Among these drugs, special attention has been paid to a known radioprotector 2-mercaptoethanolamine, butylhydroxytoluene (BHT), used as preservative in food, and analogues of vitamin B, 2-ethyl-6-methyl-3-oxypyridine.[17] However, the first drug has an unpleasant smell and is not convenient. BHT in high doses in some animal species could induce tumors in lung, esophagus, and forestomach.[20] 2-Ethyl-6-methyl-3-oxypyridine has antigonadotropic activity and is not always desirable.

Tocopherol (vitamin E), having the properties of an antioxidant, increased the life span of rats according to third type of geroprotectors and increases benign tumor incidence in rats.[21] Dubina and Razumovich[22] tested a sodium salt of ethylendiaminotetraacetate (EDTA-Na$_2$) as a geroprotector. They hypothesized that EDTA-Na$_2$ could chelate heavy metals inducing intra- and intermolecular links and might prevent their accumulation in tissues with age, thus increasing life span. And it turned out to be successful—the increase of mean (but not maximal) life span was marked, and there was a decrease in inflammatory and other intercurrent diseases in rats treated with EDTA-Na2 as compared to controls. But in old rats treated with chelating agents, the incidence of malignant tumors increased. Also, the supplementation of low level tritium oxide to the drinking water of rats gave the same effect.[23]

What measures or drugs slow down aging according to the second type of geroprotector? In 1934, McCay[24] showed that limits in food consumption might increase by nearly 50% the life span of rats in comparison with animals without food restriction. These experiments have been repeated in many laboratories throughout the world. It appeared that a caloric restricted diet increases the life span of animals more effectively in cases when it begins at weaning. Growth and puberty of animals are delayed. The analysis of survival curves showed a decrease of population aging rate according to the second type of geroprotector. It should be noted that under various conditions, the decline in the immune system and delayed diseases of old rats such as glomerulonephritis, myocardiodystrophy, arteriosclerosis and, most important, tumor development are delayed.[11,12] However, in some kinds of restricted diet (e.g., limitation in protein), no decrease of pathological processes was found and the rate at some sites (e.g., hemopoietic system) even increases. It is difficult to recommend for humans strong caloric restriction because it could be followed by a delay in puberty and blockage in the cyclic activity of ovaries.

Limitation of fat in the diet could be the most important factor, since fat causes excessive weight and risk of heart diseases and cancer.[5] It worthy of note that some antidiabetic biguanide drugs (phenformin, buformin) may lead to decrease of weight, and improvement in carbohydrate, lipid, and immune homeostasis.[15] The mean life span of mice treated with phenformin increased by 25%; besides, spontaneous tumor incidence decreased significantly.[8] The cyclic function of the reproductive system in rats exposed to long-term gavage of phenformin remained normal longer than in controls.[8]

Gerontologists should pay special attention to immune modulators that control and stimulate the function of the immune system. Many researchers considered the decrease of immune system activity with age to be a major mechanism of aging and development of age-related pathology, including cancer in the elderly. Treatment with thymic hormones could restore the immune function in old animals. In some experiments, life span prolongation was shown in rodents treated with thymic peptide preparations, e.g., thymosin V. In our experiments, thymic peptide preparation thymalin administered to mice of two strains beginning at the age of 3.5 months increased their life span and decreased spontaneous tumor incidence.[25]

A peptide preparation of bovine pineal gland was more effective as geroprotector and cancer preventive agent. Thus, long-term administration of epithalamin was followed by 25–36% increase in mean life span of mice and rats, occasional increase in maximum life span and in tumor latency, together with a decrease in tumor incidence.[25,26] It worthy of note that in rodents exposed to epithalamin, a delay in switch off of reproductive function occurred as well as a delay in decline of immune function activity, and an improvement in glucose and lipid metabolism. In fact, epithalamin was also effective when administered starting at the age 12 months in mice and 15 months in rats.[25,27] Why did this preparation prove to be effective?

All "secrets" of this gland have not yet been solved. Being a mediator between environmental signals (light, electromagnetic fields and some others) and the internal milieu of the organism, the pineal gland controls a number of principal biological processes in the organism, including water-salt metabolism and the function of neuroendocrine and immune systems. It was shown that pineal gland function decreased with age.[28] According Walker et al.,[29] the increase of life span by caloric-restricted diet is due to the delay in age-related decrease of pineal function. These data are in agreement with observations on the life span reduction in pinealectomized rats, on the one hand, and on life span prolongation due to exposure to pineal hormone (melatonin or pineal peptides) administration on the other hand.[28,30] It worthy of note that exposure of rodents to a constant light regime that suppresses pineal activity followed by impairment of cyclic function of reproductive system, caused the premature switch off of the estrous cycle and led to an increase in body weight and tumor incidence.[8]

Thus, it is possible to increase life span in laboratory animals. In some cases, the price of this is rather disproportional to profit—some pathological processes could develop, including cancer. But it coincides with the main purpose of gerontology—to add years to the life as well as to add life quality to these years. The increase of mean life span without an increase in maximum life span ("rectangularization" of the Gompertz curve; third type of aging delay) is not the best way for humans. This approach leads to an increase in age-related pathology, heart diseases, and cancer morbidity. In other words, the increase in life span achieved by the decrease in the risk of mortality in childhood and young adults is followed by an increase in probability to develop the diseases of civilization, cancer included.

We believe that further progress in modern preventive medicine requires attention to the prolongation of human life span. The unfavorable factors of environment can be expected to have only a partial solution under the conditions of the burst of industrialization, urbanization, and increase in environmental pollution. New technology and approaches for the decrease of environmental pollution must solve the serious scientific and technical problems and require substantial economic costs. It seems that the changes in human life-style (tobacco smoking, alcohol drinking, diet peculiarities, sexual, and other habits) already have been shown to be effective in decrease of cancer and some other diseases of civilization followed by a favorable effect in human longevity.

The increase of human life span could be reality despite the fact that many mechanisms of aging and carcinogenesis are still obscure. Healthy life-style, fat-restricted diet enriched with fibers and vitamins, some drugs that normalize age-related hormone-metabolic and immunologicals lesions (e.g., epithalamin and some immunomodulators) have been shown to be effective in reducing the rate of aging and should favorably affect life span with reduced rate of cancer incidence and cardiovascular diseases.[8] Taking into account the increased risk of carcinogenic factors of environment (chemical agents, ionizing and UV irradiation), attention must be paid also to antioxidants and antimutagens that prevent the genetic lesions caused by carcinogenic agents.

REFERENCES

1. 1989. Health of the Elderly. Report of a WHO Expert Committee. Technical Report Series 779. WHO. Geneva, Switzerland.
2. GAVRILOV, L. A. & N. S. GAVRILOVA. 1991. The Biology of Life Span: A Quantitative Approach. Harwood Academic Publ. Chur.
3. LUDWIC, F. C. 1980. What to expect from gerontological research? Science **209:** 1071.
4. 1990. Global Estimates for Health Situation Assessment and Projections. WHO. Geneva, Switzerland.
5. DOLL, R. & R. PETO. 1981. The cause of cancer. Quantitative estimates of avoidable risks of cancer in the United States today. J. Natl. Cancer Inst. **66:** 1193–1312.
6. 1987. Aging in Today's Environment. Committee on Chemical Toxicity and Aging. National Academy Press. Washington, D.C.
7. PAIGEN, B., P. A. HOLMES, A. MOROOW & D. MITCHELL. 1986. Effect of 3-methylcholanthrene on atherosclerosis in two congenic strains of mice with different susceptibilities to methylcholanthrene-induced tumors. Cancer Res. **46:** 3321–3324.

8. ANISIMOV, V. N. 1987. Carcinogenesis and Aging. 2. CRC Press, Inc. Boca Raton, Fla.
9. COTZIAS, G. C., S. T. MILLER, A. R. NICHOLSON, W. H. MASTON & L. C. TANG. 1974.
    Prolongation of life-span in mice adapted to large amount of L-dopa. Proc. Natl. Acad.
    Sci. USA 71: 2466–2469.
10. LA BELLA, F. S. & S. VIVIAN. 1975. Effect of beta-aminopropionitrile and prednisolone on
    survival of male LAF/J mice. Exp. Gerontol. 10: 185–188.
11. WEINDRUCH, R. H. & R. L. WALFORD. 1988. The Retardation of Aging and Disease by
    Dietary Restriction. C. C. Thomas Co. Springfield, Ill.
12. MASORO, E. J. 1992. Retardation of aging processes by nutritional means. Ann. N.Y.
    Acad. Sci. 673: 29–35.
13. PETO, R., S. E. PARISH & R. G. GRAY. 1985. There is no such thing as aging, and cancer is
    not related to it. IARC Sci. Publ. 58: 43–53.
14. BURNET, F. M. 1976. Immunology, Aging and Cancer. Medical Aspects of Mutation and
    Selection. Freeman and Co. San Francisco, Calif.
15. DILMAN, V. M. & W. DEAN. 1992. The Neuroendocrine Theory of Aging and Degenera-
    tive Disease. Center for Bio-Gerontology. Pensacola, Fla.
16. MARTIN, G. M. 1980. Genotropic theories of aging: an overview. Adv. Pathobiol. 7: 5–39.
17. EMANUEL, L. K. & N. M. EMANUEL. 1978. Types of experimental delay in aging patterns.
    Exp. Gerontol. 13: 25–29.
18. ANISIMOV, V. N. 1992. Age as a factor of risk in multistage carcinogenesis. In Geriatric
    Oncology. L. Balducci, G. H. Lyman & W. B. Ershler, Eds.: 53–59. J. B. Lippincott Co.,
    Philadelphia, Pa.
19. HARMAN, D. 1992. Role of free radicals in aging and disease. Ann. N.Y. Acad. Sci.
    673: 126–141.
20. 1986. IARC Monographs on the Evaluation of the Carcinogenic Risk of Chemicals to
    Humans. 40: 161–184. Some Naturally Occurring and Synthetic Food Components,
    Furocoumarines and Ultraviolet Radiation. IARC. Lyon, France.
21. PORTA, E. A., N. S. JOUN & R. T. NITTA. 1980. Effect of the type of dietary fat at two levels
    of vitamin E in Wistar male rats during development and aging. Life span, serum
    biochemical parameters and pathological changes. Mech. Ageing Dev. 113: 1–39.
22. DUBINA, T. L. & A. N. RAZUMOVICH. 1975. Introduction in Experimental Gerontology.
    Nauka i Tekhnika. Minsk, Byelorussia.
23. MUKSINOVA, K. N., V. S. VORONIN & E. N. KIRILLOVA. 1983. Late effect of chronic
    exposure to tritium oxide. In Biological Effects of Low Doses of Radiation. Y. I.
    Moskalev, Ed.: 70–74. Institute of Biophysics Publ.
24. MCCAY, C. M. & M. F. CROWELL. 1934. Prolonging the life span. Sci. Monthly 39: 405–
    414.
25. ANISIMOV, V. N., A. S. LOKTIONOV, V. G. MOROZOV & V. KH. KHAVINSON. 1989. Effect of
    low-molecular-weight factors of thymus and pineal gland on life span and spontaneous
    tumour development in females of different age. Mech. Ageing Dev. 49: 245–257.
26. ANISIMOV, V. N. 1988. Pineal gland, aging and carcinogenesis. In The Pineal Gland and
    Cancer. D. Gupta, A. Attanasio & R. J. Reiter, Eds.: 107–118. Brain Res. Promotion.
    London & Tubingen.
27. ANISIMOV, V. N., L. A. BONDARENKO & V. KH. KHAVINSON. 1992. Effect of pineal peptide
    preparation (epithalamin) on life span and pineal and serum melatonin level in old rats.
    Ann. N.Y. Acad. Sci. 673: 53–57.
28. ANISIMOV, V. N. & R. J. REITER. 1990. Function of pineal gland in cancer and aging. Vopr.
    Onkol. 36: 259–268.
29. WALKER, R. F., K. M. MCMAHON & E. B. PIVORUN. 1978. Pineal gland structure and
    respiration as affected by age and hypocaloric diet. Exp. Gerontol. 13: 91–99.
30. PIERPAOLI, W., A. DALL'ARA, E. PEDRINIS & W. REGELSON. 1991. The pineal control of
    aging. The effects of melatonin and pineal grafting on the survival of older mice. Ann.
    N.Y. Acad. Sci. 621: 291–313.

Evaluation of Geriforte, an Herbal Geriatric Tonic, on Antioxidant Defense System in Wistar Rats

BALKAR SINGH, S. P. SHARMA, AND RITU GOYAL

Laboratory of Nutritional Histopathology and Aging
Department of Zoology
Kurukshetra University
Kurukshetra-132 119, India

INTRODUCTION

The free radical theory of aging proposed by Harman[1] states the involvement of active oxygen species in aging. Free radical damage to membranes of the nerve cells has been suggested to be the primary cause of aging of an organism.[2] The monovalent reduction of oxygen that occurs during normal oxidative metabolism results in the production of highly reactive oxygen species including superoxide free radicals (SOR).[3]

Some oxygen free radicals are dismutated very actively by superoxide dismutase (SOD).[4] The product of the dismutation process is hydrogen peroxide (H_2O_2) which is per se less harmful to the biological molecules than the SOR[2] and is eliminated by catalase (CAT) and glutathione peroxidase (GPx).[5,6] Another highly reactive hydroxyl radical ($\cdot OH$) generated by the action of H_2O_2 and SOR via the iron-catalyzed Haber-Weiss reaction is also a potentially damaging radical. The attack of $\cdot OH$ on polyunsaturated fatty acids within the cellular membranes results in lipid peroxidation[7,8] leading ultimately to the formation of the age pigment lipofuscin, which is directly related to the age of animals.[9]

Geriforte, an herbomineral formulation, is an ideal geriatric tonic to solve the problem of aging. The oral administration of this Ayurvedic drug has been reported to inhibit the formation of lipofuscin in aging rats.[10,11] Since SOR is the root cause of lipofuscin formation, alterations in the level of SOD, CAT, and lipid peroxidation could substantially influence the process of aging. Therefore, in the present study, the Ayurvedic drug Geriforte has been evaluated for SOD, CAT, and thiobarbituric acid reactive substance in terms of malondialdehyde (MDA), a product of lipid peroxidation, in the brain of aging Wistar male rat.

MATERIAL AND METHODS

Twenty-two month old Wistar male rats used in the present experiment were obtained from the Animal House, Kurukshetra University, Kurukshetra, India. The animals were divided into experimental and control groups of 10 animals each. The experimental animals were given Geriforte powder (The Himalaya Drug Co. Bombay, India) orally by mixing it with cane sugar (1:1) at a dosage of 900 mg/kg body weight per day for two months. Another group of animals received an equal amount of sugar only, served as control. Both groups of animals received Gold Mohur rat feed (Hindustan Lever Ltd. Bombay, India) and water *ad libitum*. The animals were housed in the same room maintained at $27 \pm 2°C$ under 12 h light-dark cyclic illumination provided by Laxman Sylvania 40W fluorescent tubes.

The animals were sacrificed after anesthetizing with ether. Before sacrifice, they were observed on starvation for 12 hours. The brain was removed quickly from the skull, and the homogenate was prepared in 10 mM tris-HCl extraction buffer containing 0.32 M sucrose and 1 mM EDTA at pH 7.4. The sample was homogenized in a Teflon glass homogenizer. The crude homogenate was centrifuged at 13,600 g for 30 minutes. The supernatant (postmitochondrial) was collected and used for the determination of enzyme activities and lipid peroxidation. The cytosolic Cu-Zn SOD was estimated according to the method of Marklund and Marklund[12] by monitoring the ability of SOD to inhibit the autoxidation of pyrogallol. One unit of SOD activity is defined as the amount of enzyme required to inhibit the rate of pyrogallol autoxidation by 50% at 25°C. The activity of CAT was determined following the method of Aebi.[13] One unit of enzyme activity is defined as the amount of CAT that decomposes 1 μmol of H_2O_2 in 1 min. Lipid peroxidation in terms of MDA was estimated by using the method of Placer *et al.*[14] The data obtained in the present study were analyzed statistically using Student's t-test.

RESULTS

The data obtained from the control and Geriforte-treated Wistar male rats on SOD, CAT, and lipid peroxidation have been summarized in TABLE 1. The Geriforte-

TABLE 1. Effect of Geriforte on the Activity of Antioxidant Enzymes and Lipid Peroxidation in the Brain of Wistar Male Rats[a]

Groups	SOD (units/mg protein)	CAT (units/mg protein)	MDA (nmol/g tissue wet weight)
Control animals	8.00 ± 0.12	2.77 ± 0.98	164.89 ± 4.98
	$p < 0.01$	$p < 0.01$	$p < 0.01$
Geriforte-treated animals	9.92 ± 0.27	3.60 ± 0.08	121.87 ± 1.89

[a]Each value is the mean ± standard error of the mean of data from 10 animals.

treated rat brain had significantly ($p < 0.01$) a higher level of SOD and CAT contents than that recorded in their respective controls. The contents of SOD and CAT in Geriforte-treated brain increased by 24% and 30% respectively. However, the magnitude of MDA content is reported to be decreased significantly ($p < 0.01$) in the Geriforte-treated rat brain. The decrease in MDA content in Geriforte-treated animals was 26%.

DISCUSSION

In the present study, the Geriforte-administered rats have been found to exhibit an increased level of SOD and CAT with a decreased level of MDA.

It is now well established that the aging process is associated with an increased susceptibility of tissue to free radical damage[1] as well as elevated level of free radicals, as evidenced by the accumulation of the age pigment lipofuscin.[15] Lipid perxidation, which leads to the formation of the age pigment, has been identified as a primary deteriorative reaction in aging, caused by free radicals and SOD was shown to inhibit lipid peroxidation *in vitro*.[16] A decline in SOD level as a function of age has been studied in a variety of organs of various animals.[17-20] Thus, it would be of interest to investigate whether the present antiaging Ayurvedic Drug, Geriforte, exerts its geriatric effects by inducing the production of SOD and CAT, and inhibiting lipid peroxidation in old animals.

Geriforte, an herbomineral compound, includes a group of Rasayans such as *Centella asiatica* (Brahmi), *Phyllanthus emblica* (Amla), *Withania somnifera* (Asvagandha), and *Tinospora cardifolia* (Guduchi). Rasayans bring about balance in physiology, enhance immunity, and retard aging.[21] It seems possible that Geriforte postpones the onset of aging by inducing the production of SOD and CAT, which scavenge SOR and eliminate H_2O_2 respectively from the biological pathways. It is surmised that the Rasayanic constituents of Geriforte act synergistically to induce the higher production of SOD and CAT *in vivo*. A question to which we have no clear answer yet is, by what mechanism does this antiaging Ayurvedic drug induce the *in vivo* production of SOD and CAT.

As is evident from the present results, Geriforte has a marked potency to induce a large amount of SOD and CAT production against the damaging effects of free radicals. We can safely say that Geriforte is an ideal geriatric tonic for promoting health and longevity. However, further investigations are needed to elucidate the exact mode of action of individual ingredients of Geriforte in the aging process.

SUMMARY

Geriforte, an herbomineral compound prepared from several herbs and minerals, is being used as a restorative tonic to solve the problems of old age in India. Since active oxygen species have been proposed to be involved in the aging process of the brain, alterations in the level of enzymes involved in the defense system against free radicals and other active oxygen species could substantially influence the aging process. Therefore, in the present study, this antistress adaptogenic Ayurvedic preparation has been evaluated for the activities of superoxide dismutase (SOD) and catalase (CAT), key enzymes of the cellular defense system, in the brain of aging Wistar male rats. The present study was carried out on 22-month-old rats. They were given Geriforte powder orally at a dosage of 900 mg/kg body weight once a day for two months. The Geriforte-treated rat brain had significantly high levels of SOD and CAT activities than those recorded in their respective controls. The contents of SOD and CAT in Geriforte-administered brain increased by 24% and 30%, respectively. In the present investigation, free radical damage was assessed by measuring thiobarbituric acid reactive substance (TBARS) in postmitochondrial fractions of brain homogenate. The magnitude of TBARS has been reported to be decreased by 26% in the Geriforte-treated rat brain. In conclusion, it seems logical to suppose that Geriforte, a combination of several plant ingredients and minerals, protects the body against the damaging effects of free radicals by producing large amounts of antioxidant enzymes.

ACKNOWLEDGMENTS

One of the authors, R. Goyal, is thankful to the Pt. Thakur Dutt Sharma Dharmarth Trust for awarding a research scholarship. The authors are grateful to

Dr. J. S. Yadav, Professor and Chairman, Department of Zoology, Kurukshetra University, Kurukshetra for providing necessary research facilities. The meaningful suggestions of Dr. Bhopal Singh (Ayurveda) and Dr. Balbir Singh (Ayurveda), S. K. Govt. Ayurvedic College, Kurukshetra, are thankfully acknowledged. The generous supply of Geriforte by Dr. R. M. Captain, The Himalaya Drug. Co. Bombay, is also gratefully acknowledged.

REFERENCES

1. HARMAN, D. 1981. The aging process. Proc. Natl. Acad. Sci. USA **78**: 7124–7128.
2. Zs.-NAGY, I. 1988. The theoretical background and cellular autoregulation of biological waste product formation. *In* Lipofuscin—1987: State of the Art. I. Zs.-Nagy, Ed.: 23–50. Akademiai Kiado, Budapest & Elsevier Science Publishers, Amsterdam.
3. FRIDOVICH, I. 1978. The biology of oxygen radicals. Science **201**: 875–880.
4. McCORD, J. M. & I. FRIDOVICH. 1969. Superoxide dismutase. An enzymic function for erythrocuprein (haemocuprein). J. Biol. Chem. **224**: 6049–6055.
5. CHANCE, B. 1952. The state of catalase in the respiring bacterial cell. Science **11**: 202–204.
6. HALLIWELL, B. & J. M. C. GUTTERIDGE, Eds. 1989. Free Radicals in Biology and Medicine. 2nd Edit. Clarendon Press. Oxford, England.
7. BABBS, C. F. 1985. Role of iron ions in the genesis of reperfusion injury following successful cardiopulmonary resuscitation: preliminary data and a biochemical hypothesis. Ann. Emerg. Med. **14**: 777–783.
8. RICHARDS, R. T. & H. M. SHARMA. 1991. Free radicals in health and disease. Indian J. Clin. Pract. **2**(7): 15–26.
9. TAPPEL, A. L. 1973. Lipid peroxidation damage to cell components. Fed. Proc. **32**: 1870–1874.
10. SHARMA, S. P., T. J. JAMES, R. GOYAL, B. SINGH, R. KOCHAR & S. GUPTA. 1991. Effect of Geriforte, an Ayurvedic drug, on the spinal cord and heart of adult Wistar rats. Indian J. Gerontol. **2**(2 & 3): 24–31.
11. SHARMA, S. P., V. PANDEY, T. J. JAMES & B. SINGH. 1992. Lipofuscinolytic effect of Geriforte: a fluorescent microscopical study. Ageing Soc. **2**(4 & 5): 32–38.
12. MARKLUND, S. & G. MARKLUND. 1974. Involvement of superoxide anion radical in the autoxidation of pyrogallol and a convenient assay for superoxide dismutase. Eur. J. Biochem. **47**: 469–474.
13. AEBI, H. 1984. Catalase *in vitro*. Methods Enzymol. **105**: 121–126.
14. PLACER, Z. A., L. L. CUSHMAN & B. C. JOHNSON. 1966. Estimation of product of lipid peroxidation (malondialdehyde) in biochemical systems. Anal. Biochem. **16**: 359–364.
15. LEIBOVITZ, B. & B. V. SIEGEL. 1980. Aspects of free-radical reactions in biological systems. J. Gerontol. **35**(1): 45–56.
16. TYLER, D. D. 1975. Polarographic assay and intracellular distribution of superoxide dismutase in rat liver. Biochem. J. **147**: 493–504.
17. REISS, U. & D. GERSHON. 1976. Comparison of cytoplasmic superoxide dismutase in liver, heart and brain of aging rats and mice. Biochem. Biophys. Res. Commun. **73**(2): 255–262.
18. BENZI, G., F. MARGATICO, O. PASTORIS & R. F. VILLA. 1989. Relationship between aging, drug treatment and the cerebral enzymatic antioxidant system. Exp. Gerontol. **24**: 137–148.
19. SEMSEI, I., G. RAO & A. RICHARDSON. 1991. Expression of superoxide dismutase and catalase in rat brain as a function of age. Mech. Ageing Dev. **58**: 13–19.
20. CAND, F. & J. VERDETTI. 1989. Superoxide dismutase, glutathione peroxidase, catalase and lipid peroxidation in the major organs of the ageing rats. Free Radical Biol. Med. **7**: 59–63.
21. SHARMA, P. V. 1983. On Rasayana (promotion therapy). *In* Caraka Samhita. P. V. Sharma, Ed. **2**: 1–116. Chaukhambha Orientalia. Delhi, India.

Beneficial Effects of Vanadyl Sulfate Administration on Sugar Metabolism in the Senescent Rat[a]

E. BERGAMINI, V. DE TATA, M. NOVELLI,
G. CAVALLINI, P. MASIELLO, AND Z. GORI.

Centro di Ricerca Interdipartimentale sull'Invecchiamento
Istituto di Patologia Generale
Università di Pisa
Via Roma, 55
56100 Pisa, Italy

INTRODUCTION

The process of aging results in a progressive deterioration in most endocrine functions. With regard to the endocrine pancreatic function, it is well known that aging is associated with an impairment of glucose tolerance both in humans and in experimental animals.[1,2] The age-associated alterations of glucose homeostasis can be related both to a decline of the insulin secretory response of pancreatic islets with age[3-5] and to the loss of the normal sensitivity of peripheral tissues to insulin.[6]

In order to evaluate the relative contribution of these two mechanisms to the determinism of the age-related alterations of carbohydrate metabolism, we have investigated the effects of the oral administration of vanadyl sulfate on glucose metabolism and on the insulin responsiveness of isolated islets in senescent rats. Both vanadate and the vanadyl forms of vanadium have indeed been shown by many investigators to have insulin-like effects on glucose metabolism.[7]

MATERIALS AND METHODS

Experiments were performed on male Sprague-Dawley albino rats of 3 and 24–26 months of age fed *ad libitum* with a standard laboratory chow. Rats of both ages were divided in two groups. One group was given tapwater to drink; the second group received drinking water supplemented with 0.5 mg/ml vanadyl sulfate. Vanadyl sulfate administration caused no significant changes in body weight or food and water intake in treated rats with respect to controls during the experimental period.

After 4 days of vanadyl sulfate administration, an oral glucose tolerance test (OGTT, 2 g/kg bw) was performed in overnight fasted 3- and 24-mo-old control and vanadyl-treated rats. Blood samples were collected at 0, 15, 30, 60, 120, and 180 min after glucose administration, and plasma glucose and insulin were measured.

After 3 additional days of vanadyl sulfate treatment, muscle glycogen was determined in the extensor digitorum longus (EDL) and in the soleus (S) muscles of both fasted and fed animals by the colorimetric anthrone method.[8]

[a]This work was supported in part by grants from Ministero dell'Università e della Ricerca Scientifica e Tecnologica and Consiglio Nazionale delle Ricerche.

Islets of Langerhans were isolated by collagenase digestion[9] from the pancreases of other groups of 3- and 26-mo-old rats after 3 weeks of vanadyl sulfate treatment. After 60 min preincubation period in modified Krebs-Ringer bicarbonate (KRB) buffer containing 0.5% bovine serum albumin, 10 mM Hepes (pH 7.4) and 2.8 mM glucose, groups of 7–10 islets were incubated for 60 min at 37°C in a humidified atmosphere of 5% CO_2 in air, in 1 ml KRB-Hepes buffer containing 2.8 or 16.7 mM glucose and various other secretagogues [20 mM arginine, 20 mM 2-ketoisocaproate (2-KIC), 1 mM 3-isobutyl-1-methyl-xanthine (IBMX) and 30 mM KCl]. At the end of the incubation, the medium was collected for insulin determination. Finally, 1 ml of cold acidified ethanol (HCl 0.7 M:ethanol, 1:3, v/v) was added to the islets in order to extract their insulin content.

Plasma insulin and insulin released into the incubation medium and extracted with acidified ethanol from either the homogenized whole pancreas or the isolated islets were determined by radioimmunoassay.[10]

RESULTS AND DISCUSSION

We have investigated the age-related modifications of glucose homeostasis and its response to vanadyl sulfate administration in the rat. Two different metabolic

TABLE 1. Plasma Glucose and Insulin Levels during an Oral Glucose Tolerance Test in 3-Month-Old Control (C) and Vanadyl Sulfate–Treated (V) Rats[a]

Time (min)		0	15	30	60	120	180
Plasma glucose (mg/ 100 ml)	C	98.3 ± 1.98	147 ± 4.30	162 ± 4.87	164 ± 3.92	126 ± 5.06	106 ± 4.15
	V	92.5 ± 2.18	155 ± 4.97	159 ± 4.21	165 ± 4.08	127 ± 3.84	98.0 ± 2.92
Plasma insulin (ng/ml)	C	2.95 ± 0.28	8.07 ± 0.43	9.10 ± 0.55	7.86 ± 0.61	4.21 ± 0.63	3.62 ± 0.40
	V	3.26 ± 0.23	7.90 ± 0.64	8.95 ± 1.07	7.08 ± 0.76	3.87 ± 0.76	3.29 ± 0.28

[a]Means of 10 cases ± standard error (SE) for each point are given. Statistical analysis, see TABLE 2.

parameters have been considered: the tolerance to an oral glucose load, and the postprandial ability of skeletal muscles to accumulate glycogen. TABLE 1 shows that vanadyl sulfate administration (0.5 mg/ml in the drinking water for 4 days) has no significant effects on plasma glucose and insulin levels in younger rats after the intragastric administration of a glucose load (2 g/kg bw). On the other hand, vanadyl sulfate administration improves remarkably the OGTT in senescent animals. TABLE 2 shows that in control senescent rats the oral glucose load induces a significant rise in plasma glucose levels which still remain significantly elevated above the basal values after 120 and 180 min.

Concomitantly there is a significant increase in plasma insulin concentration which peaks after 15 min, still remaining above basal values after 120 and 180 min. In vanadyl sulfate–treated animals, the plasma glucose levels after the oral glucose load peak earlier and after 180 min they do not differ significantly from the basal values. Likewise, 180 min after the glucose load, insulin appears to be significantly lower in vanadyl-treated rats than in controls.

FIGURE 1 shows that muscle glycogen levels exhibit age-related changes that are different in fasted and fed rats, vary with the type of muscle, and are affected by vanadyl sulfate administration (0.5 mg/ml in the drinking water for 7 days). One of the most prominent age-related changes, mainly in the slow-twitch soleus muscle, is the reduced capability to refill glycogen stores in the postprandial time in agreement with De Tata et al.[11] In 24-mo-old rats, vanadyl sulfate treatment restores the postprandial ability of skeletal muscles to accumulate glycogen, which becomes quantitatively similar to that observed in young rats. In 3-mo-old rats, vanadyl sulfate treatment has no effect on the basal or on the postprandial muscle glycogen levels.

Vanadyl sulfate does not modify plasma glucose and insulin levels, nor does pacreatic insulin content, in both young and old rats (data not shown).

Most of the age-related alterations of the normal glucose homeostasis have been attributed to the loss of the normal sensitivity to insulin, since both insulin binding and maximal insulin-stimulated glucose transport are reduced in adipocytes isolated from old rats[12,13] and in hindlimb preparations from 12-mo-old rats.[14] Our finding

TABLE 2. Plasma Glucose and Insulin Levels during an Oral Glucose Tolerance Test in 24-Month-Old Control (C) and Vanadyl Sulfate-Treated (V) Rats[a]

Time (min)		0	15	30	60	120	180
Plasma glucose (mg/ 100 ml)	C	84.3 ± 3.93	115 ± 7.28	129 ± 8.75	143 ± 6.35	135 ± 4.21	128 ± 5.02
	V	84.8 ± 6.69	99.1 ± 5.80	131 ± 8.61	117 ± 8.20^b	113 ± 9.39^b	94.0 ± 9.67^c
Plasma insulin (ng/ml)	C	2.62 ± 0.26	6.11 ± 1.12	5.36 ± 0.63	5.88 ± 0.52	5.13 ± 0.58	4.32 ± 0.25
	V	2.25 ± 0.42	5.73 ± 0.97	7.13 ± 1.42	5.47 ± 1.05	4.44 ± 0.72	2.69 ± 0.63^b

[a]Means of 10 (for glucose) or 5 (for insulin) cases $\pm$ SE are given. Statistical analysis (ANOVA, F test) showed that: *Plasma glucose:* the response to the glucose load ($p < 0.01$), the effect of age ($p < 0.01$), and of vanadate ($p < 0.01$) and the interactions between response to the glucose load and age ($p < 0.01$), and age and vanadate ($p < 0.01$) are significant. All other interactions are not significant. *Plasma insulin:* the response to the glucose load ($p < 0.01$), the effect of age ($p < 0.01$) are significant. All other effects and interactions are not significant. The symbols[b] and [c] indicate that the difference between vanadyl treated and control is significant with the paired *t* test ($p < 0.05$ and $p < 0.01$ respectively).

that the oral administration of vanadyl sulfate has a beneficial effect on both the examined indicators of glucose metabolism in senescent rats can be considered in this perspective. In our conditions, we have detected no apparent signs of toxicity of the vanadyl sulfate: body weight gain and daily food and water intake are not significantly modified by the treatment (in agreement with Sakurai et al.).[15] Moreover, vanadyl sulfate administration does not produce any significant modification of the ability of liver to accumulate glycogen in response to feeding (data not shown). If we take into account the facts that blood glucose is the only source of glucose for glycogen synthesis in muscle and that vanadyl sulfate does not induce any significant change in the plasma levels of both glucose and insulin, perhaps we may conclude that the beneficial effect of vanadyl sulfate on sugar metabolism in senescent rats can be attributed to a restoration of the ability of peripheral tissues to respond efficiently to circulating insulin. Thus, insulin target tissues themselves can be the site of vanadate action, and augmentation of peripheral glucose utilization can be the major determinant of the antidiabetic action of vanadate.[16-21]

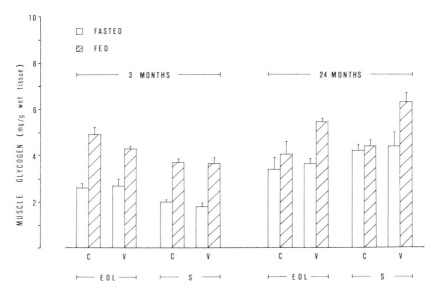

FIGURE 1. Glycogen content of EDL and S muscles of fasted and fed controls (C) and vanadyl sulfate–treated (V) rats of 3 and 24 months of age. Means ± standard error of 5 cases are given. The statistical analysis (ANOVA, F test) showed that the effect of different age, feeding, and interaction between age and feeding, age and vanadate, vanadate and feeding, and age and vanadate and feeding were significant with both muscles (EDL: $p < 0.05$; $p < 0.01$; $p < 0.01$; $p < 0.05$; $p < 0.01$; $p < 0.01$; S: $p < 0.01$; $p < 0.01$; $p < 0.05$; $p < 0.01$; $p < 0.01$; $p < 0.01$; $p < 0.05$, respectively). The effect of vanadate was significant ($p < 0.05$) in the S muscle only.

On the other hand, it should be remembered that insulin secretory function in response to metabolic demand appears to be impaired with increasing age in animals.[3–5] In order to explore the effect of the oral administration of vanadyl sulfate on the functional decline of beta cells, we have investigated the "*in vitro*" insulin secretory response of islets isolated from 26-mo-old rats treated with vanadyl sulfate (0.5 mg/ml in the drinking water) for 3 weeks.

TABLE 3. Insulin Release from Isolated Islets of Control (C) and Vanadyl Sulfate–Treated (V) Rats of 26 Months of Age[a]

	IRI Release (ng × islet^{-1} × h^{-1})				
	2.8 mM Glucose	16.7 mM Glucose	16.7 mM Glucose + 1 mM IBMX	16.7 mM glucose +20 mM arginine	16.7 mM Glucose + 20 mM 2-KIC
C	1.85 ± 0.39 (5)	3.94 ± 0.79 (5)	8.04 ± 1.86 (5)	7.44 ± 1.28 (4)	7.86 ± 1.56 (5)
V	2.91 ± 0.25 (4)	4.25 ± 0.49 (5)	11.05 ± 0.39 (4)	4.99 ± 0.55 (4)	6.34 ± 0.67 (5)

[a]Islets were incubated for 60 min in the presence of the indicated substances. Results are given as mean ± standard error of the mean number of observations indicated in parentheses. No significant change was observed between islets of control and vanadyl sulfate-treated rats (unpaired Student's *t*-test). IRI = immunoreactive insulin; IBMX = isobutylmethylxanthine; 2-KIC = 2-ketoisocaproate.

TABLE 3 shows that the secretory response of islets isolated from vanadyl sulfate–treated 26-mo-old rats is similar to that of islets taken from nontreated animals of the same age.

In conclusion, our results suggest that the oral administration of vanadyl sulfate has a beneficial effect on the glucose tolerance of senescent animals, restores the ability of skeletal muscles to accumulate glycogen efficiently in response to circulating insulin, and may compensate for the age-related loss of hormone sensitivity in the peripheral tissues. On the other hand, vanadyl sulfate treatment does not affect the insulin responsiveness of isolated islets in aging rats.

REFERENCES

1. DAVIDSON, M. B. 1979. The effect of aging on carbohydrate metabolism: a review of the English literature and a practical approach to diagnosis of diabetes mellitus in the elderly. Metabolism **8:** 688–705.
2. DE FRONZO, R. A. 1981. Glucose intolerance and aging. Diabetes Care **4:** 493–501.
3. REAVEN, E. P., G. GOLD & G. M. REAVEN. 1979. Effect of age on glucose-stimulated insulin release by beta-cells of the rat. J. Clin. Invest. **64:** 591–599.
4. SARTIN, J. L., M. CHAUDHURI, S. FARINA & R. C. ADELMAN. 1986. Regulation of insulin secretion by glucose during aging. J. Gerontol. **41:** 30–35.
5. BERGAMINI, E., M. BOMBARA, V. FIERABRACCI, P. MASIELLO & M. NOVELLI. 1991. Effect of different regimens of dietary restriction on the age-related decline in insulin secretory response of isolated rat pancreatic islets. Ann. N.Y. Acad. Sci. **621:** 327–336.
6. REAVEN, E. P., D. WRIGHT, C. E. MONDON, R. SOLOMON, H. HO & G. M. REAVEN. 1983. Effect of age and diet on insulin secretion and insulin action in the rat. Diabetes **32:** 175–180.
7. SHECTHER, Y. 1990. Insulin-mimetic actions of vanadate: possible implications for future treatments of diabetes. Diabetes **39:** 1–5.
8. HASSID, W. Z. & S. ABRAHAM. 1966. Chemical procedure for analysis of polisaccharides. Methods Enzymol. **8:** 34–37.
9. LACY, P. E. & M. KOSTIANOVSKY. 1967. Method for the isolation of intact islets of Langerhans from the rat pancreas. Diabetes **16:** 35–39.
10. HERBERT, V., K. S. LAU, C. W. GOTTLIEB & S. J. BLEICHER. 1965. Coated charcoal immunoassay of insulin. J. Clin. Endocrinol. **25:** 1375–1384.
11. DE TATA, V., G. CAVALLINI, P. MASIELLO, M. POLLERA, Z. GORI & E. BERGAMINI. 1991. Age-related changes in muscle glycogen metabolism. Aging **3:** 408–410.
12. OLEFSKY, J. M. & G. M. REAVEN. 1975. Effect of age and obesity on insulin binding to isolated rat adipocytes. Endocrinology **96:** 1486–1498.
13. OLEFSKY, J. M. 1976. The effects of spontaneous obesity in insulin binding, glucose transport and glucose oxidation in isolated rat adipocytes. J. Clin. Invest. **57:** 842–851.
14. NARIMIYA, M., S. AZHAR, C. B. DOLKAS, C. E. MONDON, C. SIMS, D. W. WRIGHT & G. M. REAVEN. 1984. Insulin resistance in older rats. Am. J. Physiol. **246:** E397–E404.
15. SAKURAI, H., K. TSUCHIYA, M. NUKATSUKA, M. SOFUE & J. KAWADA. 1990. Insulin-like effect of vanadyl ion on streptozotocin-induced diabetic rats. J. Endocrinol. **126:** 451–459.
16. MEYEROVITCH, J., Z. FARFEL, J. SACK & Y. SHECHTER. 1987. Oral administration of vanadate normalizes blood glucose levels in streptozotocin-treated rats. Characterization and mode of action. J. Biol. Chem. **262:** 6658–6662.
17. GIL, J., M. MIRALPEIX, J. CARRERAS & R. BARTRONS. 1988. Insulin-like effects of vanadate on glucokinase activity and fructose-2, 6-biphosphate levels in the liver of diabetic rats. J. Biol. Chem. **263:** 1868–1871.
18. BLONDEL, O., D. BAILBE & B. PORTHA. 1989. In vivo insulin resistance in streptozotocin-diabetic rats: evidence for reversal following oral vanadate treatment. Diabetologia **32:** 185–190.
19. BENDANAYAN, M. & D. GINGRAS. 1989. Effect of vanadate administration on blood

glucose and insulin levels as well as on the exocrine pancreatic function in streptozotocin-diabetic rats. Diabetologia **32:** 561–567.

20. PEDERSON, R. A., S. RAMANADHAM, A. M. J. BUCHAM & J. H. MCNEILL. 1989. Long-term effects of vanadyl treatment on streptozotocin-induced diabetes in rats. Diabetes **38:** 1390–1395.

21. VENKATESAN, N., A. AVIDAN & M. B. DAVIDSON. 1991. Antidiabetic action of vanadyl in rats independent of in vivo insulin-receptor kinase activity. Diabetes **40:** 492–498.

Pharmacological Interventions for the Changes of Chloride Channel Conductance of Aging Rat Skeletal Muscle[a]

A. DE LUCA, S. PIERNO, AND D. CONTE CAMERINO[b]

Unit of Pharmacology
Department of Pharmacobiology
Faculty of Pharmacy
University of Bari
Via Orabona 4, Campus
70125 Bari, Italy

INTRODUCTION

The decrease of muscle performance described in aged humans and animals is due to a series of concurrent events such as a loss of muscle mass,[1] a reduced protein synthesis,[2] and an impaired regenerating ability.[3] The impaired protein synthesis may play a crucial role, i.e., it may account for the reduced volume and Ca^{2+}-ATPase activity of sarcoplasmic reticulum (SR)[4] with consequent prolongation of Ca^{2+} reuptake by SR and half-relaxation time[4] and shift of the voltage for mechanical activation towards more negative potentials.[5] We have recently demonstrated that during aging, important changes also occur in membrane electrical properties. In particular, we observed a specific reduction of resting membrane conductance to chloride ions (G_{Cl}) occurring at a high rate in skeletal muscle of 29-month-old rats with consequent changes of the excitability characteristics related to this parameter.[6] Indeed, the large G_{Cl} controls membrane stability and a decrease of G_{Cl} is responsible for the pathological signs of myotonic syndromes.[7] Up to now, little biophysical and biochemical information can be obtained about the channels responsible for the large muscle G_{Cl}[8,9] and the changes they undergo in various situations as aging. Thus, from recent pharmacological investigations we proposed that the age-related decline of muscle G_{Cl} may be due to the presence of different isoforms of chloride channels.[10] Also, we have described that phorbol esters, specific activators of protein kinase C (pKC), are 20 times more potent in decreasing G_{Cl} in aged with respect to adult rats,[11] suggesting an age-related impairment of the intracellular modulatory pathways controlling channel state. However, a decrease in the number of conductive channels as a consequence of the reduced protein synthesis may also play an important role. The reduced protein synthesis can be likely related to a reduced level of growth hormone (GH) and related insulin-like growth factor 1 (IGF-1) found in serum of old humans and animals.[3,12] Indeed, administration of GH to old subjects increases lean body mass and restores IGF-1 levels in serum.[3,13] Also, this hormonal treatment counteracts the reduced protein synthesis in skeletal muscle from aged rats.[2] The present study was aimed at gaining insight into pharmacological treatments able to ameliorate the reduction of chloride conductance in skeletal muscle

[a]This work was supported by Italian CNR (P. F. Invecchiamento no. 93.1.333).
[b]Author to whom correspondence should be addressed.

undergoing aging, thus improving muscle performance. In particular, we have evaluated *in vitro* the effects of compounds that through various mechanisms can directly modify muscle chloride channel conductance, as well as the possible protective effect of an *in vivo* chronic treatment with therapeutic doses of GH on such an age-related decrease of G_{Cl}.

METHODS

Aged (23–29 month old) and adult (6–9 month old) male and female Wistar (Charles River, Calco, Italy) rats were used for all the experiments. For *in vitro* pharmacological studies, the extensor digitorum longus (EDL) muscles were removed from the rats under urethane anesthesia (1.2 g/kg ip), and placed in a muscle bath at 30°C and superfused with normal and chloride-free physiological solutions[6,10] with or without the tested compounds. To evaluate the effect of chronic GH treatment on membrane electrical properties, aged female rats of the Wistar Kyoto strain were treated from the age of 21 months with 150 μg/kg biosynthetic human GH (Genotropin 4 IU sterile powder-Kabi Vitrum, Stockholm, Sweden) sc 6 days a week for 6–8 weeks. Untreated aged rats received 0.1 ml distilled H_2O sc daily for the whole period of treatment. The electrophysiological experiments were made *in vitro* at the end of the treatment period. The normal physiological solution had the following composition (in mM): NaCl 148; KCl 4.5; $CaCl_2$ 2.0; $MgCl_2$ 1.0; $NaHCO_3$ 12; NaH_2PO_4 0.44; and glucose 5.55. The chloride-free solution was made by equimolar substitution of methylsulfate salts for NaCl and KCl and nitrate salts for $CaCl_2$ and $MgCl_2$. All solutions were gassed with 95% O_2 and 5% CO_2 (pH 7.2–7.4). The compounds tested *in vitro* were R-(+) 2-(*p*-chlorophenoxy) propionic acid (synthesized in our laboratories), taurine, glibenclamide, forskolin, and calcium ionophore A23187 (Sigma, St. Louis, Mo.). The component ionic conductances were calculated from membrane resistance (R_m) values in normal and chloride-free solutions[6,10] by cable analysis with the two intracellular microelectrode current clamp method in which a hyperpolarizing square current pulse is passed through one electrode and the membrane voltage response is monitored at two distances from the current electrode.[6,10] Current pulse generation, acquisition of voltage records, and calculation of fiber constants were done under computer control, as described in detail elsewhere.[14] The total membrane conductance, G_m, was considered to be $1/R_m$ in the normal physiological solution. The potassium conductance, G_K, was $1/R_m$ in the chloride-free physiological medium. The mean chloride conductance, G_{Cl}, was calculated as the mean G_m minus the mean G_K. The data are expressed as mean ± standard error (SE). The estimates of SE of absolute and normalized G_{Cl} values were obtained as described by Green and Margerison.[15] The excitability characteristics were determined by recording the intracellular membrane potential response to square-wave constant current pulses. In each fiber, the membrane potential was set by a steady holding current to −80 mV, before passing the depolarizing pulses.[6] Significance between groups of mean was evaluated by unpaired Student's *t*-test.

RESULTS

Component Ionic Conductances during Aging

Resting component conductances to chloride (G_{Cl}) and potassium (G_K) ions of skeletal muscle membrane undergo remarkable changes during the aging process. As previously described, G_{Cl} is significantly decreased with respect to the value of adulthood.[6] Such a decrease is a constant phenomenon of aged muscles; in fact we observed this decrease in EDL muscles of rats of either inbred and outbred strains (FIGURE 1). The potassium conductance, G_K, showed a tendency to increase (FIGURE 1). The increased value of G_K could be reduced by *in vitro* application of glibenclamide (50 μM), a specific blocker of ATP-sensitive potassium channels,[16] suggesting the possible involvement of these channels, and therefore metabolic changes of muscle cells, during aging.

Effects of Compounds Acting with Receptor-Mediated Mechanisms on Chloride Conductance

Very few compounds are able to increase muscle G_{Cl}, thus having an important therapeutic role in situations characterized by abnormally low G_{Cl} such as aging. Among these there are the R-(+) enantiomers of clofibric acid derivatives. In fact we have already demonstrated that opposite enantiomers of this class of compounds have opposite effects on muscle G_{Cl}, leading us to propose the presence of two stereospecific binding sites controlling channel state.[17] In particular, the R-(+) isomers of this series are able to produce a peculiar biphasic effect on chloride conductance by increasing G_{Cl} at low concentrations (1–10 μM) and decreasing this parameter, but never by more than 25%, at concentrations higher than 10 μM.[17] The biphasic effect of the R-(+) isomer of the most potent derivative known so far, 2-p-chlorophenoxy propionic acid (CPP), on G_{Cl} of adult EDL muscle is shown in

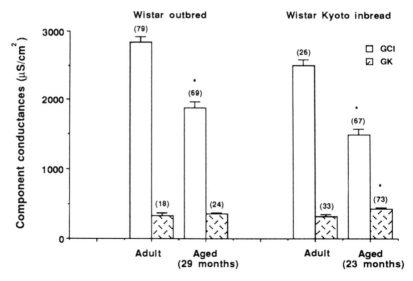

FIGURE 1. Absolute values of resting membrane component conductances to chloride (G_{Cl}) and potassium (G_K) ions of extensor digitorum longus muscle fibers from adult (6–9 month old) and aged (23 or 29 month old) Wistar rats of either outbred (left) and inbred (right) strains. Each bar is the mean ± SE from the number of fibers in brackets above the bars. *Significantly different with respect to the adult value of the related strain. $p < 0.05$ and less.

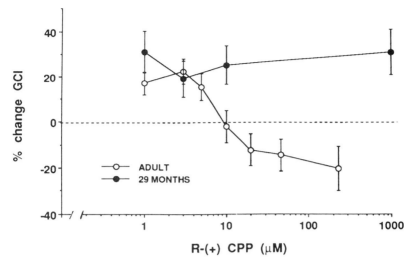

FIGURE 2. Normalized percent change of chloride conductance produced by *in vitro* application of increasing concentrations of R-(+) isomer of 2-(p-chlorophenoxy) propionic acid (CPP) to extensor digitorum longus muscle fibers from adult (6–9 month old) and aged (29 month old) rats. Each value is the mean ± SE from 27–56 normalized fibers.

FIGURE 2. We tested the effect of this compound on skeletal muscle of aged rats. We found that the R-(+) CPP applied *in vitro* on EDL muscle from 29-month-old rats produced the expected increase of G_{Cl} at low concentrations (1–3 μM); surprisingly the enhancing effect on G_{Cl} was observed also at higher concentrations, up to 1 mM (FIGURE 2). Thus, in aging muscles, the biphasic effect by R-(+) CPP was missing, supporting an age-related change of the receptors' nearby chloride channel[10] and suggesting a potential role of this compound in counteracting the decrease of G_{Cl} of aged muscle.

We have previously shown that *in vitro* application of taurine decreases membrane excitability of skeletal muscle by specifically increasing muscle G_{Cl}.[18] This effect could be mediated by the direct interaction of taurine with a low-affinity binding site, described in other tissues,[19] near the channel. We evaluated the effect of *in vitro* application of taurine on muscle fibers from 18-month-old rats and compared these effects with those produced in adulthood. Taurine increased G_{Cl} in both adult and aging muscle fibers, although these preliminary results suggest a higher potency of the amino acid on aging muscles than on adult ones, especially at the higher concentrations tested (TABLE 1). Indeed, at 30 mM, taurine increases G_{Cl} by 38.9 ± 8% and 48.4 ± 13% in adult and aging muscle fibers, respectively.

Effects of Compounds Acting on Intracellular Modulatory Pathways of the Chloride Channel

It has been described that chloride channels of various tissues, such as airway epithelia and cardiomyocytes, can be opened by activation of a cAMP-dependent protein kinase A (pKA).[20] We tested whether the activation of this enzymatic

TABLE 1. Effects of Taurine on Chloride Conductance of Extensor Digitorum Longus Muscle Fibers from Adult and Aged Rats[a]

Experimental Conditions	Dose (mM)	n	G_{Cl} ($\mu S/cm^2$)	Percent Increase G_{Cl}
6–9 months		64	2667 ± 95	
Taurine	0.45	34	3085 ± 142[b]	15.7 ± 4.7
	4.5	26	3340 ± 140[b]	25.2 ± 4.8
	18	17	3678 ± 245[b]	37.9 ± 7.3
	30	31	3705 ± 257[b]	38.9 ± 8.3
18 months		13	2287 ± 216	
Taurine	0.45	11	2661 ± 274	16.3 ± 11.5
	4.5	9	2942 ± 219	28.6 ± 11.4
	18	12	3248 ± 172[b]	42.0 ± 12.3
	30	13	3394 ± 122[b]	48.4 ± 13.2

[a]The columns from left to right are as follows: experimental conditions and age of the rat used; dose of taurine tested *in vitro* on EDL muscle fibers; n, number of fibers sampled; G_{Cl}, resting conductance to chloride ions; percent increase G_{Cl}, percent effect of taurine on G_{Cl} of adult and aged muscle fibers. [b]Significantly different from control values ($p < 0.05$ or less).

pathway could be useful in increasing muscle G_{Cl}, in particular during aging. Thus, we tested the effect of forskolin, a specific activator of adenilate cyclase, on G_{Cl} of adult and aged EDL muscle fibers. Forskolin (1.5 μM) applied *in vitro* on aged EDL fibers did not produce any significant increase or change of G_{Cl} (FIGURE 3). On adult skeletal muscle, forskolin was without any increasing effect on G_{Cl} and, by the use of concentrations as large as 50 μM, we actually observed a modest 20% decrease of

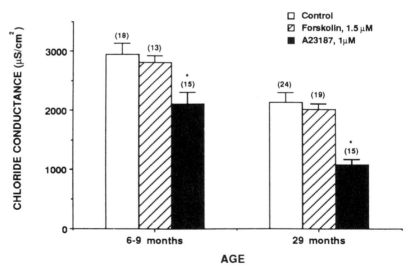

FIGURE 3. Absolute values of chloride conductance of adult (6–9 month old) and aged (29 month old) EDL muscle in the absence and in the presence of forskolin and calcium ionophore A23187. Each bar is the mean ± SE from the number of fibers in brackets above the bars. *Significantly different with respect to age-related controls ($p < 0.05$ and less).

G_{Cl}, suggesting a marginal role of pKA in the control of the muscle chloride channel. Also, intracellular calcium has been found to open chloride channels of various tissues.[21] We tested the effect of an increase of cytosolic calcium by *in vitro* application of the calcium ionophore A23187 on G_{Cl} of adult and aged muscle fibers. As it can be seen in FIGURE 3 in both adult and aged muscles, 1 μM A23187 did not increase but actually decreased G_{Cl}. The decrease of G_{Cl} by A23187 was more pronounced in aged than in adult muscle fibers, being about 50% and 30%, respectively, as expected by the proposed higher cytosolic calcium concentration in muscle fibers undergoing aging.[4,5]

Effects of Chronic Treatment with Growth Hormone on Ionic Conductances of Aged Muscles

In the 23-month-old female rats of the Wistar Kyoto strain that in the preceeding 6–8 weeks received a chronic treatment with 150 μg/kg GH, we observed a significant improvement of resting ionic conductances. In particular, G_{Cl} was signifi-

TABLE 2. Effects of a 6–8 Week Daily Treatment with GH on Component Ionic Conductances and Excitability Characteristics of Extensor Digitorum Longus Muscle Fibers from Aged Female Rats[a]

Age	n	G_{Cl} (μS/cm²)	G_K (μS/cm²)	n'	I_{th} (nA)	Lat (ms)
6–9 months	33	2492 ± 93	316 ± 31	10	110 ± 9.0	6.5 ± 0.5
23 months	73	1482 ± 79[b]	422 ± 22[b]	35	58 ± 2.4[b]	14 ± 1.3[b]
23 months + GH	78	1942 ± 78[c]	315 ± 19[c]	32	123 ± 10[c]	9.5 ± 1.6[c]

[a]Age, of the rats in months; GH was administered daily for 6–8 weeks as described in Methods; n, number of fibers sampled for component conductances to chloride (G_{Cl}) and potassium (G_K) ions; n', number of fibers sampled for I_{th}: threshold current to elicit one action potential; and Lat, latency of action potential, i.e., the delay between the application of the current pulse and the onset of the action potential. Values are mean ± SE. Significantly different [b]from adult control ($p < 0.05$ and less) and [c]from aged untreated rats ($p < 0.001$).

cantly restored toward the adult value; indeed it was increased by about 40% with respect to the untreated age-matched controls. Also, the GH treatment fully restored potassium conductance G_K down to the adult value (TABLE 2). In GH-treated aged rats, in parallel to the restoration of membrane ionic conductances, we observed a significant improvement of membrane excitability. In particular the threshold current to elicit the first action potential (I_{th}) was complitely restored and the latency of the action potential was significantly shortened toward the adult value (TABLE 2).

DISCUSSION

The large contribution of macroscopic G_{Cl} to the total membrane conductance is important to maintain appropriate muscle performance. Indeed myotonic muscle, where the genetic defect involves specifically chloride channels so that G_{Cl}, if any, is abnormally low,[22,23] experiences abnormal membrane hyperexcitability and prolonged contractures.[7] Similar signs are observed when G_{Cl} of healthy muscles is decreased by specific myotonia inducer drugs.[17] The aging process of skeletal muscle is characterized by a specific and recurrent decrease of G_{Cl}[6,11] which may in part account for the impairment of muscle performance.[1] As already described, such a decrease may be due to a change as well as to a decrease in the number of conductive channels.[6,10,11] However, the changes of G_{Cl}, and therefore of chloride channels, related to the aging process seem to be different from those occurring in myotonic muscles in terms of pharmacological approach and therefore possibility of improvement. Indeed, compounds able to increase G_{Cl}, such as $R(+)$ CPP and taurine, fail to increase G_{Cl} in myotonic muscle,[14] as expected by a genetic defect leading to a complete lack of functional chloride channels. On the contrary, these compounds are effective on G_{Cl} of aged muscle fibers and actually they increase G_{Cl} more in aged than in adult muscle. The different pharmacological response between adult and aged muscle fibers corroborates the hypothesis of different chloride channels contributing to the low G_{Cl} during aging. Also, the higher responsivity of aged muscles to drugs able to increase G_{Cl} opens further interesting therapeutic possibilities. These compounds have been, however, tested *in vitro,* and the real possible utility of them upon *in vivo* treatment remains to be tested. This possibility should be checked in particular for taurine, which is a natural amino acid normally occurring in high concentration in excitable tissues such as skeletal muscle and actually lacking relevant side effects.[19] In this regard, it should also be taken into account that taurine content in serum and in some tissues has been found to be reduced in aged Fisher 344 rats.[24] In contrast, the attempt we made to increase G_{Cl} through the intracellular modulatory pathways did not reveal any interesting results, mostly because in skeletal muscle, in contrast with other tissues,[20,21] chloride conductance seem to be controlled only in a negative direction by the pathways tested so far. As already proposed,[11] it is possible that the decrease of G_{Cl} is due to an overactivity of some of these pathways. However, compounds able to remove excessive phosphorylation, such as phosphatase activators, may be helpful to verify this hypothesis, but with very little interest from a therapeutic point of view. Interesting results have been observed with the chronic *in vivo* treatment of aged rats with growth hormone. Skeletal muscle is among the tissues most sensitive to GH; i.e., a treatment with the hormone stimulates both DNA and protein synthesis in adult and aged rats.[2,3,25] Myopathic reactions are observed in cases of hormone deficiency as well as its hyperproduction as in acromegaly.[26] Thus, the decreased secretion of GH observed in aged humans and animals[12] may cause important impairment of muscle function. In aged subjects, GH administration restores the lowered plasmatic levels of IGF-1,[3,13] the peptide that mediates most of the peripheral actions of GH. Also, exogenous GH administration to aged rats restores the impaired protein synthesis of skeletal muscle.[2,3] We found that a 6–8 week chronic treatment with GH increased G_{Cl} toward the adult value. The easiest explanation for the effects on G_{Cl} observed after chronic GH treatment may be an increase in the number of conductive channels consequent to a restored protein synthesis. The few studies available on the GH/IGF stimuli on cell membranes are in favor of a protein synthesis mediated effect. Indeed, GH increases the Na^+-K^+ pump synthesis in adult rat skeletal muscle.[25] Also, IGFs, with a receptor mediated process, increase paracellular permeability of T84 cell monolayer; this effect is due to the increased protein synthesis since it is prevented by cycloheximide.[27] Further interest in the treatment of aging subjects with GH also resides in the general beneficial effect of membrane electrical properties we observed in the treated aged rats, i.e., the complete restoration of G_K. Such restoration of G_K could be related to mechanisms other than protein synthesis. For instance it is known that GH stimulates cellular anabolism; thus, the effect of the hormone on G_K can result from a general improvement of cellular state of aged muscle fibers and a consequent closure of the ATP sensitive and/or Ca^{2+} sensitive K^+ channels[16] which may both contribute to the large macroscopic G_K recorded in aged muscle fibers.[4–6]

REFERENCES

1. GRIMBY, G. & B. SALTIN. 1983. The aging muscle. Clin. Physiol. **3**: 219–218.
2. SONNTAG, W. E., V. W. HYLKA & J. MELTAS. 1985. Growth hormone restores protein synthesis in skeletal muscle of old male rats. J. Gerontol. **40**: 689–694.
3. ULLMAN, M., A. ULLMAN, H. SOMMERLAND, A. SKOTTNER & A. OLDFORS. 1990. Effects of growth hormone on muscle regeneration and IGF-1 concentration in old rats. Acta Physiol. Scand. **140**: 521–525.
4. LARSSON, L. & G. SALVIATI. 1989. Effects of age on calcium transport activity of sarcoplasmic reticulum in fast- and slow-twitch rat muscle fibers. J. Physiol. **419**: 253–264.
5. DE LUCA, A. & D. CONTE CAMERINO. 1992. Effects of aging on the mechanical threshold of rat skeletal muscle fibers. Pflügers Arch. **420**: 407–409.
6. DE LUCA, A., M. MAMBRINI & D. CONTE CAMERINO. 1990. Changes in membrane ionic conductances and excitability characteristics of rat skeletal muscle during aging. Pflügers Arch. **415**: 642–644.
7. RÜDEL, R. & F. LEHMANN-HORN. 1985. Membrane changes in cells from myotonia patients. Physiol. Rev. **65**: 310–356.
8. CHUA, M. & W. I. BETZ. 1991. Characterization on the surface membrane of adult rat skeletal muscle. Biophys. J. **59**: 1251–1260.
9. STEINMEYER, K., C. ORTLAND & T. J. JENTSCH. 1991. Primary structure and functional expression of a developmentally regulated skeletal muscle chloride channel. Nature **354**: 301–304.
10. DE LUCA, A., V. TORTORELLA & D. CONTE CAMERINO. 1992. Chloride channels of skeletal muscle from developing, adult and aged rats are differently affected by enantiomers of 2-(*p*-chlorophenoxy) propionic acid. Naunyn-Schmiedeberg's Arch. Pharmacol. **346**: 601–606.
11. DE LUCA, A., D. TRICARICO, S. PIERNO & D. CONTE CAMERINO. 1992. Changes of chloride channel regulation in rat skeletal muscle during aging. Ann. N.Y. Acad. Sci. **673**: 154–159.
12. COCCHI, D. 1992. Age-related alterations in gonadotropins, adrenocorticotropin and growth hormone secretion. Aging Clin. Exp. Res. **4**: 103–113.
13. RUDMAN, D., A. G. FELLER, H. S. NAGRAY, G. A. GERGANS, P. Y. LALITHA, A. F. GOLDBERG, R. A. SCHLENKER, L. COHN, I. W. RUDMAN & D. E. MATTSON. 1990. Effects of human growth hormone in men over 60 years old. N. Engl. J. Med. **28**: 485–493.
14. BRYANT, S. H. & D. CONTE CAMERINO. 1991. Chloride channel regulation in the skeletal muscle of normal and myotonic goats. Pflügers Arch. **417**: 605–610.
15. GREEN, J. R. & D. MARGERISON, Eds. 1978. Statistical Treatment of Experimental Data: 86–88. Elsevier. New York, N.Y.
16. BERNARDI, H., J. N. BIDARD, M. FOSSET, M. HUGUES, C. MOURRE, C. REHM, G. ROMEY, H. SCHMID-ANTOMARCHI, H. SCHWEITZ, J. R. DE WEILLE & M. LAZDUNSKI. 1989. Molecular properties of potassium channels. Arzneim.-Forsch. Drug Res. **89**: 159–163.
17. DE LUCA, A., D. TRICARICO, R. WAGNER, S. H. BRYANT, V. TORTORELLA & D. CONTE CAMERINO. 1992. Opposite effects of enantiomers of clofibric acid derivative on rat skeletal muscle chloride conductance: antagonism studies and theoretical modeling of two different receptor site interactions. J. Pharmacol. Exp. Ther. **260**: 364–368.
18. CONTE CAMERINO, D., F. FRANCONI, M. MAMBRINI, F. BENNARDINI, P. FAILLI, S. H. BRYANT & A. GIOTTI. 1987. The action of taurine on chloride conductance and excitability characteristics of rat skeletal muscle fibers. Pharmacol. Res. Commun. **19**: 685–701.
19. HUXTABLE, R. J. 1992. The physiological actions of taurine. Physiol. Rev. **72**: 101–163.
20. NAGEL, G., T. C. HWANG, K. L. NASTIUK, A. C. NAIR & D. C. GADSBY. 1992. The protein

kinase A–regulated cardiac chloride channel resembles the cystic fibrosis transmembrane conductance regulator. Nature **360:** 81–84.

21. PACAUD, P., G. LOIRAND, J. L. LAVIE, C. MIRONNEAU & J. MIRONNEAU. 1989. Calcium-activated chloride current in rat vascular smooth muscle cells in short-term primary culture. Pflügers Arch. **413:** 629–636.

22. KOCH, M. C., K. STEINMEYER, C. LORENZ, K. RICKER, F. WOLF, M. OTTO, B. ZOLL, F. LEHMANN-HORN, K. H. GRZESCHIK & T. J. JENTSCH. 1992. The skeletal muscle chloride channel in dominant and recessive human myotonia. Science **257:** 797–800.

23. STEINMEYER, K., R. KLOCKE, C. ORTLAND, M. GRONEMEIER, H. JOCKUSCH, S. GRÜNDER & T. J. JENTSCH. 1991. Inactivation of muscle chloride channel by transposon insertion in myotonic mice. Nature **354:** 304–308.

24. DAWSON, R. & D. R. WALLACE. 1992. Taurine content in tissues from aged Fischer 344 rats. Age **15:** 73–81.

25. DØRUP, I., A. FLYVBJERG, M. E. EVERTS & H. ØRSKOV. 1992. Effects of growth hormone on growth and muscle Na^+-K^+ pump concentration in K^+-deficient rats. Am. J. Physiol. **262:** E511–E517.

26. MASTAGLIA, F. L. 1983. Pathological changes in skeletal muscle in acromegaly. Lancet **2:** 907.

27. McROBERTS, J. A. & N. E. RILEY. 1992. Regulation of T84 cell monolayer permeability by insuline-like growth factors. Am. J. Physiol. **262:** C207–C213.

Apparent Retardation of Aging in *Drosophila melanogaster* by Inhibitors of Reverse Transcriptase

CHRISTOPHER J. I. DRIVER AND DARREN J. VOGRIG

Deakin University
Rusden Campus
662 Blackburn Road
Clayton, VIC 3168, Australia

INTRODUCTION

Transposable elements are discrete regions of DNA that occur in every eukaryotic organism and that behave as if they were parasitic. Many are closely related to integrated forms of retro viruses and lack only a functional *env* gene. Others are more distantly related to viruses. These sequences are capable of intracellular replication using a viruslike particle as an intermediate and are capable of spreading rapidly through a population by non-Mendelian inheritance in which all the offspring of a carrier usually are also carriers. Reinsertion of the DNA, and nuclease activity associated with the elements, are responsible for extensive chromosomal fragmentation and remodeling. In *Drosophila,* most spontaneously occurring new mutations are a result of transposable elements. In addition, many of the commonly investigated elements are capable of causing mutations in somatic cells.[1]

Two elements, LINE-1 and *alu,* have been intensively studied in humans. They constitute a significant fraction of the chromosomal DNA and are associated with the G/Q and R banding patterns seen in stained metaphase cells.[2] Several germ line mutations produced by insertion of one or the other of these elements have been described. A neurofibromatosis type 1 *de novo* mutation has been reported that was produced by an *alu* element insertion.[3] A similar mutation at the cholinesterase gene has also been reported,[4] as have LINE-1 insertion germ line mutations at the Haemophilia A locus.[5] In addition human DNA contains a large number of endogenous proviruses and related sequences that are potentially capable of transposition.[6]

As well as germ line transposition, the *alu* and LINE-1 elements are also capable of somatic transposition. Transposition of *alu* elements has been shown in a number of human leukemias[7] and in human carcinoma cells.[8] In addition, insertion into new sites in somatic cells by LINE-1 elements has been shown in several animal and human cancers.[9]

Somatic transposition may be an important feature of aging. Age-associated changes indicating transposition of the IAP element has been shown in rodents.[10] In *Drosophila melanogaster,* the transposable elements *copia* and *412* increase in copy number in aged adult tissue.[11] Furthermore induction of transposition of a P element construct shortened life span.[11,12] As a result of findings such as these, several authors have suggested that transposable elements may induce sufficient cell damage to be responsible for aging.[10,11,13,14]

To test this model of aging, flies were treated with drugs that are likely to inhibit transposition. Transposable elements in *Drosophila* replicate using the enzyme reverse transcriptase.[1] Therefore drugs that can inhibit reverse transcriptase were tested for their ability to retard aging.

METHODS AND MATERIALS

Drosophila melanogaster strains used in these experiments were the wild-type strain Canton-S and the mutant strain *white* (white eyed).

Control media was as described previously for the high carbohydrate-low fat diet.[15] Phosponoformic acid (PFA) or dideoxyadenosine (ddI) was dissolved in 0.2 cm^3 of $NaHCO_3$ to vials containing 7 g of medium, mixed, and allowed to stand one week to allow to dry.

Fecal pellet density, an indirect measure of food intake, was determined as described previously.[15]

Activity was measured in the vials containing up to 10 flies, using a Perkin Elmer spectophotometer with a chart recorder. The cuvette carrier was removed and the tube placed in the light beam. The wavelength was set to 700 nm to minimize the visibility of the beam to the flies. When flies walked or flew into the beam the event was registered as a spike on the chart recorder. The number of such spikes obtained in ten minutes was used as a measure of activity.

RESULTS

Survey of Drugs with Reverse Transcriptase Inhibitor Activity

In the first set of experiments, three drugs able to inhibit reverse transcriptase were fed to flies at several concentrations. The drugs were fed to the flies for their entire life. The effects of these drugs are shown in FIGURE 1. Both ddI and PFA produced a modest but significant life span extension.

One criterion of aging is that the process is irreversible. Therefore we tested for an effect on an irreversible process by discontinuing the drug at a time before significant deaths occurred, and testing for a persistent effect on life span. In addition, it seemed likely that older flies should be more sensitive to toxicity than young flies. Accordingly, the effects of toxicity could be minimized by feeding the drugs at a time when death was not highly probable. For this reason also, the drugs were fed only in a part of the life span. The period of feeding used in these experiments was in the adult life preceding the loss of 10% of the population. Mortality was subsequently scored in each group. FIGURE 2 shows the effect of this protocol on life span with a range of concentrations of ddI and PFA. An extension of life span approximately equal to or greater than shown in FIGURE 2 was obtained under these circumstances, even though the flies were exposed to the drug for a shorter period of time.

Further Investigations on PFA

The drug with the greater effect, PFA, was selected for further study.

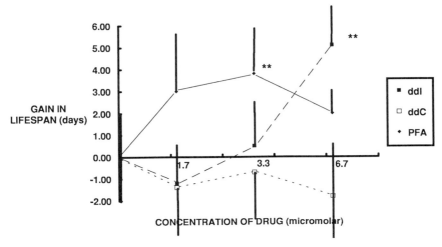

FIGURE 1. Tests of the effects of inhibitors of reverse transcriptase on life span of *Drosophila*. A logarithmic scale for concentration is used. The control is indicated at the origin. The drugs were added to the food in the final concentration shown in the table, and given for the whole of the life of the fly. Bars indicate standard error of the mean. The number of flies in each group was 100–250. Where these bars would overlap, only one arm is shown. Differences significantly different from the control are indicated (**$p < 0.01$; Students t-test).

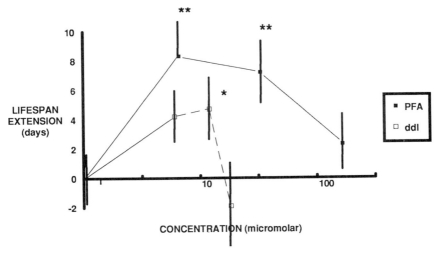

FIGURE 2. The effect of PFA and ddI addition at several concentrations to the medium, on the lifespan of *Drosophila*. A logarithmic scale for concentration is used as previously. In these experiments flies were treated for five weeks with PFA or six weeks with ddI and then transferred to control medium. Approximately 100–200 flies were used for each group. In this time, less than 10% of the flies had died in each set of experiments. The bars shown are standard errors of these differences. The points significantly different from the control are indicated thus: *$p < 0.05$ and **$p < 0.01$, student's t-test.

A Test for a PFA-Sensitive, Infectious Agent

PFA is active against a number of viruses including retro viruses and, at higher concentrations, RNA viruses and Herpes viruses, and it is potentially toxic to other infectious agents.[16] Was there such a PFA-responsive infectious agent present in this strain that shortened life span? One possible test would be to test other strains for responsiveness to PFA. The mutant strain *white* was also tested for its response to PFA. Its responses are very similar to Canton-S (TABLE 1).

In addition, if such infectious agents were present, it might be expected that flies should have had less of these agents after six weeks of PFA treatment than control flies. In that case, exposure of treated flies to untreated flies should reinfect the treated flies with the putative infectious agent, and reduce or eliminate the life span extension. We have shown that the life span of *white* and its response to PFA is very similar to the Canton-S strain. Therefore these two strains were used in an experiment in which flies were given different treatments and subsequently mixed. In the mixture of flies, each group could be distinguished because of the different eye colour.

In this experiment, flies were initially cultured 10 to a vial. One group of flies were raised on control medium and the second group of flies on PFA. When the drug

TABLE 1. The Effect of PFA on the Life Span of the Mutant Strain *White*[a]

	Control	PFA Fed
Canton-S	78.6 ± 1.9 (58)	82.7 ± 2.0 (49)
white	75.1 ± 2.6 (43)	80.6 ± 1.6 (39)

[a]The flies were treated with 6 µM PFA for 6 weeks, and then transferred to a control diet. The life spans are in days. The standard error of the mean of the lifespans is shown after the ±, and the number of flies in each groups is shown in parentheses. The effect of PFA is significant for each strain. ($p < 0.01$, Student's t-test).

was discontinued at six weeks, half of the control flies were mixed with half of the PFA-treated flies and the survival of each group counted separately in the same tube. The other flies within the other two groups were pooled so that the density of flies was 20 per vial as with the combined group. To control for any small differences on longevity associated with eye color, a second set of flies was also used in which the colors were reversed. The results for each strain were pooled. The results are shown in FIGURE 3. PFA treated flies lived just as long whether they were exposed to other PFA flies or untreated flies. In addition, the life span of control flies was not altered by exposure to PFA treated or untreated flies.

Does PFA Induce Undereating?

An increase in life span could be obtained by inducing the flies to eat rather less food. *Drosophila,* like many other animals, will live longer if the food intake is slightly reduced.[17] Food intake was measured indirectly by counting the number of fecal pellets.[15] TABLE 2 shows that the food intake of both strains used in these experiments is not reduced by PFA.

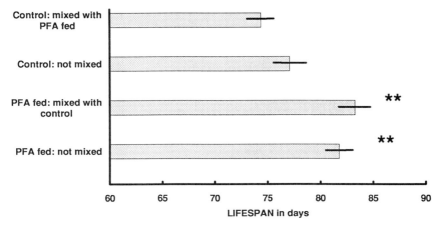

FIGURE 3. A test for the possibility of PFA responsive infectious agents. Canton S and *white* flies were cultured as described in FIGURE 3. At six weeks, groups of PFA-treated flies were mixed with untreated flies and the subsequent life span of each group was determined within that mixture. The origin of each fly in the group could be determined because the flies could be distinguished by the eye color. The bar labeled "Control:mixed with PFA fed" refers to these controls. The bar labeled "PFA fed: mixed with control" refers to this PFA fed group. Control groups consisted only of untreated flies or of PFA treated flies that were pooled to the same density without mixing. The bars relating to these groups are labeled "not mixed." The error bars shown are standard errors of the means. The points indicated (**) are significantly different from the control of the same strain ($p < 0.01$, student's t-test). The life spans of each control group are not significantly different from each other and also the life spans of each PFA group are not significantly different from each other. The increase of life span is significant ($p < 0.01$) for mixed and unmixed flies, and the increase for flies that are mixed is not less than that obtained when the flies are not mixed. This indicates that an infectious agent that would reduce or eliminate the life span increase is not transferred from control flies to PFA-treated flies.

Deterioration of Activity

Locomotor activity falls rapidly with age.[17] FIGURE 4 shows that PFA substantially retards this fall. PFA was most effective at 12 μM and was less effective at higher concentrations. A similar concentration dependence was observed for the effect of PFA on life span (FIGURE 2). This suggests that the same process is being affected.

TABLE 2. The Effect of PFA on Food Intake, Measured Indirectly by Estimation of Fecal Pellet Production[a]

	Control	Plus PFA
Canton-S	119 ± 11 (10)	133 ± 28 (11)
white	74 ± 5 (12)	77 ± 5 (12)

[a] Pellet density was measured in vials that had housed flies for one week, by counting within 1 cm squares on the walls of the vials as described by Driver and Lamb.[19] Measurements were taken within the first two weeks of adult life. The errors shown are standard errors of the mean, the numbers in parentheses are numbers of vials counted. There is no significant difference between control and experimental groups for either strain (Student's t-test).

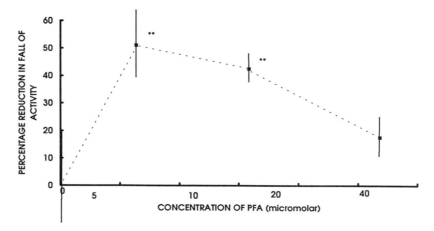

FIGURE 4. The effect of PFA on the decline of activity. Flies were treated with several concentrations of PFA for six weeks as described in FIGURE 2. Activity was measured during these six weeks, and the mean rate of decline of activity determined. The bars shown are standard errors of the means. The points indicated (**) are significantly different from the control ($p < 0.01$, student's t-test).

Lack of an Effect of Chemical Analogues that Are Not Reverse Transcriptase Inhibitors

To control for nonspecific effects, flies were treated with a variety of related compounds. Pyrophosphate and oxalate are structural analogues of phosponoformic acid that have considerably less effect on reverse transcriptase (RT).[20] FIGURE 5

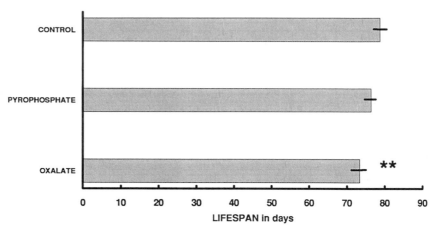

FIGURE 5. The effect of analogues of PFA on life span. Sodium pyrophosphate (6 μM) or sodium oxalate (6 μM) was used for treatment of flies for six weeks as described in FIGURE 2 and 5. The concentration used is that found to be optimal for PFA as shown in FIGURE 2 and 5. The bars shown are standard errors of the means. The points indicated (**) are significantly different from the control ($p < 0.01$, student's t-test). Pyrophosphate is without effect in life span whereas oxalate reduces the life span slightly.

shows that pyrophosphate does not increase the life span at a concentration at which PFA is effective whereas oxalate decreases the life span by about six days.

DISCUSSION

The hypothesis tested in this work was that inhibitors of reverse transcriptase may slow aging by inhibition of replication of transposable elements. The results produced are consistent with this possibility. However a number of other possibilities must be considered.

PFA and ddI are antiviral agents that act on reverse transcriptase and, with less effect, on a number of other viral DNA polymerases.[16] Thus the possibility should be considered that PFA is acting on an infective virus, thereby extending the life span. A life span significantly shorter than that obtained by other workers may indicate an unusual disease process. The life span of the control group in these studies (60–80 days) compares favorably with life spans of wild-type strains published by other laboratories (25–80 days, median 45 days).[19] This shows that these flies have been maintained in a good state of health. Microscopic examination of flies raised under these conditions indicates age-associated changes that are very similar to those previously published.[20] While it would be desirable to repeat the experiment in a virus-free condition, such a condition is very difficult to verify. Therefore the experiment in FIGURE 3 was used to test whether such an agent was acting in these experiments. This experiment indicates that PFA-sensitive infectious agents did not contribute significantly to mortality.

The effect appears to be chemically specific. Two unrelated compounds that are both inhibitors of reverse transcriptase will retard aging. Furthermore, pyrophosphate and oxalate, which are analogues of PFA with no effect on reverse transcriptase,[18] were unable to increase longevity at similar concentrations.

To test an agent that may alter aging, it is desirable to test both life span and physiological deterioration. In this paper, deterioration of activity was assayed. PFA was able to reduce the rate of loss of activity in these test conditions. PFA was most effective at 6 μM to 12 μM and less effective at higher concentrations. A similar concentration effect was observed on life span. This suggests that the same process was altered in both systems.

Life span may be changed by altering the rate of deterioration, by altering environmental stress, or by altering the ability to cope with environmental stress. One criterion of aging is that the process is irreversible. Therefore, we tested for an effect on an irreversible process by discontinuing the drug at a time before significant deaths occurred, and allowed deaths to occur in untreated flies in an environment apparently identical to the control environment.

Aging is not inhibited 100% under these conditions. If aging were inhibited completely, the life span would have been extended for exactly the same time as the flies were exposed to the drug. It is possible to calculate the reduction in aging by using the ratio of the life span extension to the time of drug treatment. Using this calculation procedure, the maximum inhibition of aging achieved in these experiments was only 23%. It seems likely that to completely inhibit transposition of all elements, it will be necessary to use a combination of drugs: this possibility is currently being investigated.

These limited initial measurements on *Drosophila* support the hypothesis that aging may be, at least partly, a result of the action of transposable elements. Agents capable of inhibiting replication of these elements merit further investigation as a class of antiaging agents.

SUMMARY

It is proposed that aging is induced by somatic replication of transposable elements (TEs). Most transposable elements in *Drosophila* reproduce by reverse transcription. Therefore inhibitors of reverse transcriptase were tested for their ability to retard aging in *Drosophila melanogaster*. Two inhibitors, phosphonoformic acid (PFA) and dideoxyinosine (ddI), were capable of prolonging life span when administered for the first half of the adult life. PFA was investigated further. It also produced a reduction in the rate of decline of behavior. PFA appeared not to act on an infectious agent in these experiments, nor did it alter the food intake. Analogues unable to inhibit RT had no life span prolonging effect at similar concentrations to that of PFA.

ACKNOWLEDGMENTS

The authors would like to thank Ms. Kaylene Patterson, Ms. Tracy Marsh, and Mr. Patrick Driver for technical assistance at several stages of this work.

REFERENCES

1. FINNEGAN, D. J. & D. H. FAWCETT. 1986. Transposable elements in *Drosophila melanogaster*. In *Oxford Surveys on Eukaryotic Genes 3*. Academic Press. London & New York.
2. KORENBERG, J. & M. C. RYKOWSKI. 1988. Human genome organisation: *Alu*, LINES, and the molecular structure of metaphase bands. Cell **53:** 391–400.
3. WALLACE, M. R., L. B. ANDERSEN, A. M. SAULINO, P. E. GREGORY, T. W. GREGORY, T. W. GLOVER & F. S. COLLINS. 1991. A *de novo Alu* insertion results in neurofibromatosis. Nature **353:** 864–866.
4. MURATANI, K., T. HADA, Y. YAMAMOTO, T. KANEKO, Y. SHIGETO, T. OHUE, J. FURUYAMA & K. HIGSHINO. 1992. Inactivation of the cholinesterase gene by *alu* insertion—possible mechanism for human gene transposition. Proc. Natl. Acad. Sci. USA **88**(24): 11315–11319.
5. KAZAZIAN, H. H., C. WONG, H. YOUSSOUFIAN, A. F. SCOTT, D. G. PHILLIPS & S. K. ANTONARAKIS. 1988. Haemophilia A resulting from *de novo* insertion of the L1 sequences represents a novel mechanism for mutation in man. Nature **332:** 164–166.
6. LIEBMOSCH, C., M. BACHMANN, R. BRACWERNER, T. WERNER, V. ERFLE & R. HEHLMANN. Expression and significance of human endogenous retro viral sequences. Leukemia **6**(S3): S72–S75.
7. FILATOV, L. V., S. E. MAMAYEVA & N. V. TOMILIN. 1991. *Alu* family variation in neoplasia. Cancer Genet. Cytogenet. **56**(1): 11–22.
8. LIN, C. S., D. A. GOLDTHWAIT & D. SAMOIS. 1988. Identification of *Alu* transposition in human lung carcinoma cells. Cell **54:** 153–159.
9. RECHAVI, G., N. KATZIR & D. GIVOL. 1988. Insertional mutagenesis and breast carcinoma. Nature **335:** 595–596.
10. BROWN, A. R., P. O. P. TSO & R. G. CUTLER. 1991. Expression of the intracisternal-A particle endogenous retro-virus genes over the lifetime of mouse and syrian hamster. Arch. Gerontol. Geriatrics **13:** 15–30.
11. DRIVER, C. J. I. & S. W. MCKECHNIE. 1992. Transposable elements as a factor in aging of *Drosophila melanogaster*. Ann. N.Y. Acad. Sci. **673:** 83–91.
12. KIRKWOOD, T. B. L. 1989. DNA, mutations and aging. Mutat. Res. **219:** 1–7.
13. WOODRUFF, R. C. 1992. Transposable DNA and life history traits. 1. Transposition of P DNA elements in somatic cells reduces the lifespan of *Drosophila melanogaster*. Genetica **86:** 143–154.
14. MURREY, V. 1990. Hypothesis: are transposons a cause of ageing? Mutat. Res. **237:** 59–63.

15. DRIVER, C. J. I. & M. J. LAMB. 1979. Metabolic changes in ageing *Drosophila melanogaster*. Exp. Gerontol. **14:** 95–100.
16. OBERG, B. 1983. Antiviral effects of phosphonoformate (PFA, Foscarnet Sodium). Pharmacol. Ther. **19:** 387–415.
17. DRIVER, C. J. I., R. WALLIS, G. COSOPODIOTIS & G. ETTERSHANK. 1986. Is a fat metabolite the major diet dependent accelerator of ageing? Exp. Gerontol. **14:** 497–507.
18. VRANG, L. & B. OBERG. 1986. PPi analogs as inhibitors of human T-lymphotropic virus type III reverse transcriptase. Antimicrob. Agents Chemother. **29:** 867–872.
19. BAKER, G. T., III, M. JACOBSON & G. MOKRYNSKI. 1985. Aging in *Drosophila*. *In* Handbook of Cell Biology and Aging. V. Cristofalo, Ed.: 511–578. CRC. Boca Raton, Florida.
20. MIQUEL, J. 1971. Aging of male *Drosophila melanogaster:* histological, histochemical and ultrastructural observations. Adv. Gerontol. Res. **3:** 39–71.

Restorative Effect of *Bacillus subtilis* Spores on Interferon Production in Aged Mice[a]

G. GRASSO,[b,e] P. MIGLIACCIO,[b] C. TANGANELLI,[c]
M. A. BRUGO,[d] AND M. MUSCETTOLA[c]

*Institutes of Human Anatomy[b] and
General Physiology[c]
53100 Siena, Italy*

[d]*Sanofi Winthrop SpA
Milan, Italy*

INTRODUCTION

Cytokines are autocrine, paracrine, and endocrine regulatory (glyco)proteins that interact with specific cell receptors and have pleiotropic effects. They affect the activation state, proliferation, differentiation, maturation, and function of other cell types in the immune system as well as those in the major organ systems. It is well known that immune function declines with age in humans and experimental animals.[1] One important component of this decline is reduced cytokine production, primarily murine interleukin-1 (IL-1),[2–4] IL-2,[5,6] and increased IL-3[7,8] and IL-4[7] secretion. Information about age-related production of another group of cytokines, the interferons (IFNs), is contradictory. The amount of IFN in the serum induced by Newcastle disease virus decreased with aging of the animal.[9,10] Another report shows an age-related decline in IFN-γ production in PHA- and ConA-stimulated mouse spleen cells,[11] and two reports demonstrate an increase of this cytokine in ConA-stimulated murine splenocytes.[12,13] It is well established that *Bacillus subtilis* spores have immunomodulatory and immunostimulatory activities in experimental animals and man.[14–21] Intravenous injection of *B. subtilis* in mice is reported to induce plasma IFN-γ production[22] and oral administration of *B. subtilis* spores in rabbits to induce high levels of plasma IFN-like activity.[23] Because peritoneal and spleen cells from mice fed with *B. subtilis* spores produce significantly higher IFN-β and -γ levels than those of controls,[24] we evaluated the influence of age on IFN production and the effect of oral administration of *B. subtilis* spores in restoring IFN production in aged mice.

MATERIALS AND METHODS

Twelve young (7-week-old), 19 middle-aged (11-month-old), and 10 old (22-month-old) female Balb/c mice were randomly allocated to two different groups (control and treated). The mice were maintained at a constant temperature

[a]Work supported in part by 60% funds from MURST, Rome, Italy.
[e]Address for correspondence: Institute of Human Anatomy, Via Del Laterino 8, 53100 Siena, Italy.

(22°C ± 2°C) on a 12 h light/dark cycle and fed with a standard diet and water *ad libitum*. The treated animals were fed *B. subtilis* spores suspended in saline at a concentration of 2.5 × 10⁶ spores per day per animal for 14 days (young mice) and for 8 weeks (middle-aged and old mice). The mice were sacrificed by cervical dislocation. Peritoneal cells were harvested by washing the peritoneal cavity with RPMI 1640 medium–10% heat inactivated fetal calf serum. The spleen was removed and teased in RPMI 1640. After washing, the splenocytes were stimulated for 72 h with ConA (5 µg/ml at 37°C) and PHA (2 µg/ml). Peritoneal cells were stimulated for 24 h with LPS (2 µg/ml at 26°C).[25,26] The microplaque reduction assay, described elsewhere,[27] was used throughout for the titration of IFN activity using L929 cells as indicator cells and vesicular stomatitis virus as challenge virus. Each assay included the international standards for mouse IFN-α, -β, and -γ to check the sensitivity and reproducibility of our test system. Samples were tested at least twice in quadruplicate. IFN activity was expressed in IU/ml, and typing was carried out using specific anti-IFN monoclonal antibodies. The data were processed by ANOVA. Differences were considered statistically significant for $p < 0.05$.

RESULTS

The body weight of control mice did not differ in the three age groups (FIGURE 1), but in treated animals there was a small increase in young and middle-aged mice and a significantly higher increase ($p < 0.05$) in old mice with respect to controls. Spleen weight of control mice increased with age, the highest weight occurring in middle-aged animals; in old treated animals, there was a significant ($p < 0.05$) increase with respect to controls. IFN-γ production by ConA- and PHA-stimulated spleen cells from control and treated mice of the three age groups is shown in FIGURES 2 and 3. ConA- and PHA-stimulated splenocytes from middle-aged and old mice produced lower IFN-γ levels than those of young mice. *B. subtilis* spores completely restored and increased IFN-γ production ($p < 0.001$). IFN-β production by LPS-stimulated peritoneal cells from control and treated mice of three age groups is shown in FIGURE 4. LPS-stimulated peritoneal cells from middle-aged and old mice also produced significantly lower IFN-β levels than those of young mice ($p < 0.001$), and the treatment completely restored and increased IFN-β production ($p < 0.001$).

DISCUSSION

Since several cytokines are critically involved in the induction and expression of immunological function, age-related alterations in cytokine production and response may play an important role in the senescence of the immune response. In line with previous data,[11] the present findings demonstrate that ConA- and PHA-stimulated spleen cells from aged mice produce significantly lower IFN-γ levels than those of young mice. LPS-stimulated peritoneal cells from aged mice also produced significantly lower IFN-β levels than those of young mice. This result is in agreement with reports of an age-related decline in IFN-α and IFN-γ production[28] by human peripheral blood mononuclear cells. Because IL-2 regulates IFN-γ production in humans[29-31] and rodents,[32-33] and IFN-γ, in turn, induces the expression of IL-2 receptors,[34] our data are consistent with the observation of age-related defects of IL-2 secretion[5,6] and IL-2 receptor expression[35] by mitogen-activated cells.

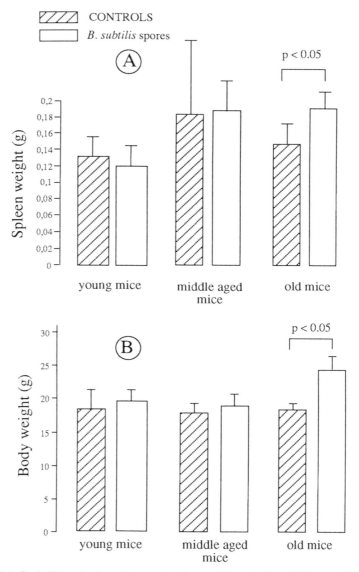

FIGURE 1. Body (B) and spleen (A) weights of young (7-week-old), middle-aged (11-month-old), and old (22-month-old) mice fed with *B. subtilis* spores. Young mice fed for 14 days; middle-aged and old mice fed for 8 weeks.

The precise mechanism of impaired IFN production with aging is still not clear. It has recently been suggested that aging may lead to a defect in signal transduction during the mitogenic activation of T lymphocytes. Decreased Ca^{2+} mobilization,[36–38] reduced production of inositol phosphates, and defective protein kinase C activa-

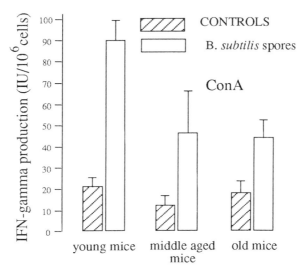

FIGURE 2. IFN-γ production *ex vivo* by ConA-stimulated spleen cells from young (7-week-old), middle-aged (11-month-old), and old (22-month-old) mice fed with *B. subtilis* spores. Young mice fed for 14 days; middle-aged and old mice fed for 8 weeks.

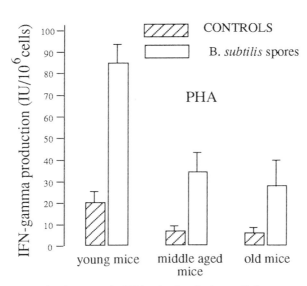

FIGURE 3. IFN-γ production *ex vivo* by PHA-stimulated spleen cells from young (7-week-old), middle-aged (11-month-old), and old (22-month-old) mice fed with *B. subtilis* spores. Young mice fed for 14 days; middle-aged and old mice fed for 8 weeks.

tion[36] were found in ConA-stimulated T lymphocytes from old mice, suggesting a possible defect in phospholipase C–induced hydrolysis of phosphatidyl-inositol 4,5-bisphosphate. Since lectin-induced transmembrane signaling is mediated by the inositol-phospholipid pathway with subsequent coordinate expression of IL-2 and IFN-γ genes,[39,40] and because Ca^{2+} mobilization and protein kinase C activation play a crucial role in the production of IL-2 and the expression of IL-2 receptors,[41-44] a defect in transmembrane signaling would result in decreased synthesis of these cytokines. Another finding of interest in mice is the demonstration, with limiting dilution analysis, that the decline in IL-2 production reflects a decrease, with age, in

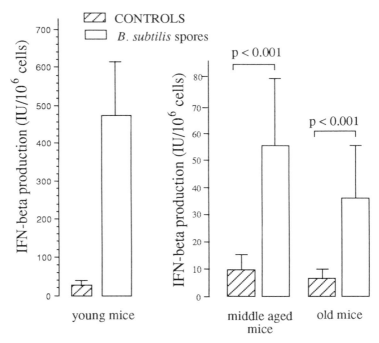

FIGURE 4. IFN-β production *ex vivo* by LPS-stimulated peritoneal cells from young (7-week-old), middle-aged (11-month-old), and old (22-month-old) mice fed with *B. subtilis* spores. Young mice fed for 14 days; middle-aged and old mice fed for 8 weeks.

the number of precursors for IL-2-producing helper cells.[45] Furthermore mouse helper T cells can be distinguished by their cytokine production patterns. Two distinct, mutually exclusive cytokine production profiles were proposed. Type 1 T helper (T_H1) cells produce IL-2, IFN-γ, and TNF-β, whereas type 2 T helper (T_H2) cells secrete IL-4, IL-5, IL-6, and IL-10.[46,47] Therefore the lower IL-2 and IFN-γ levels found in aged mice agree with the reduced number of IL-2-producing cells.

If the age-related decline in immune function is due, at least in part, to reduced synthesis of some immunoregulatory cytokine, the administration of substances that increase cytokine production could have restorative effects on immune response in old mice. Two observations in particular are consistent with this supposition. First, recent evidence suggests that T cell reactivities to mitogens and alloantigens by Peyer's patch cells of aged mice were generally retained at high levels with respect to their young counterparts.[48] Secondly, oral administration of *B. subtilis* spores in young mice increased IFN production by mitogen-stimulated spleen cells.[24] Both demonstrations led us to test the possibility that these spores could restore IFN secretion in old mice. The results show that *B. subtilis* spores completely restore and also increase IFN-γ and -β production respectively in spleen and peritoneal cells from aged mice with respect to young controls. This increased IFN-γ production is in line with immunostimulatory activities of *B. subtilis* spores such as enhanced macrophage-mediated cytotoxicity, increased lymphocyte proliferation in response to PHA and ConA, raised NK cell function,[15] stimulated secretion of IgA,[14,20] increase in mean survival time, and delay of tumoral growth in mice transplanted with compatible leukemic and solid tumor cells.[15] Moreover, clinical improvement in patients with chronic diarrhea with a selective IgA deficiency has been found after spore administration.[16] Finally, long-term oral administration of *B. subtilis* spores significantly reduced the frequency of urinary tract infections in older subjects.[18] Although the immunostimulating mechanism of *B. subtilis* spores is not clear, the above results suggest the involvement of the cytokines, particularly IFN-γ, and confirm that antigens introduced into the small intestine can induce both local and systemic responses. These findings also extend previous data on the stimulating effect of zinc[49] and certain thymic hormones[50] on IFN-γ production *in vitro* and on normalization of this cytokine by splenocytes from old mice fed with zinc and/or thymomodulin[11] and *Lactobacillus bulgaricus* and *Streptococcus thermophilus*.[51]

The intestine, continually exposed to harmless food constituents, commensal microbes, and enteropathogenic microorganisms, contains most of the lymphoid cells of the body, collectively named the gut-associated lymphoid tissue (GALT).[52] GALT largely consists of lymphoid aggregates, known as Peyer's patches, characterized by a specialized follicle-associated epithelium overlying lymphoid follicle domes which includes special follicle enterocytes and M cells, the latter differentiated for the uptake and transport of intestinal antigens to the underlying lymphoid tissue. Nonpathogenic as well as pathogenic organisms are effective in stimulating follicle development, and the proportion of M cells has been shown to increase after exposure of specific pathogen-free mice to a normal environment.[53] M cells are able to translocate indigenous enteric bacteria[54] and whole noninvasive enteropathogen bacteria[55] from the intestinal lumen to underlying lymphoid tissue, suggesting that normal enteric microflora also undergoes transepithelial migration.[51] We are currently investigating whether a similar translocation also operates for *B. subtilis,* which efficiently colonizes mice and human intestine. Preliminary results show that the proportion of M cells and lymphocytes observed in the basolateral pocket was significantly higher in animals fed with *B. subtilis* than controls. Light microscopy also showed increased lymphocyte traffic in Peyer's patches of treated animals with the perinodular lymphatic sinuses expanded and full of lymphocytes (data not shown). Furthermore, recent studies[56] demonstrate an increase in M-cell numbers and the CD4+/CD8+ ratio in Peyer's patch follicle-associated epithelium after oral administration of nonpathogenic *Salmonella typhimurium aroA⁻* in germ-free mice. A large proportion of intestinal intraepithelial lymphocytes, which together with epithelial cells are the first line of defense against intestinal antigens, express αβ or γδ T-cell receptors. Localization of murine γδT cells to intestinal epithelium is independent of normal microbial colonization;[57] in contrast, αβT cells increase after microbial colonization in germ-free mice.[58] It has been proposed that γδT cells reside in the spaces between epithelial cells, where they produce IFN-γ,[59] and that they do not recirculate, mediating immunological surveillance of the epithelia. In contrast, αβT cells recirculate continuously from blood to lymph for surveillance of the internal milieu.[60] Another interesting result is the change in glycolipid composition[61] and differential induction of major histocompatibility complex (MHC) class II molecules[62] of the intestinal epithelial cells in mice in relation to cell differentiation and bacterial association. Finally, the translocation of Enterobacteriaceae and lactobacilli into mesenteric lymph node has been observed after microbial colonization in germ-free mice.[58]

The above changes in the local subepithelial immune environment, or humoral mediators locally produced, could expand M-cell population with a subsequent rapid increase in antigen-transporting capacity.[56] One of these mediators could be IFN-γ, and several lines of evidence are consistent with this suggestion: (1) intestinal intraepithelial γδT cells produce IFN-γ;[59] (2) cyclosporin-A, which inhibits IFN-γ production,[63] reduces M-cell numbers in antigen-stimulated mouse Peyer's patches;[64] (3) IFN-γ enhances expression of secretory component, thus playing an important role in enhancing external transport of dimeric IgA and pentameric IgM;[65] (4) surface receptors for IFN-γ are found in epithelial cells,[66] and this cytokine directly affects the barrier function of cultured intestinal epithelial monolayers;[67] (5) M-cells express class II MHC determinants on the basolateral plasma membrane, and this expression is enhanced by pretreatment with IFN-γ;[68] (6) finally, the traffic of mature lymphocytes and their normal localization within various organs are of considerable importance to the initiation and propagation of the immune response. The mucosa-associated lymphoid tissues are major sites of lymphoid cell migration. Moreover, adhesion of lymphocytes to high endothelial venule cells is the first essential step for cell migration from the blood into the tissue. Tissue-specific lymphocyte surface receptors, termed homing receptors, and tissue-specific vascular addressins control the extravasation of lymphocyte subsets.[69] An endothelial cell differentiation antigen, involved in lymphocyte traffic, is selectively induced by IFN-γ,[70] and, besides, the lymphocyte adhesion to cultured Peyer's patch high endothelial venule cells is mediated by organ-specific homing receptors and can be regulated by IFN-γ.[71]

Taken together, these studies suggest that *B. subtilis,* which efficiently colonizes the mouse intestine, competes with enteropathogenic microorganisms in the adhesion to M-cells and subsequent transport to the basolateral pocket and underlying lymphoid tissue to stimulate mucosal immune responses. The antigen challenge increases M-cell numbers with consequent local production of IFN-γ,[23] which in turn expands M-cell population with subsequent rapid amplification of bacterial translocation. IFN-γ could also increase the expression of a Peyer's patch–specific endothelial addressin which promotes lymphocyte adhesion, resulting in increased lymphocyte traffic into the organ. The entire array of antigens derived from *B. subtilis* could induce an efficient mucosal immune response against potentially harmful intestinal microflora and enteropathogenic microorganisms.

In conclusion, this study is in line with previous data on the age-related decline in IFN production. It confirms the immunostimulating effects of *B. subtilis* spores on cytokine production[22–24] and demonstrates that oral administration may restore IFN production in aged mice. It also confirms the local and systemic immunomodulatory activities of *B. subtilis* spores and justifies their therapeutic use in the elderly.

REFERENCES

1. MILLER, R. A. 1991. Aging and immune function. Int. Rev. Cytol. **124:** 187–215.
2. BRULEY-ROSSET, M. & I. VERGNON. 1984. Interleukin-1 synthesis and activity in aged mice. Mech. Ageing Dev. **24:** 247–254.

3. INAMIZU, T., M.-P. CHANG & T. MAKINODAN. 1985. Influence of age on the production and regulation of interleukin-1 in mice. Immunology **55**: 447–455.
4. SAUDER, D. N., U. PONNAPPAN & B. CINADER. 1989. Effect of age on cutaneous interleukin 1 expression. Immunol. Lett. **20**: 111–114.
5. THOMAN, M. L. & W. O. WEIGLE. 1981. Lymphokines and ageing: interleukin-2 production and activity in aged animals. J. Immunol. **127**: 2102–2106.
6. MILLER, R. A. & O. STUTMAN. 1981. Decline in aging mice of the anti-2,4,6 trinitrophenyl (TNP) cytotoxic T cell response attributable in loss of Lyt-2-, interleukin-2 producing helper cell function. Eur. J. Immunol. **11**: 751–756.
7. KUBO, M. & B. CINADER. 1990. Polymorphism of age-related changes in interleukin (IL) production: differential changes of T helper subpopulations, synthesizing IL 2, IL 3, IL 4. Eur. J. Immunol. **20**: 1289–1296.
8. KUBO, M. & B. CINADER. 1990. IL-3 production as a function of age and its correlation with splenomegaly: age versus disease-related change. Immunol. Lett. **24**: 133–136.
9. DE MAYER, E. & J. DE MAYER-GUIGNARD. 1968. Influence of animal genotype and age on the amount of circulating interferon induced by Newcastle disease virus. J. Gen. Virol. **2**: 445–449.
10. BLACH-OLSZEWSKA, Z., M. CEMBRZYNSKA-NOWAK & E. KWASNIEWSKA. 1984. Age-related synthesis of spontaneous interferon in BALBtc mice. Contr. Oncol. **20**: 224–232.
11. GRASSO, G., M. MUSCETTOLA, R. STECCONI, M. MUZZIOLI & N. FABRIS. 1992. Restorative effect of thymomodulin and zinc on interferon-gamma production in aged mice. Ann. N.Y. Acad. Sci. **673**: 256–259.
12. HEINE, J. W. & W. H. ADLER. 1977. The quantitative production of interferon by mitogen-stimulated mouse lymphocytes as a function of age and its effect on the lymphocytes proliferative response. J. Immunol. **118**: 1366–1369.
13. SAXENA, R. K., Q. B. SAXENA & W. H. ADLER. 1988. Lectin-induced cytotoxic activity in spleen cells from young and old mice. Age-related changes in types of effector cells, lymphokine production and response. Immunology **64**: 457–461.
14. BONOMO, R., G. LUZI, A. FRIELINGSDORF & F. AIUTI. 1980. Ruolo delle IgA secretorie nelle funzioni dell'immunità locale dell'apparato digerente. Impiego delle spore di *B. subtilis* in alcune forme morbose con deficit di IgA e ipogammaglobulinemia. Chemioter. Antimicrob. **4**: 237–240.
15. SPREAFICO, F., N. POLENTARUTTI, A. VECCHI, S. FILIPPESCHI, A. TAGLIABUE, M. SIRONI & M. L. MORAS. 1980. L'effetto immunostimolatore delle spore di *Bacillus subtilis* aspetti sperimentali. Chemioter. Antimicrob. **3**: 259–266.
16. DAMMACCO, F., M. TRIGGIANI, M. T. VENTURA & L. BONOMO. 1980. L'immunomodulazione nelle sindromi da deficienza immunologica primitiva. Chemioter. Antimicrob. **3**: 288–296.
17. BENEDETTINI, G., G. DE LIBERO, R. PIEROTTI, M. CAMPA & G. FALCONE. 1983. Immunomodulation by *Bacillus subtilis* spores. Boll. Ist. Sieroter. Milan **62**: 509–516.
18. MERONI, P. L., R. PALMIERI, W. BARCELLINI, G. DE BARTOLO & C. ZANUSSI. 1983. Effect of long-term treatment with *Bacillus subtilis* on the frequency of urinary tract infections in older patients. Chemioterapia **2**: 142–144.
19. NOVELLI, A., A. ULIVELLI, E. F. REALI, F. MANNELLI, L. TROMBI, C. BELCARI, R. SPEZIA & P. PERITI. 1984. *Bacillus subtilis* spores as a natural pro-host oral agent. Preliminary data in children. Chemioterapia **3**: 152–155.
20. FIORINI, G., C. CIMMINIELLO, R. CHIANESE, G. P. VISCONTI, D. COVA, T. UBERTI & A. GIBELLI. 1985. *Bacillus subtilis* selectively stimulates the synthesis of membrane bound and secreted IgA. Chemioterapia **4**: 310–312.
21. CIPRANDI, G., A. SCORDAMAGLIA, D. VENUTI, M. CARIA & G. W. CANONICA. 1986. *In vitro* effect of *Bacillus subtilis* on the immune response. Chemioterapia **5**: 404–407.
22. NOZAKI-RENARD, J. 1978. Induction d'interféron par *Bacillus subtilis*. Ann. Microbiol. (Inst. Pasteur) **129A**: 525–543.
23. MUSCETTOLA, M., G. GRASSO, P. MIGLIACCIO & V. C. GALLO. 1991. Plasma interferon-like activity in rabbits after oral administration of *Bacillus subtilis* spores. J. Chemotherapy **3** (Suppl. 3): 130–132.
24. MUSCETTOLA, M., G. GRASSO, Z. BLACH-OLSZEWSKA, P. MIGLIACCIO, C. BORGHESI-

NICOLETTI & V. C. GALLO. 1992. Effects of *Bacillus subtilis* spores on interferon production. Pharmacol. Res. **26** (Suppl. 2): 176–177.

25. CEMBRZYNSKA-NOWAK, M. 1986. Interferons from mouse lymphocytes produced at various temperatures (26°C and 37°C). Arch. Immunol. Ther. Exp. **34**: 525–532.

26. GESSANI, S., F. BELARDELLI, A. PECORELLI, P. PUDDU & C. BAGLIONI. 1989. Bacterial lipopolysaccharide and gamma interferon induce transcription of beta interferon mRNA and interferon secretion in murine macrophages. J. Virol. **63**: 2785–2789.

27. MUSCETTOLA, M. & G. GRASSO. 1990. Somatostatin and vasoactive intestinal peptide reduce interferon gamma production by human peripheral blood mononuclear cells. Immunobiology **180**: 419–430.

28. ABB, J., H. ABB & F. DEINHARDT. 1984. Age-related decline of human interferon alpha and interferon gamma production. Blut **48**: 285–289.

29. KASAHARA, T., J. J. HOOKS, S. F. DOUGHERTY & J. J. OPPENHEIM. 1983. Interleukin 2 (IL 2)–mediated immune interferon (IFN-γ) production by human T cells and T cell subsets. J. Immunol. **130**: 1784–1789.

30. REEM, G. H. & N.-H. YEH. 1984. Interleukin 2 regulates expression of its receptor and synthesis of γ-interferon by human T lymphocytes. Science **225**: 429–430.

31. VILCEK, J., D. HENRIKSEN-DESTEFANO, D. SIEGEL, A. KLION, R. J. ROBB & J. LE. 1985. Regulation of IFN-γ induction in human peripheral blood cells by exogenous and endogenously produced interleukin 2. J. Immunol. **135**: 1851–1856.

32. TORRES, B. A., W. L. FARRAR & H. M. JOHNSON. 1982. Interleukin 2 regulates immune interferon (IFN gamma) production by normal and suppressor cell cultures. J. Immunol. **128**: 2217–2219.

33. KLEIN, J. R. & J. BEVAN. 1983. Secretion of immune interferon and generation of cytotoxic T cell activity in nude mice are dependent on interleukin 2: age-associated endogenous production of interleukin 2 in nude mice. J. Immunol. **130**: 1780–1783.

34. JOHNSON, H. M. & W. L. FARRAR. 1983. The role of a gamma interferon-like lymphokine in the activation of T cells for expression of interleukin-2 receptors. Cell. Immunol. **75**: 154–159.

35. PROUST, J. J., D. S. KITTUR, M. A. BUCHHOLZ & A. A. NORDIN. 1988. Restricted expression of mitogen-induced high affinity IL-2 receptors in aging mice. J. Immunol. **141**: 4209–4216.

36. PROUST, J. J., C. R. FILBURN, S. A. HARRISON, M. A. BUCHHOLZ & A. A. NORDIN. 1987. Age-related defect in signal transduction during lectin activation of murine T lymphocytes. J. Immunol. **139**: 1472–1478.

37. MILLER, R. A., B. JACOBSON, G. WEIL & E. R. SIMONS. 1987. Diminished calcium influx in lectin stimulated T cells from old mice. J. Cell. Physiol. **132**: 337–342.

38. LERNER, A., B. PHILOSOPHE & R. A. MILLER. 1988. Defective calcium influx and preserved inositol phosphate generation in T cells from old mice. Aging: Immunol. Infect. Dis. **1**: 149–157.

39. WISKOCIL, R., A. WEISS, J. IMBODEN, R. KAMIN-LEWIS & J. STOBO. 1985. Activation of a human T cell line: a two-stimulus requirement in the pretranslational events involved in the coordinate expression of interleukin 2 and γ-interferon genes. J. Immunol. **134**: 1599–1603.

40. FARRAR, W. L., M. C. BIRCHENALL-SPARKS & H. B. YOUNG. 1986. Interleukin induction of interferon γ mRNA synthesis. J. Immunol. **137**: 3836–3840.

41. DEPPER, J. M., W. J. LEONARD, M. KRONKE, P. D. NOGUCHI, T. A. CUNNINGHAM, T. A. WALDMANN & W. C. GREENE. 1984. Regulation of interleukin 2 receptor expression: effects of phorbol diester, phospholipase C, and reexposure to lectin or antigen. J. Immunol. **133**: 3054–3061.

42. ALBERT, F., C. HUA, A. TRUNEH, M. PIERRES & A.-M. SCHMITT-VERHULST. 1985. Distinction between antigen receptor and IL-2 receptor triggering events in the activation of alloreactive T cell clones with calcium ionophore and phorbol ester. J. Immunol. **134**: 3649–3655.

43. FARRAR, W. L. & W. B. ANDERSON. 1985. Interleukin-2 stimulation of protein kinase C plasma membrane association. Nature **315**: 233–235.

44. FARRAR, W. L. & F. W. RUSCETTI. 1986. Association of protein kinase C activation with IL receptor expression. J. Immunol. **136**: 1266–1273.

45. MILLER, R. A. 1984. Age-associated decline in precursor frequency for different T cell–mediated reactions, with preservation of helper or cytotoxic effect per precursor cell. J. Immunol. **132:** 63–68.
46. MOSMANN, T. R., H. CHERWINSKI, M. W. BOND, M. A. GIEDLIN & R. L. COFFMAN. 1986. Two types of murine helper T cell clone. I. Definition according to profiles of lymphokine activities and secreted proteins. J. Immunol. **136:** 2348–2357.
47. CHERWINSKI, H. M., J. H. SCHUMACHER, K. D. BROWN & T. R. MOSMANN. 1987. Two types of mouse helper T cell clone. III. Further differences in lymphokine synthesis between TH1 and TH2 clones revealed by RNA hybridization, functional monospecific bioassays and monoclonal antibodies. J. Exp. Med. **166:** 129–144.
48. ERNST, D. N., W. O. WEIGLE & M. L. THOMAN. 1987. Retention of T cell reactivity to mitogens and alloantigens by Peyer's patche cells of aged mice. J. Immunol. **138:** 26–31.
49. SALAS, M. & H. KIRCHNER. 1987. Induction of interferon-γ in human leukocyte cultures stimulated by Zn^{2+}. Clin. Immunol. Immunopathol. **45:** 139–142.
50. RENTZ, E. & W. DIEZEL. 1983. Influence of thymic hormones on mitogen-induced interferon production in lymphocytes. I. Augmentation of mitogen-induced immune interferon production by thymosin. Arch. Geschwulstforsch. **53:** 547–550.
51. MUSCETTOLA, M., L. MASSAI, C. TANGANELLI & G. GRASSO. Effects of lactobacilli on interferon production in young and aged mice. Ann. N.Y. Acad. Sci. (This volume.)
52. BIENENSTOCK, J. & A. D. BEFUS. 1980. Mucosal immunology. Immunology **41:** 249–270.
53. SMITH, M. W., P. S. JAMES & D. R. TIVEY. 1987. M cell numbers increase after transfer of SPF mice to a normal animal house environment. Am. J. Pathol. **128:** 385–389.
54. BERG, R. D. & A. W. GARLINGTON. 1979. Translocation of certain indigenous bacteria from the gastrointestinal tract to the mesenteric lymph nodes and other organs in a gnotobiotic mouse model. Infect. Immun. **23:** 403–411.
55. OWEN, R. L., N. F. PIERCE, R. T. APPLE & W. C. CRAY, JR. 1986. M cell transport of *Vibrio cholerae* from the intestinal lumen into Peyer's patches: a mechanism for antigen sampling and for microbial transepithelial migration. J. Infect. Dis. **153:** 1108–1118.
56. SAVIDGE, T. C., M. W. SMITH, P. S. JAMES & P. ALDRED. 1991. Salmonella-induced M-cell formation in germ-free mouse Peyer's patch tissue. Am. J. Pathol. **139:** 177–184.
57. BANDEIRA, A., T. MOTA-SANTOS, S. ITOHARA, S. DEGERMANN, C. HEUSSER, S. TONEGAWA & A. COUTINHO. 1990. Localization of γ/δ T cells to the intestinal epithelium is independent of normal microbial colonization. J. Exp. Med. **172:** 239–244.
58. UMESAKI, Y., H. SETOYAMA, S. MATSUMOTO & Y. OKADA. 1993. Expansion of αβ T-cell receptor-bearing intestinal intraepithelial lymphocytes after microbial colonization in germ-free mice and its independence from thymus. Immunology **79:** 32–37.
59. TAGUCHI, T., W. K. AICHER, K. FUJIHASHI, M. YAMAMOTO, J. R. MCGHEE, J. A. BLUESTONE & H. KIYONO. 1991. Novel function for intestinal intraepithelial lymphocytes. Murine CD3+, γ/δ TCR+ T cells produce IFN-γ and IL-5. J. Immunol. **147:** 3736–3744.
60. JANEWAY, C. A., B. JONES & A. HAYDAY. 1988. Specificity and function of T cells bearing γδ receptors. Immunol. Today **9:** 73–76.
61. UMESAKI, Y. 1984. Immunohistochemical and biochemical demonstration of the change in glycolipid composition of the intestinal epithelial cell surface in mice in relation to cell differentiation and bacterial association. J. Histochem. Cytochem. **32:** 299–304.
62. MATSUMOTO, S., H. SETOYAMA & Y. UMESAKI. 1992. Differential induction of major histocompatibility complex class II molecules on the mouse intestine by bacterial colonization. Gastroenterology **103:** 1777–1782.
63. ESPEVIK, T., I. S. FIGARI, M. R. SHALABY, G. A. LACKIDES, G. D. LEWIS, H. M. SHEPARD & M. A. PALLADINO, JR. 1987. Inhibition of cytokine production by cyclosporin A and transforming growth factor β. J. Exp. Med. **166:** 571–576.
64. SAVIDGE, T. C. & M. W. SMITH. 1990. Cyclosporin-A reduces M cell numbers in antigen-stimulated mouse Peyer's patches. J. Physiol. **422:** 84P.
65. SOLLID, L. M., D. KVALE, P. BRANDTZAEG, G. MARKUSSEN & E. THORSBY. 1987. Interferon-γ enhances expression of secretory component, the epithelial receptor for polymeric immunoglobulins. J. Immunol. **138:** 4303–4306.
66. UCER, U., H. BARTSCH, P. SCHEURICH & K. PFIZENMAIER. 1985. Biological effects of gamma interferon on human tumour cells. Int. J. Cancer **36:** 103–108.

67. MADARA, J. L. & J. STAFFORD. 1989. Interferon-γ directly affects barrier function of
     cultured intestinal epithelial monolayers. J. Clin. Invest. **83:** 724–727.
68. ALLAN, C. H., D. L. MENDRICK & J. S. TRIER. 1993. Rat intestinal M cells contain acidic
     endosomal-lysosomal compartments and express class II major histocompatibility
     complex determinants. Gastroenterology **104:** 698–708.
69. BERG, E. L., L. A. GOLDSTEIN, M. A. JUTILA, M. NAKACHE, L. J. PICHER, P. R. STREETER,
     N. W. WU, D. ZHOU & E. C. BUTCHER. 1989. Homing receptors and vascular
     addressins: cell adhesion molecules that direct lymphocyte traffic. Immunol. Rev.
     108: 5–18.
70. DUIJVESTIJN, A. M., A. B. SCHREIBER & E. C. BUTCHER. 1986. Interferon-γ regulates an
     antigen specific for endothelial cells involved in lymphocyte traffic. Proc. Natl. Acad.
     Sci. USA **83:** 9114–9118.
71. CHIN, Y.-H., J.-P. CAI & K. JOHNSON. 1990. Lymphocyte adhesion to cultured Peyer's
     patch high endothelial venule cells is mediated by organ-specific homing receptors and
     can be regulated by cytokines. J. Immunol. **145:** 3669–3677.

Potential Interaction between Prolonged Cyclosporin Administration and Aging in the Rat Kidney

Z. GREENFELD,[a] I. PELEG,[b] , M. BREZIS,[a]
S. ROSEN,[c] AND S. PISANTY[d]

[a]Department of Medicine
Hadassah-University Hospital
Mt. Scopus
Jerusalem, Israel

[b]Connective Tissue Research Laboratory
Hadassah School of Dental Medicine
Jerusalem, Israel

[c]Department of Pathology
Beth Israel Hospital
Harvard Medical School
Boston, Massachusetts

[d]Department of Diagnosis and Oral Medicine
Hadassah School of Dental Medicine
Jerusalem, Israel

Cyclosporin (CsA) is a very potent immunosuppressive and therefore the drug of choice in prevention of solid organ allograft rejection and graft-versus-host disease.[1] Unfortunately, nephrotoxicity may develop during the treatment, as reflected by reversible reduction in glomerular filtration and/or irreversible interstitial fibrosis formation.[2] The mechanisms responsible for these toxic effects are not yet fully understood. We have previously shown that chronic CsA administration leads to tubulointerstitial damage (tubular atrophy and associated interstitial fibrosis) to the renal tissue in the rat, a process accelerated by a salt-depletion diet.[3] A reminiscent structural alteration occurs in the renal medulla of the aging rat (casts, tubular atrophy, and interstitial fibrosis).[4] Moreover, the mRNA levels of collagen type I, the main constituent of fibrotic tissue, are increased in cortex and outer medulla of old relative to young rat kidneys, providing at least a partial explanation to the increase in renal collagen content.[5] Therefore, fibrosis formation seems to be a common feature to aging and long-term CsA in the rat kidney. In addition, both conditions are known to reduce glomerular filtration. Thus, CsA and aging may interact synergistically, and this possibility was investigated in the present study by evaluating various renal parameters: kidney function, tissue collagen content, mRNA levels of interstitial collagen (types I and III), and extent of tubulointerstitial damage. This issue is of clinical relevance, as the age of both recipients and donors of kidney transplants has increased during recent years and CsA is being used as a principal component of postoperative immunosuppressive therapy.

Male Sprague-Dawley rats were used. Eight old (age 20 months) and 5 young (age 3 months) were injected subcutaneously with CsA (12.5 mg/kg body weight/day) for 10 weeks. An additional 5 old and 5 young rats served as controls, being

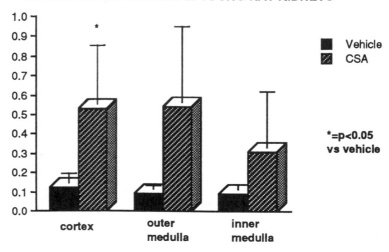

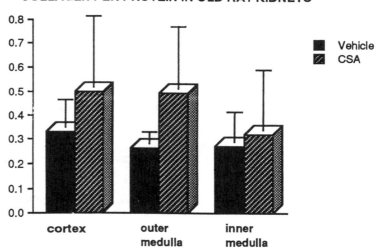

FIGURE 1. Collagen per protein (μg/μg) in the various kidney regions of young and old rats treated with CsA or vehicle.

similarly treated with the vehicle (cremaphore) and being pair fed. At the conclusion of the experiment, all rats were transferred to metabolic cages for urine collection. The right kidney was dissected into cortex and outer and inner medulla to determine the tissue collagen content (by hydroxyproline evaluation) and the steady-state mRNA levels of interstitial collagen types I and III (by dot-blot method), as previously described.[5] The left kidney was perfused-fixed with 1.25% glutaraldehyde solution for morphological examination.[3] Urine albumin and plasma creatinine were measured to assess renal function.

CsA treatment elevated plasma creatinine values (from 55 ± 1 to 82 ± 5 μmol/l in young and from 76 ± 11 to 109 ± 18 μmol/l in old rats, $p < 0.05$ for both

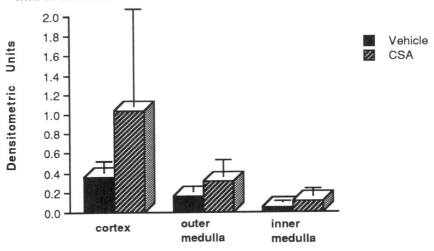

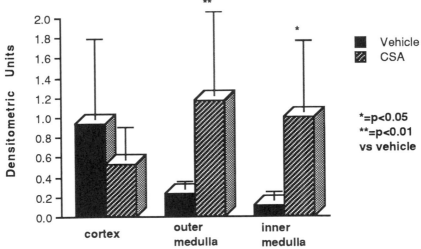

FIGURE 2. Steady-state mRNA levels of collagen types I + III in the various kidney regions of young and old rats treated with CsA or vehicle.

comparisons), suggesting reduced glomerular filtration by CsA in both age groups. Albuminuria was also increased (from 8.3 ± 1 to 15.8 ± 4.6 mg albumin/24 h in young rats, $p < 0.05$, and from 22.3 ± 7.5 to 230.5 ± 250.0 mg/24 h in old rats). The amount of collagen per protein, as measured in cortex and outer and inner medulla, was increased by CsA in both young and old animals (ANOVA, $p < 0.05$) (FIGURE 1). At the molecular level, CsA increased moderately the steady-state mRNA values of interstitial collagen (types I + III) in all renal regions in young rats (ANOVA, $p < 0.02$) (FIGURE 2). In old rats, by contrast, collagen mRNA levels were not changed in the cortex, but were clearly increased in outer ($p < 0.01$) and inner ($p < 0.05$) medulla (FIGURE 2). The amount of tubulointerstitial damage was increased by CsA (semiquantitative scoring on a scale from 0 to 3, from 0 to 0.59 ± 0.10 in young and from 0.70 ± 0.35 to 1.33 ± 0.91 in old rats, $p < 0.01$ for both comparisons). In the liver, morphological changes, examined after hematoxylin-eosin staining, or collagen changes, using Masson's trichrome staining, were unremarkable, suggesting specific nephrotoxicity of CsA.

The experimental conditions approximate the clinical circumstances of the older donor, in whom phases of age-associated alterations occur in the kidney, facing then CsA treatment, as part of the immunosuppressive protocol received by the recipient. In old compared to young rats, prolonged CsA administration has a resembling effect on renal function (decline in glomerular filtration), collagen content (augmented), and morphology (tubulo-interstitial injury). These findings support the notion that advanced donor age is not a contraindication in renal transplants.[6] On the other hand, the change with aging in the collagen mRNA response to CsA (FIGURE 2) indicates that further investigation is needed.

To conclude, the present study showed that prolonged CsA treatment seems to interact with aging in the rat kidney: CsA accelerates the aging damage, while the collagen mRNA response to CsA is altered by aging.

REFERENCES

1. HESS, A. D., P. M. COLOMBANI & A. H. ESA. 1986. Cyclosporine and the immune response: basic aspects. Crit. Rev. Immunol. **6**: 123–132.
2. KOPP, J. B. & P. E. KLOTMAN. 1990. Cellular and molecular mechanisms of cyclosporin nephrotoxicity. J. Am. Soc. Nephrol. **1**: 162–179.
3. ROSEN, S., Z. GREENFELD & M. BREZIS. 1990. Chronic cyclosporine-induced nephropathy in the rat. Transplantation **49**(2): 445–452.
4. STILLMAN, I. E., Z. GREENFELD, M. BREZIS & S. ROSEN. 1991. Correlation of medullary changes with progressive renal dysfunction in the aging kidney. J. Am. Soc. Nephrol. **2**: 691.
5. PELEG, I., Z. GREENFELD, H. COOPERMAN & S. SHOSHAN. 1993. Type I and type III collagen mRNA levels in kidney regions of old and young rats. Matrix **13**: 281–287.
6. O'CONNOR, K. J., J. W. BRADLEY & S. I. CHO. 1988. Extreme donor age in kidney transplantation. Transplant. Proc. **20**(5): 770–771.

Functional Significance
of Pharmacological Blocking
# of Renal Thromboxane in Old
and Young Rat Kidneys

Z. GREENFELD, M. RATHAUS,[a] AND M. BREZIS

Department of Medicine
Hadassah-University Hospital
Mt. Scopus
Jerusalem, Israel

[a]Department of Nephrology
Meir Hospital
Kfar-Saba, Israel

Arachidonic acid metabolites are autacoids that in the kidney modulate renal function.[1] Among them, the vasoconstrictor thromboxane (TXA) is produced in increased amounts in various renal diseases.[1] We have previously found that old rat kidneys synthesize more TXA than young rat kidneys in all renal regions (glomeruli, cortical tubules, outer and inner medulla).[2] In addition, glomerular TXA closely and negatively correlated with creatinine clearance [a measure of glomerular filtration rate (GFR), $r = -0.91$, $p < 0.002$].[3] A decline in GFR is characteristic of renal aging. Therefore, if TXA were involved in this phenomenon, then pharmacological blocking of TXA would increase GFR (FIGURE 1).

Nine old (age 22 months) and nine young (age 4 months) Sprague-Dawley male rats were administered a selective thromboxane synthase inhibitor, UK 38,485 (dazmegrel, Pfizer Inc.), for one week. The cumulative dose was 15 mg/kg body weight per day. The rats were injected intraperitoneally (ip) three times over 12 hours each day. The creatinine clearance was calculated before and at the conclusion of the treatment, after measuring urine and plasma creatinine. The urine was collected in metabolic cages. Creatinine clearance was slightly increased by UK 38,485 in old rats and clearly increased in young rats ($p < 0.01$) (FIGURE 2). Sodium and potassium excretion, a measure of renal tubular function, was not altered by the treatment in neither of the age groups. The selective action of UK 38,485 on TXA was confirmed by measuring various prostaglandins in the urine, before and after treatment, by a method previously described.[2] Only the levels of TXA, but not of the other prostaglandins, were lowered by dazmegrel in both old and young rats. In a separate set of experiments, a TXA receptor antagonist (SQ 29,548, Squibb) was added to the perfusate of isolated perfused kidney. This experimental device mimics renal function *ex vivo*.[4] The GFR was measured by the clearance of ^{3}H-Inulin and was evaluated before and 40 minutes after SQ 29,548 addition to the perfusate (10^{-7} M). The perfusion medium consisted of a Krebs-Ringer-Henseleit solution, 6.7 g/dl bovine serum albumin and 5 mM glucose. Experiments were performed in 3 old and 4 young rats. In all perfusions, the drug did not affect GFR (FIGURE 3).

In conclusion, in old rat kidneys, the relation between increased glomerular

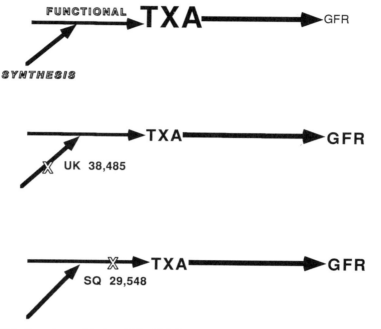

FIGURE 1. Experimental design. If the high TXA production in the old rat kidney is involved in reduction of GFR, then pharmacological blocking of functional TXA would restore, at least in part, GFR levels.

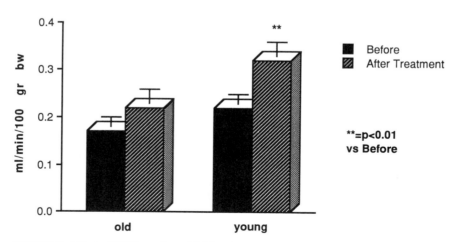

FIGURE 2. Effect of TXA synthase inhibitor UK 38,485 on GFR (measured by creatinine clearance) in old and young rats.

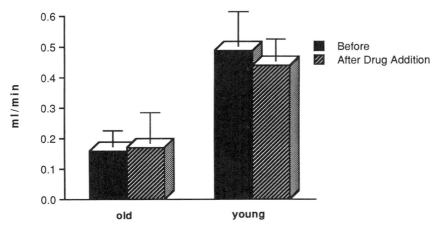

FIGURE 3. Effect of TXA receptor antagonist SQ 29,548 on GFR of old and young isolated perfused rat kidneys.

production of thromboxane and decreased GFR seems to be an associative rather than a causal one.

REFERENCES

1. COLLINS, D. M., T. M. COFFMAN & P. E. KLOTMAN. 1991. The role of thromboxane in the pathogenesis of acute renal failure. *In* Acute Renal Failure. K. Solez & L. C. Racusen, Eds.: 13–47. Marcel Dekker, Inc. New York, N.Y.
2. RATHAUS, M., Z. GREENFELD, E. PODJARNY, M. BREZIS, J. GREEN & J. BERNHEIM. 1992. Altered prostaglandin synthesis and impaired sodium conservation in the kidneys of old rats. Clin. Sci. **83**(3): 301–306.
3. GREENFELD, Z., E. PODJARNY, M. RATHAUS, J. SHAPIRA, J. BERNHEIM & M. BREZIS. 1990. Prostanoid synthesis in kidneys of old rats. J. Am. Soc. Nephrol. **1**: 442.
4. ROSS, B. D., F. H. EPSTEIN & A. LEAF. 1973. Sodium reabsorption in the perfused rat kidney. Am. J. Physiol. **225**: 1165–1171.

Prostaglandin Cytoprotection of Galactosamine-Incubated Hepatocytes Isolated from Young and Old Rats

ZBIGNIEW KMIEC

Department of Histology
Medical School Gdansk
80-210 Gdansk, Poland

INTRODUCTION

The aging process is associated with changes at cellular and tissue levels that may lead to deterioration of organ functions. Numerous age-related alterations in liver structure and functions were found. However, under basal conditions, the majority of hepatic functions are well compensated due to the great reserve capacity of this organ.[1–3] On the other hand, under exogenous or endogenous stimulation, age-related functional decrease in hepatic functions might become evident.[1,4,5] There is a higher frequency of adverse drug reactions in the elderly,[6–8] and clinical evidence suggests more severe course of hepatic failure in old patients.[9,10] Therefore any improvement in the treatment of hepatic disfunction in the elderly could be of a potentially great importance.

The cytoprotective actions of prostaglandins (PGs) were first found in experimental studies of ulcer disease.[11] However, it soon became clear that these compounds could also decrease or abolish damage caused by various noxious agents to liver[12] and other organs.[13] The cytoprotective effects of PGE_2[14,15] and of prostacyclin[16–20] elicited in isolated or cultured hepatocytes indicate that they are due to direct cellular actions of PGs. It was shown in human studies that PGE_1 improved the outcome of fulminant hepatic failure[21] and of primary graft nonfunction in liver transplant.[22] Because hepatoprotective activities of PGs have not yet been studied in old animals, we decided to determine the effects of PGE_1 and two prostacyclin analogues, 9β-methylcarbacyclin[17,19] (9MC) and TRK-100,[23] on the isolated hepatocytes of young and old rats incubated with galactosamine (GalN), a model hepatotoxin.[24]

MATERIALS AND METHODS

Animals

Male Wistar rats 4–6 and 24–29 months old ("young" and "old" respectively) were used. This strain of rats has been used in our laboratory for several years, and the characteristics of the animals have been described.[25] Animals were fed a commercial stock diet (LSM diet, Bacutil, Poland) *ad libitum* and had free access to water. The mean weight of young rats was 285 ± 5 ($n = 29$) and of old ones 373 ± 7 ($n = 28$).

Chemicals

Prostaglandin E_1 (*Prostin VR Pediatric*) was from Upjohn (Kalamazoo, Mich.). 9β-Methylcarbacyclin was a gift of Wellcome Res. Labs. (Beckenham, United Kingdom), and TRK-100 (sodium-(1R*,2R*,3aS*,8bS*)-2,3,3a,8b,-tetrahydro-2-hydroxy-1- [(E)(3S*)-3-hydroxy-4-methyl-1-octen-6-ynyl] -1H-cyclopenta-[*b*]benzofuran-5-butyrate was donated by Toray Res. Labs. (Osaka, Japan). Collagenase type IV, glucagon, and forskolin were purchased from Sigma (St. Louis, Mo.).

Preparation and Incubation of Isolated Hepatocytes

Isolated hepatocytes were prepared by *in situ* collagenase perfusion of rat liver as described previously:[19,25] $3–6 \times 10^6$ hepatocytes (>85% excluding trypan blue) were incubated at 37°C in a shaking water bath in the total volume of 2 ml of Krebs Ringer bicarbonate buffer (KRB), pH 7.4, containing 10 mM glucose, 1% dialyzed bovine serum albumin, and 0.5 μCi ^{3}H-leucine (Amersham Buchler, Germany). The rate of protein synthesis (dependent on endogenous stores of amino acids) was measured by the incorporation of ^{3}H-leucine tracer into acid precipitable material.[19,26]

The supernatant from a 0.5 ml aliquot of cell suspension was stored at −20°C for determination of lactate dehydrogenase (LDH) activity as described previously.[26] Total LDH content was determined after mixing 0.2 ml of cell suspension with 1.8 ml 0.5% Triton X-100 to lyse the cells.

Treatment of Hepatocytes with D-Galactosamine and Prostaglandins

D(+)-Galactosamine hydrochloride (Sigma) and 9β-methylcarbacyclin were prepared as described previously.[19] TRK-100 was prepared as a stock solution in sterile 0.9% NaCl (1 mg/ml) and stored at −20°C until use. Aliquots of PGE_1 (0.5 mg/ml) were lyophylized, stored at −70°C and dissolved in KRB immediately before use. Prostaglandins were added to vials at the same time as liver cells. When hepatocytes were incubated with both prostaglandin and galactosamine, the cells were preincubated with the prostaglandin for 15 min before the addition of GalN. ^{3}H-leucine was added with hepatocytes.

Determination of Adenine Nucleotides, Cyclic AMP, and Protein Content

Samples (0.8 ml) of cell suspensions were extracted at 4°C with 30 μl of 12 M perchloric acid. The precipitates were centrifuged, supernatant was neutralized with 2 M KOH to pH 6.6–8.0, and stored at −70°C. The amount of adenine nucleotides was determined by reverse-phase high-performance liquid chromatography (HPLC).[27]

Cyclic 3′,5′-adenosine-mononophosphate (cAMP) content in isolated hepatocytes was measured with radiocompetitive assay (Amersham Buchler, Germany) according to the manufacturer's instruction.

Protein was determined by the method of Lowry.[28]

Expression of Results and Statistics

Because the protein content of isolated liver cells of young and old rats was similar (2.53 ± 0.12 and 2.89 ± 0.14 mg protein $\times 10^6$ cells), all results have been expressed *per* mg protein as the mean ± standard error of the mean (SEM). Statistical significance was determined by Student's *t*-test.

RESULTS

Properties of Isolated Hepatocytes

At the beginning of incubation, mean viability (trypan bue exclusion) of hepato-cytes isolated from young and old rats was 89.7 ± 3.4% ($n = 28$) and 91.3 ± 3.9%, respectively, and did not decrease more than 10% after 2-hour long incubation. The basal LDH activity in the initial cell suspension was 0.049 ± 0.004 and 0.061 ± 0.005 U/mg cell protein in hepatocytes of young and old rats, respectively, which was equivalent to 4.73% and 5.30% of total LDH activity. The LDH release from control cells after 90 min of incubation was 8.11% and 9.35%, and after 180 min 19.82% and 17.83% of total LDH activity of hepatocytes of young and old rats, respectively.

The rate of ^{3}H-leucine incorporation into hepatocytes was linear in hepatocytes of both young and old rats for 120 min of incubation (FIGURE 1). There was a tendency towards smaller values of protein synthesis in liver cells of old rats. However, these differences were statistically significant only at one time point.

The Effects of GalN on Isolated Hepatocytes

Different concentrations of galactosamine (2.5–100 mmoles/l) were used to compare its effect on the rate of protein synthesis and LDH release in hepatocytes of young and old rats.

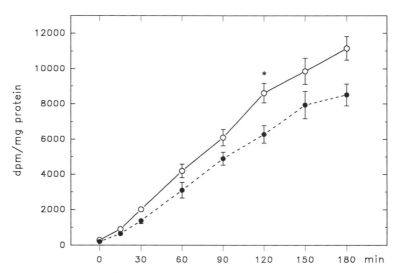

FIGURE 1. Time course of ^{3}H-leucine incorporation into isolated hepatocytes of young (open symbols) and old (filled symbols) rats. *$p < 0.05$, $n = 7$. The description of symbols is the same for all figures.

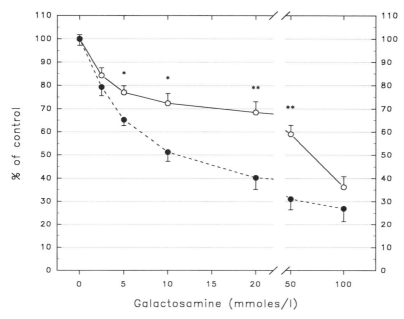

FIGURE 2. Effect of different galactosamine concentrations on ³H-leucine incorporation into cell protein. *$p < 0.05$, young vs. old, $n = 7$. Hepatocytes were incubated for 75 min with GalN.

³H-leucine incorporation into cell protein was significantly lower in hepatocytes of old rats as compared to young ones at the galactosamine concentrations of 5–50 mM (FIGURE 2). As the depression of protein synthesis in cells of old rats at the 10 mM GalN was almost twice as big as in hepatocytes of young ones, this concentration of aminosugar was chosen for the studies of prostaglandin effects on isolated liver cells.

Contrary to its effect on protein synthesis, galactosamine at 2.5–100 mmoles/l increased LDH release to a similar extent (in the range 135–360% of control values) in hepatocytes of both young and old rats.

Effects of Prostaglandins on Hepatocytes Incubated with Galactosamine

The preincubation of hepatocytes for 15 min with 9β-methylcarbacyclin before adding 10 mM GalN reduced degree of protein synthesis inhibition from 47.5% (only 10 mM GalN present) to 86.5% (82 nM 9MC and 10 mM GalN) of control values in hepatocytes of old rats, and from 72.1% (GalN only) to 85.5% of control in hepatocytes of young ones (FIGURE 3). This protective effect of 9MC was dose dependent (41–560 nM) in liver cells of old rats and was observed only at 82 nM 9MC in hepatocytes of young ones.

Preincubation of hepatocytes with 10 or 100 nM PGE₁ also led to smaller GalN-induced inhibition of ³H-leucine incorporation into isolated hepatocytes of both young and old rats (FIGURE 4). However, recovery of protein synthesis was, as in

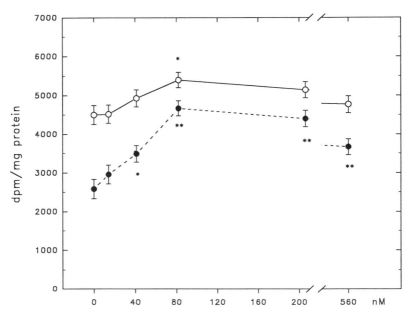

FIGURE 3. Effect of different concentrations of 9MC on protein synthesis in hepatocytes incubated for 1 h with 10 mM galactosamine. Control values (no GalN) were 6260 ± 830 and 5480 ± 760 dpm/mg/75 min for hepatocytes of young and old rats, respectively. *,**$p < 0.05$ and $p < 0.001$ vs. 10 mM GalN only, $n = 7$.

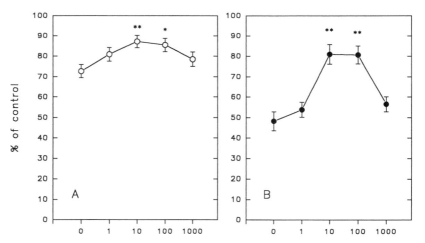

FIGURE 4. Effect of PGE$_1$ on protein synthesis in hepatocytes of (A) young and (B) old rats incubated for 1 h with 10 mM GalN. *,**$p < 0.05$ and $p < 0.001$ vs. 10 GalN only, $n = 7$.

the case of 9MC, not complete, and reached 80% of control values in hepatocytes of old, and 85% in cells of young rats.

TRK-100, another prostacyclin analogue, did not influence GalN-related depression of protein synthesis in isolated hepatocytes of either old or young rats (data not shown).

The preincubation of isolated liver cells of young and old rats with prostaglandins before adding 10 mM galactosamine did not affect the rate of LDH release from the cells (data not shown).

None of the prostaglandins tested changed the rate of LDH release or ³H-leucine incorporation into control hepatocytes of young or old rats (data not shown).

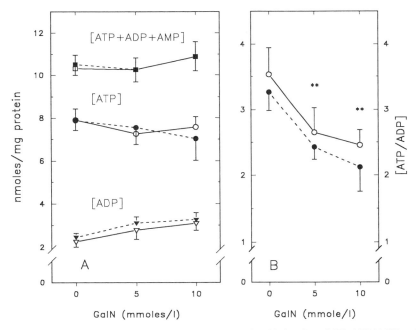

FIGURE 5. Effect of galactosamine on (A) adenine nucleotide levels and (B) ATP/ADP ratio in hepatocytes of young and old rats. Symbols represent means ± standard deviation. *$p < 0.01$ vs. control, $n = 4$.

Adenine Nucleotide Content in Hepatocytes Incubated with Galactosamine

Galactosamine at the concentrations of 5 and 10 mM significantly increased ADP and AMP, and decreased ATP content in hepatocytes of young and old rats (FIGURE 5A). As a result, there was a significant decrease in the ATP/ADP ratio (FIGURE 5B) which, however, was not age related. None of the prostaglandins used affected adenine nucleotide content of hepatocytes incubated with galactosamine (data not shown).

The Effects of Prostaglandins on Cyclic AMP Content of Hepatocytes

As shown in FIGURE 6 both PGE_1 and 9β-methylcarbacyclin increased cAMP level in isolated liver cells of young, but not of old, rats. This effect was rather small as compared to glucagon-induced rise in intracellular cyclic AMP. TRK-100 did not influence cAMP content in hepatocytes of either young or old rats. Forskolin increased cAMP content to a similar extent in hepatocytes of both young and old rats.

DISCUSSION

Galactosamine has been widely used as a model hepatotoxin because it produces reversible liver damage that morphologically and biochemically resembles human

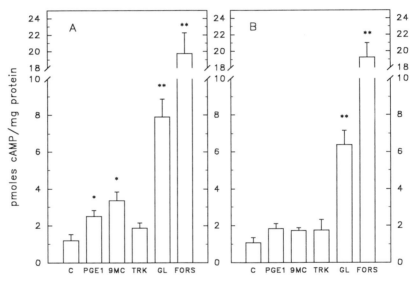

FIGURE 6. Effect of PGE_1 (0.1 μM), 9MC (0.2 μM), TRK-100 (0.1 μM), glucagon (GL, 0.1 μM), and forskolin (FORS, 10 μM) on cyclic AMP content of isolated hepatocytes of (A) young and (B) old rats. *,**$p < 0.05$ and $p < 0.001$ vs. control (C), respectively.

hepatitis.[24] Biochemical lesions induced in liver by GalN involve depletion of uridine nucleotides and accumulation of UDP-sugars resulting in the inhibition of transcription and translation, and supression of glycogen and UDP-glucuronic acid synthesis.[29] Additionally, activation of macrophages and neutrophils plays also a prominent role in the development of galactosamine-hepatitis.[29,30]

Despite frequent use of GalN in toxicological studies, the effect of aging on GalN hepatotoxicity has been investigated by only few authors. Platt *et al.*[31] found increased hepatocellular damage caused by GalN in old female Wistar rats as compared to young animals. In contrast, Rikans[32] reported similar extent of GalN-induced liver damage in young, middle-aged, and old male Fischer 344 rats. In an *in vitro* system, Abdul and Mehendale[33] added 5 mM galactosamine to cultured hepatocytes of 14- and 24-month-old male Sprague-Dawley rats for 12, 24, 48, or 60 hours and measured percentage of nonviable cells (trypan blue exclusion), LDH leakage, and uridine nucleotide levels. They found that cultured hepatocytes of old rats were less sensitive to toxic effects of GalN than the cells of adult ones. However, a careful reexamination of their data reveals that control hepatocytes of adult rats in 24- and 48-hour-old cultures already showed about 3 times higher LDH release and 3 times smaller viability than control cells of old rats. After recalculation, their data show that in fact GalN affected LDH release and cell viability to a similar extent in cultured hepatocytes of both age groups.[33] The data on uridine nucleotide levels in cells cultured in the presence of GalN[33] suggest that, to some extent, a dedifferentiation process would have to take place as the levels of UTP were rather high (50% of control) as compared to the *in vivo* GalN action on the liver.[24] It is likely that the discrepancy between results of Abdul and Mehendale[33] and results of the present study is caused by different methodology and differences in strains of rats used. Although cellular levels of uridine nucleotides were not measured in the present investigation, it was shown by other authors[34] that UTP, UDP, and UMP levels dropped rapidly in isolated hepatocytes of young rats incubated with 4 mM GalN. It is therefore not possible that differences in the content of uridine nucleotides or adenine nucleotides (FIGURE 5) could explain greater inhibition of protein synthesis in GalN-exposed hepatocytes of old rats. Probably some age-related changes in translation apparatus might be responsible for this effect.

The observations showing hepatoprotective effects of some prostaglandins[12,14–20] in young animals have been extended in the present investigation on hepatocytes isolated from old rats. This *in vitro* system allows us to exclude extrahepatic (i.e., vasoactive or immunomodulatory) effects of prostaglandins.[35,36] None of the prostaglandins tested decreased GalN-induced LDH leakage, which suggests that they did not interfere with mechanisms leading to the ultimate cell injury in about 15% of all incubated hepatocytes. However, preincubation of cells with 9β-methylcarbacyclin and PGE$_1$ improved the rate of protein synthesis in the remaining partially damaged hepatocytes of young and old rats (FIGURES 3 and 4). The cytoprotective effects of prostaglandins on liver cells of old rats were not reported earlier. As the GalN-induced supression of protein synthesis was higher in liver cells of old rats, this protective effect of PGs was more prominent in those cells. However, some factors responsible for the inhibition of translation by GalN did not respond to prostaglandins, as the reversal of protein synthesis inhibition was not complete.

It was suggested that cyclic AMP might protect rat hepatocytes from immunologically mediated injury.[37] Although PGE$_1$ and prostacyclin activate adenylate cyclase in many cell systems,[35] the way(s) through which PGE$_1$ and 9β-methylcarbacyclin exerted cytoprotective action in our experimental system must involve other mechanisms. Both PGs protected hepatocytes of young and old rats but increased cyclic AMP levels only in cells of young animals. It should be noted that the reactivity of hepatocytes from old rats to glucagon, which stimulates adenyl cyclase through another receptor system, and to forskolin, which directly stimulates adenyl cyclase, was well preserved (FIGURE 6). Lack of hepatocytoprotective effect of TRK-100 demonstrates that cytoprotective properties of PGs might be pronounced in some[23] but not in all experimental models.

On the basis of the obtained data, it is not possible to determine the mechanisms involved in the improvement of protein synthesis in hepatocytes preincubated with prostaglandins. Nevertheless, the data provide strong evidence that some prostaglandins and their analogues exert direct cytoprotective effects on hepatocytes of old animals. The results substantiate the need for further research on possible therapeutical use of prostaglandins in hepatic failure of the elderly.

SUMMARY

The aim of the study was to investigate the effect of aging on cytoprotective properties of prostaglandins. Hepatocytes were obtained by collagenase perfusion of livers of young (4–6 mo) and old (24–28 mo) male Wistar rats. Cells were incubated for 1.5 h in Krebs-Ringer-bicarbonate buffer containing glucose and ^{3}H-leucine in the presence of galactosamine (2.5–100 mM), PGE_1, or two prostacyclin analogues: 9β-methylcarbacyclin and TRK-100. Cell damage was assessed by decrease in the rate of protein synthesis measured as ^{3}H-leucine incorporation into acid precipitable material, and by increase in lactate dehydrogenase release into the medium. Hepatocytes from old rats were more susceptible to supression of protein synthesis by GalN than cells of young ones. Preincubation of cells for 15 min with 9MC (41–560 nM) or PGE_1 (10–100 nM), but not with TRK-100, before adding 10 mM GalN, led to a partial recovery of protein synthesis in both age groups. GalN increased LDH release and decreased ATP/ADP ratio to a similar extent in hepatocytes of young and old rats; both parameters were not altered by preincubation of cells with PGs. PGE_1 and 9MC, but not TRK-100, elevated cyclic AMP content in hepatocytes of young but not old rats. Glucagon and forskolin similarly increased cyclic AMP content in cells of both young and old animals. These *in vitro* results suggest that PGE_1 and some prostacyclin analogues might protect hepatocytes of both young and old rats from chemical damage, and stress the necessity for further research on cyto- and hepatoprotection in the elderly.

ACKNOWLEDGMENTS

The author is greatly indebted to Professor A. Mysliwski for his continuous encouragement and valuable criticism.

REFERENCES

1. KITANI, K. 1991. Arch. Gerontol. Geriatr. **12:** 133–154.
2. POPPER, H. 1986. *In* Progress in Liver Disease. H. Popper & F. Schaffner, Eds. **8:** 659–683. Greene and Stratton. Orlando, Fla.
3. WOODHOUSE, K. & H. A. WYNNE. 1992. Drugs Aging **2:** 243–255.
4. KMIEC, Z. & A. MYSLIWSKI. 1983. Exp. Gerontol. **18:** 173–184.
5. MYSLIWSKI, A. & Z. KMIEC. 1992. Arch. Gerontol. Geriatr. **14:** 85–92.
6. DURNAS, CH., CH. LOI & B. CUSACK. 1990. Clin. Pharmacokinet. **19:** 359–389.
7. FARRELL, G. C. 1986. Therapeutics **145:** 600–604.
8. RODRIGUEZ, L. A. G., S. P. GUTTHANN, A. M. WALKER & L. LUECK. 1992. Br. Med. J. **305:** 865–868.
9. TAGGART, H. M. A. & J. M. ALDERICE. 1982. Br. Med. J. **284:** 1372–1378.
10. O'GRADY, J. G., G. J. M. ALEXANDER, K. M. HAYLLAR & R. WILLIAMS. 1989. Gastroenterology **97:** 439–445.
11. ROBERT, A. 1979. Gastroenterology **77:** 761–767.
12. STACHURA, J., A. TARNAWSKI, J. SZCZUDRAWA, J. BOGDAL, T. MACH, B. KLIMCZYK & S. KIRCHMAYER. 1980. Folia Histochem. Cytochem. **18:** 311–318.
13. HOHLFELD, T., H. STROBACH & K. SCHROR. 1992. J. Pharmacol. Exp. Therap. **264:** 397–405.
14. FUNK-BRENTANO, C., M. TINEL & C. DEGOTT. 1984. Biochem. Pharmacol. **33:** 89–96.
15. NASSERI-SINA, P., C. E. SEDDON, A. R. BOOBIS & D. S. DAVIES. 1987. Biochem. Soc. Trans. **16:** 641–642.

16. GUARNER, F., M. FREMONT-SMITH & J. PRIETO. 1985. Liver 5: 35–39.
17. NODA, Y., R. D. HUGHES & R. WILLIAMS. 1986. J. Hepatol. 2: 53–64.
18. NASSERI-SINA, P., D. J. FAWTHROP, J. WILSON, A. R. BOOBIS & D. S. DAVIES. 1992. Br. J. Pharmacol. 105(2): 417–423.
19. GOVE, C. D., R. D. HUGHES, Z. KMIEC, Y. NODA & R. WILLIAMS. 1990. Prostagl. Leukotr. Essent. Fatty Acids 40: 73–77.
20. BURSCH, W., H. S. TAPER, M. P. SOMER, S. MEYER, B. PUTZ & R. SCHULTE-HERMANN. 1989. Hepatology 9: 830–838.
21. BLENDIS, L. M. & G. A. LEVY. 1991. In Acute Liver Failure. R. Williams & R. D. Hughes, Eds.: 53–56. Smith Kline Beecham. Welwyn Garden, England.
22. MOLLISON, L. C., P. W. ANGUS & R. M. JONES. 1991. Med. J. Austr. 155: 51–53.
23. SAKAI, A., M. YAJIMA & S. NISHIO. 1990. Life Sci. 47: 711–719.
24. DECKER, K. & D. KEPPLER. 1974. Rev. Physiol. Biochem. Pharmacol. 71: 78–106.
25. KMIEC, Z. & A. MYSLIWSKI. 1985. Exp. Gerontol. 20: 271–277.
26. GOVE, C. D., R. D. HUGHES & R. WILLIAMS. 1982. Br. J. Exp. Pathol. 63: 547–553.
27. SMOLENSKI, R., D. R. LACHNO, S. J. M. LEDINGHAM & M. H. YACOUB. 1990. J. Chromatogr. 527: 414–420.
28. LOWRY, O. H., N. J. ROSENBROUGH, A. L. FARR & R. J. RANDALL. 1951. J. Biol. Chem. 193: 265–275.
29. MACDONALD, J. R., J. H. BECKSTAED & E. A. SMUCKLER. 1987. Br. J. Exp. Pathol. 68: 189–199.
30. KMIEC, Z., R. D. HUGHES, K. P. MOORE, N. SHERON, C. D. GOVE, K. T. NOURI-ARIA & R. WILLIAMS. 1993. Hepato-Gastroenterol. 40: 259–261.
31. PLATT, D., K. FORSTER & L. C. FORSTER. 1978. Mech. Age. Dev. 7: 183–188.
32. RIKANS, L. E. 1984. Toxicol. Appl. Pharmacol. 73: 243–249.
33. ABDUL-HUSSAIN, S. K. & H. M. MEHENDALE. 1991. Toxicol. Appl. Pharmacol. 107: 504–513.
34. STERMANN, R., S. R. WAGLE & K. DECKER. 1978. Eur. J. Biochem. 88: 79–85.
35. MONCADA, S., R. J. FLOWER & J. R. VANE. 1986. In The Pharmacological Basis of Therapeutics, A. G. Gilman, Ed.: 660–673. Macmillan Publishing. New York, NY.
36. ZURIER, R. B. 1990. Adv. Prostagl. Thrombox. Leukotr. Res. 21: 947–953.
37. KUREBAYASHI, Y. & Y. HONDA. 1991. Hepatology 14: 545–550.

Effects of Lactobacilli on Interferon Production in Young and Aged Mice[a]

M. MUSCETTOLA,[b,d] L. MASSAI,[b] C. TANGANELLI,[b]
AND G. GRASSO[c]

*Institutes of General Physiology[b] and
Human Anatomy[c]
53100 Siena, Italy*

INTRODUCTION

It is well established that yogurt bacteria have immunomodulatory and immuno-stimulating activities in experimental animals and man. In mice, a diet supplemented with yogurt containing viable lactobacilli induces an increase in antibody production, a modification of splenocyte surface antigens, and an increase in their proliferative response to PHA and ConA.[1,2] Furthermore, it potentiates the host's cell-mediated immune response by increasing the percentage of B lymphocytes and the PHA- and LPS-induced proliferative responses of Peyer's patch cell suspensions.[3] *In vitro* lactobacilli increase interferon-γ (IFN-γ) production by ConA-stimulated human peripheral blood mononuclear cells and NK activity.[4] The mechanism responsible for these immunomodulatory properties of lactobacilli is not clear, nor are their effects on IFN production *in vivo*.

Because reduction of cytokine production with age, primarily IFN-γ,[5,6] IFN-β,[6] interleukin-1 (IL-1),[7-9] and IL-2,[10,11] has been well documented, in the present study, we evaluated the effect on IFN production of supplementing the diet of young and aged mice with live *Lactobacillus bulgaricus* and *Streptococcus thermophilus*.

MATERIALS AND METHODS

Sixty young (7-week-old) and 16 old (19-month-old) female Balb/c mice were randomly allocated to two different groups (control and treated). The mice were housed at a constant temperature (22°C ± 2°C) with a 12 h light/dark cycle and a standard diet and water *ad libitum*. The treated animals drank water with 2% glucose containing viable or heat-killed (90°C for 15 min) *Lactobacillus bulgaricus* and *Streptococcus thermophilus* (1:1) at a concentration of 8×10^8 bacteria per day per animal for 7 and 15 days. The controls drank only water with 2% glucose. The mice were sacrificed by cervical dislocation. The spleen was removed and teased in RPMI 1640. After washing, the splenocytes were stimulated for 72 h with ConA (5 μg/ml at 37°C) and for 24 h with LPS (2 μg/ml at 26°C).[12] The microplaque reduction assay, described elsewhere,[13] was used throughout for the titration of IFN activity using L929 cells as indicator cells and vesicular stomatitis virus as challenge virus. Each assay included the international standards for mouse IFN-α, -β, and -γ to check the

[a]Work supported in part by 40% and 60% funds from MURST, Rome, Italy.

[d]Address for correspondence: Institute of General Physiology, Via Del Laterino 8, 53100 Siena, Italy.

TABLE 1. Body and Spleen Weights in Young and Aged Mice Fed with 8×10^8 Live and Heat-Killed Lactobacilli per Day per Animal for 7 Days (Mean ± Standard Deviation)

	Body Weight (g)		
	Before Treatment	After Treatment	Spleen Weight (g)
Aged controls ($n = 8$)[a]	16.10 ± 2.97	16.32 ± 3.44	0.146 ± 0.04
Aged mice ($n = 8$)			
fed with live lactobacilli	16.05 ± 3.45	16.42 ± 3.34	0.147 ± 0.03
Young controls ($n = 10$)	15.26 ± 1.06	17.02 ± 1.2	0.065 ± 0.01
Young mice ($n = 10$)			
fed with live lactobacilli	15.31 ± 0.99	15.97 ± 1.06	0.063 ± 0.01
Young mice ($n = 10$)			
fed with dead lactobacilli	14.71 ± 0.95	15.45 ± 0.92	0.064 ± 0.01

[a]n: numbers of mice.

sensitivity and reproducibility of our test system. Samples were tested at least twice in quadruplicate. IFN activity was expressed in IU/ml, and typing was carried out using specific anti-IFN monoclonal antibodies. The data were processed by ANOVA. Differences were considered statistically significant for $p < 0.05$.

RESULTS

The body weight of control and treated mice, before and after treatment, is shown in TABLE 1. Spleen weight of control mice increased with age. IFN-γ production by ConA-stimulated splenocytes from control and treated mice of the two age groups is shown in FIGURE 1. IFN-α production by LPS-stimulated spleen cells from control and treated mice is shown in FIGURE 2. IFN-γ and IFN-α production in young mice fed with live and killed lactobacilli for 15 days is shown in FIGURE 3. Splenocytes from aged mice produced significantly lower IFN-γ and

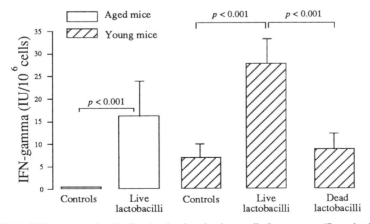

FIGURE 1. IFN-γ production by ConA-stimulated spleen cells from young (7-week-old) and old (19-month-old) mice fed with 8×10^8 live and dead lactobcilli per day for 7 days.

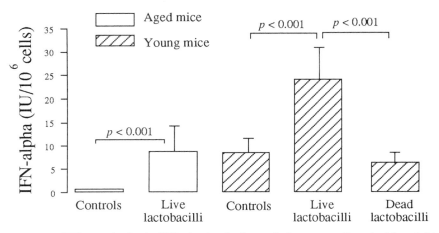

FIGURE 2. IFN-α production by LPS-stimulated spleen cells from young (7-week-old) and old (19-month-old) mice fed with 8×10^8 live and dead lactobcilli per day for 7 days.

IFN-α levels than those of young mice. Viable lactobacilli in the diet for 7 days completely restored IFN production in aged mice and significantly increased IFN production in young mice compared to controls ($p < 0.001$). Viable lactobacilli in the diet for 15 days significantly increased IFN production in young mice compared to controls ($p < 0.001$). Dead bacteria had no effect. Transmission electron microscopy of Peyer's patches (FIGURES 4 and 5) showed that many bacteria adhered selectively to the luminal surface of the M cells, specialized cells that take up gut luminal antigens and deliver them to underlying lymphoid cells in the dome region.

DISCUSSION

This study confirms and extends results previously reported by us[5,6] and others[14,15] on age-related decline in IFN production. In fact, it demonstrates that mitogen-stimulated spleen cells from aged mice produce significantly lower IFN-γ and -α levels than those of young mice. These findings are in agreement with reports of an age-related alteration in IFN-β,[6] IL-1,[7-9] IL-2,[10,11] IL-3,[16,17] and IL-4[16] production, suggesting that cytokines may play an important role in the decline of immune function.[6]

Because lactobacilli have immunomodulatory activities and increase IFN-γ production by human peripheral blood mononuclear cells *in vitro,*[4] we evaluated the influence of oral administration of *L. bulgaricus* and *S. thermophilus* on *ex vivo* IFN-α and -γ production and on the restoration of IFN levels in aged mice. The results show that a diet supplemented with lactobacilli for 7 and 15 days significantly increased IFN-α and -γ production in young mice and completely restored the cytokine levels in aged animals with respect to controls. This increased IFN-γ production is in line with immunostimulatory activities of lactobacilli such as increased proliferation of splenocytes and Peyer's patch cell suspensions in response to PHA, ConA, and LPS[2,3] and enhanced NK cell function.[4] Although the mechanism responsible for these immunostimulatory properties of lactobacilli is not clear, the available data suggest the involvement of IFN-γ and confirm that antigens introduced into the small intestine induce both local and systemic responses.

Peyer's patches are lymphoid aggregates located along the small intestine. They are characterized by a specialized follicle-associated epithelium which includes M cells differentiated for the uptake and transport of intestinal antigens to the underlying lymphoid cells in the dome region. M cell numbers increase after transfer of specific pathogen-free mice to a normal animal house environment[18] or after oral administration of nonpathogenic *Salmonella typhimurium aroA* ⁻.[19] M cells are able to translocate indigenous enteric bacteria[20] and whole noninvasive enteropathogen bacteria[21] from the intestinal lumen to underlying lymphoid tissue. Our preliminary results show that the proportion of M cells and lymphocytes observed in the

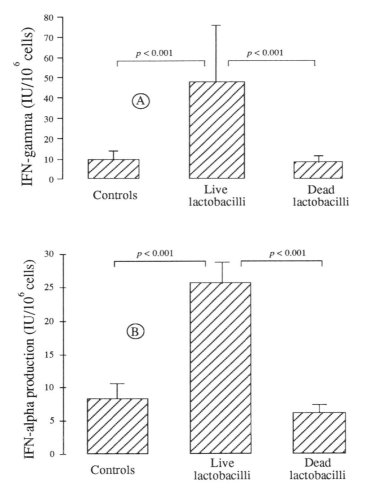

FIGURE 3. IFN-γ and -α production by spleen cells from young mice fed with live and dead lactobacilli for 15 days.

basolateral pocket was significantly higher in mice fed with live lactobacilli than in controls (data not shown). The immunogenicity of intestinal bacteria depends on the degree of mucosal adhesive properties,[22] and killed bacteria are inefficient antigens when given orally.[23] In our experiments, heat-killed bacteria had no effect on cytokine production, probably due to their rapid clearance from the small intestine. Transmission electron microscopy of ileal Peyer's patches from mice fed with viable lactobacilli showed numerous bacteria, particularly S. thermophilus, selectively adhering to luminal surface of M cells. This selective association with M cells suggests that there is translocation of lactobacilli to underlying lymphoid tissue. In fact, lactobacilli have recently been observed in mesenteric lymph node after microbial colonization in germ-free mice.[24] Lactobacilli reaching the dome region of Peyer's patches stimulate mucosal immune response, with local production of IFN-γ by γδT cells.[25] This may increase the M cell population[6] with subsequent rapid amplification of bacterial translocation. Finally, IFN-γ enhances expression of the secretory component, thus playing an important role in increasing external transport of dimeric IgA.[26] The entire array of antigens derived from lactobacilli could induce an efficient mucosal immune response against potentially harmful intestinal microflora and enteropathogenic microorganisms.

In conclusion, this study is in line with previous data on the age-related decline in IFN production. It confirms the immunostimulating effects of live *Lactobacillus bulgaricus* and *Streptococcus thermophilus* on cytokine production, suggesting that such effects can be partially modulated by increased secretion of these cytokines. It

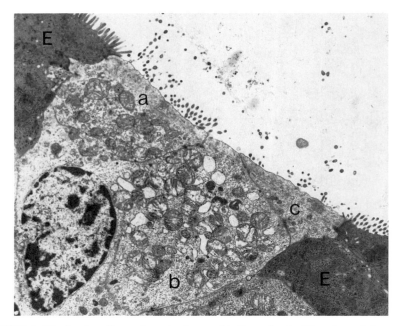

FIGURE 4. Distribution of bacteria on the dome epithelium of an ileal Peyer's patch from mice fed with viable lactobacilli. Numerous bacteria selectively adhere to luminal surface of three M cells (*a, b, c*). Note absence of microvilli in M cells compared with the two adjacent enterocytes. Transmission electron micrograph: × 4500.

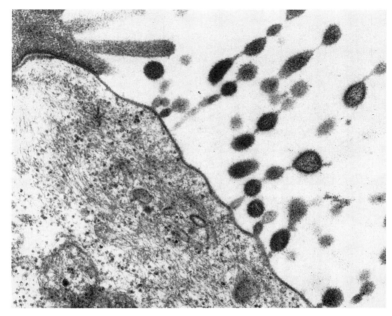

FIGURE 5. Apical cytoplasm of an M cell (cell *a* of FIGURE 4) and an enterocyte (*upper left corner*). Note selective association of *Streptococcus thermophilus* with M cells. Transmission electron micrograph: × 30,000.

also demonstrates that oral administration may restore IFN production in aged mice. Moreover it confirms the local and systemic immunomodulatory activity of live *Lactobacillus bulgaricus* and *Streptococcus thermophilus* and justifies their therapeutic use in the elderly.

REFERENCES

1. CONGE, G. A., P. GOUACHE, J. P. DESORMEAU-BEDOT, F. LOISILLIER & D. LEMONNIER. 1980. Effects comparés d'un regime enrichi en yoghourt vivant ou thermisé sur le système immunitaire de la souris. Repr. Nutr. Dev. **20:** 929–937.
2. VESELY, R., R. NEGRI, B. BIANCHI SALVADORI, D. LAVEZZARI & C. DE SIMONE. 1985. Influence of a diet additioned with yogurt on the mouse immune system. EOS J. Immunol. Immunopharmacol. **1:** 30–35.
3. DE SIMONE, C., R. VESELY, R. NEGRI, B. BIANCHI SALVADORI, S. ZANZOGLU, A. CILLI & L. LUCCI. 1987. Enhancement of immune response of murine Peyer's patches by a diet supplemented with yogurt. Immunopharmacol. Immunotoxicol. **9:** 87–100.
4. DE SIMONE, C., B. BIANCHI SALVADORI, R. NEGRI, M. FERRAZZI, L. BALDINELLI & R. VESELY. 1986. The adjuvant effect of yogurt on production of gamma-interferon by ConA-stimulated human peripheral blood lymphocytes. Nutr. Rep. Int. **33:** 419–433.
5. GRASSO, G., M. MUSCETTOLA, R. STECCONI, M. MUZZIOLI & N. FABRIS. 1992. Restorative effect of thymomodulin and zinc on interferon-gamma production in aged mice. Ann. N.Y. Acad. Sci. **673:** 256–259.
6. GRASSO, G., P. MIGLIACCIO, C. TANGANELLI, M. A. BRUGO & M. MUSCETTOLA. Restor-

ative effect of *Bacillus subtilis* spores on interferon production in aged mice. Ann. N.Y. Acad. Sci. (This volume.)

7. BRULEY-ROSSET, M. & I. VERGNON. 1984. Interleukin-1 synthesis and activity in aged mice. Mech. Ageing Dev. **24:** 247–254.

8. INAMIZU, T., M.-P. CHANG & T. MAKINODAN. 1985. Influence of age on the production and regulation of interleukin-1 in mice. Immunology **55:** 447–455.

9. SAUDER, D. N., U. PONNAPPAN & B. CINADER. 1989. Effect of age on cutaneous interleukin 1 expression. Immunol. Lett. **20:** 111–114.

10. THOMAN, M. L. & W. O. WEIGLE. 1981. Lymphokines and ageing: interleukin-2 production and activity in aged animals. J. Immunol. **127:** 2102–2106.

11. MILLER, R. A. & O. STUTMAN. 1981. Decline in aging mice of the anti-2,4,6 trinitrophenyl (TNP) cytotoxic T cell response attributable in loss of Lyt-2-, interleukin-2 producing helper cell function. Eur. J. Immunol. **11:** 751–756.

12. CEMBRZYNSKA-NOWAK, M. 1986. Interferons from mouse lymphocytes produced at various temperatures (26°C and 37°C). Arch. Immunol. Ther. Exp. **34:** 525–532.

13. MUSCETTOLA, M. & G. GRASSO. 1990. Somatostatin and vasoactive intestinal peptide reduce interferon gamma production by human peripheral blood mononuclear cells. Immunobiology **180:** 419–430.

14. DE MAYER, E. & J. DE MAYER-GUIGNARD. 1968. Influence of animal genotype and age on the amount of circulating interferon induced by Newcastle disease virus. J. Gen. Virol. **2:** 445–449.

15. BLACH-OLSZEWSKA, Z., M. CEMBRZYNSKA-NOWAK & E. KWASNIEWSKA. 1984. Age-related synthesis of spontaneous interferon in BALBtc mice. Contr. Oncol. **20:** 224–232.

16. KUBO, M. & B. CINADER. 1990. Polymorphism of age-related changes in interleukin (IL) production: differential changes of T helper subpopulations, synthesizing IL 2, IL 3, IL 4. Eur. J. Immunol. **20:** 1289–1296.

17. KUBO, M. & B. CINADER. 1990. IL-3 production as a function of age and its correlation with splenomegaly: age versus disease-related change. Immunol. Lett. **24:** 133–136.

18. SMITH, M. W., P. S. JAMES & D. R. TIVEY. 1987. M cell numbers increase after transfer of SPF mice to a normal animal house environment. Am. J. Pathol. **128:** 385–389.

19. SAVIDGE, T. C., M. W. SMITH, P. S. JAMES & P. ALDRED. 1991. Salmonella-induced M-cell formation in germ-free mouse Peyer's patch tissue. Am. J. Pathol. **139:** 177–184.

20. BERG, R. D. & A. W. GARLINGTON. 1979. Translocation of certain indigenous bacteria from the gastrointestinal tract to the mesenteric lymph nodes and other organs in a gnotobiotic mouse model. Infect. Immun. **23:** 403–411.

21. OWEN, R. L., N. F. PIERCE, R. T. APPLE & W. C. CRAY, JR. 1986. M cell transport of *Vibrio cholerae* from the intestinal lumen into Peyer's patches: a mechanism for antigen sampling and for microbial transepithelial migration. J. Infect. Dis. **153:** 1108–1118.

22. TSE, S.-K. & K. CADEE. 1991. The interaction between interstitial mucus glycoproteins and enteric infections. Parasitol. Today **7:** 163–172.

23. PIERCE, N. F., J. B. KAPER, J. J. MEKALANOS, W. C. CRAY, JR. & K. RICHARDSON. 1987. Determinants of the immunogenicity of live virulent and mutant *Vibrio cholerae* O1 in rabbit intestine. Infect. Immun. **55:** 477–481.

24. UMESAKI, Y., H. SETOYAMA, S. MATSUMOTO & Y. OKADA. 1993. Expansion of $\alpha\beta$ T-cell receptor–bearing intestinal intraepithelial lymphocytes after microbial colonization in germ-free mice and its independence from thymus. Immunology **79:** 32–37.

25. TAGUCHI, T., W. K. AICHER, K. FUJIHASHI, M. YAMAMOTO, J. R. McGHEE, J. A. BLUESTONE & H. KIYONO. 1991. Novel function for intestinal intraepithelial lymphocytes. Murine CD3+, γ/δ TCR+ T cells produce IFN-γ and IL-5. J. Immunol. **147:** 3736–3744.

26. SOLLID, L. M., D. KVALE, P. BRANDTZAEG, G. MARKUSSEN & E. THORSBY. 1987. Interferon-γ enhances expression of secretory component, the epithelial receptor for polymeric immunoglobulins. J. Immunol. **138:** 4303–4306.

The Effect of Aging and Acetyl-L-carnitine on the Function and on the Lipid Composition of Rat Heart Mitochondria[a]

G. PARADIES, F. M. RUGGIERO, G. PETROSILLO, M. N.
GADALETA, AND E. QUAGLIARIELLO

*Department of Biochemistry and Molecular Biology
and C.N.R. Unit for the Study of Mitochondria and Bioenergetics
University of Bari
Bari, Italy*

INTRODUCTION

Aging is associated with alterations of various aspects of cell functions. It is a common observation that aged animals tend to be less energetic. The molecular basis of this age-linked decline in energy metabolism is still not well understood.[1] At the cardiac level, aging is associated with a decline in functional competence. Mitochondrial membranes are considered a likely subcellular locus of the age-linked decline of energy metabolism due to their central role in the energy transduction pathways. In fact, the metabolism of the mitochondrion occurs within a membrane of highly restrictive permeability properties, which has the effect of erecting barriers across the pathways of metabolism.

The well-recognized age-dependent decrements in heart performance may be related to age-related changes in the mitochondrial membrane lipids which influence the activities of diverse membrane-bound enzymes.[2–4] Changes in membrane lipid content, lipid composition, and lipid protein interaction may occur with aging. For example, the activities of cardiac mitochondrial transport systems including adenine nucleotide, acyl-carnitine, pyruvate, and phosphate decrease with aging.[4,5–9] These changes in transporting activity have been related, at least in part, to alteration of mitochondrial membrane lipids.

Cytochrome oxidase is the terminal enzyme complex of the mitochondrial electron transport chain and catalyzes electron transfer from reduced cytochrome c to molecular oxygen. This enzyme is a vital component of cellular energy transduction responsible for virtually all oxygen consumption in mammals. The activity of this enzyme complex is controlled by the physicochemical status of the phospholipid of the mitochondrial membrane. Particularly, cytochrome oxidase is highly dependent on cardiolipin for maximal activity.[10,11]

Acetyl-L-carnitine is a natural biomolecule which acts by stimulating energy metabolism,[12] although its molecular mechanism of action is still not well known. However, many different effects of acute treatment of aged rats with this compound have been reported.[13–16] We have recently found that mitochondrial content of cardiolipin is decreased with aging and that the treatment of aged rats with acetyl-L-carnitine restores the normal level of this phospholipid in the inner mitochon-

[a]This work has been accomplished with funds from Ministero Pubblica Istruzione (60%) and Consiglio Nazionale delle Ricerche (P. F. "Invecchiamento" cod. no. 931334).

233

drial membrane.[17] These changes in cardiolipin content were associated with parallel changes in the activity of the mitochondrial phosphate carrier.

In this work, the effect of aging on the activity of cytochrome c oxidase and on membrane lipid composition in rat heart mitochondria was examined. The effects of treatment of aged animals with acetyl-L-carnitine on the activity of cytochrome oxidase and adenine nucleotide translocase, on respiratory activity, and on membrane lipid composition were also examined.

MATERIALS AND METHODS

Animals

Male Fisher rats of 5–7 (young) or 26–28 (aged) months were used throughout these studies. Young and aged rats were injected intraperitoneally with 300 mg/kg bw of acetyl-L-carnitine[17] and killed three hours after.

Rat heart mitochondria were prepared by differential centrifugation of heart homogenates essentially as described previously.[18]

Mitochondrial protein concentration was measured by the usual biuret method using serum albumin as standard.

Kinetic Studies of Cytochrome c Oxidase Activity

Cytochrome oxidase activity in freshly isolated mitochondria was measured polarographically with an oxygen electrode at 25°C. The medium was 100 mM KCl, 20 mM Na-Hepes, and 5 mM $MgCl_2$ (pH 7.4). For K_m determinations, 10 mM ascorbate, 0.05 Triton X-100, 1 mM TMPD ($NNN'N$-tetramethyl p-phenylenediamine), varying concentrations of cytochrome c (1 to 100 μM), and 0.15–0.20 mg of mitochondrial protein were present in a final volume of 1 ml. Horse heart cytochrome c (type VI, Sigma St. Louis, Mo.) was used for all experiments. Rates of oxygen uptake were corrected for autooxidation measured in the absence of mitochondria. Kinetic parameters were determined graphically from Lineweaver-Burk double reciprocal plots.

Determination of Mitochondrial Cytochrome aa₃ Content

Heme aa_3 content was determined from ΔA_{605} of reduced-minus-oxidized difference spectra.[19] Extinction coefficent values of 24 $mM^{-1}cm^{-1}$ were used.[20]

Determination of ADP Transport

The transport of ADP in mitochondria was measured by the inhibitor stop method, essentially as described in Reference 21.

Analysis of Lipids in Mitochondrial Membranes

Phospholipids and fatty acids were analyzed by high pressure liquid chromatography (HPLC) using a Beckman 344 gradient liquid chromatograph. Lipids from heart mitochondria were extracted with chloroform/methanol by the procedure used by Bligh and Dyer.[22] Phospholipids were separated by the HPLC method previously described[23] with an Altex ultrasil-Si column (4.6 × 250 mm).

To analyze fatty acids, heart mitochondria were saponified with 5% HOH in 50% aqueous methanol for 40 min at 90°C. After acidification, the solution was first extracted with chloroform, next dried, and then esterified with m-methoxyphenancyl-bromide for HPLC analysis.

Results are expressed as mean ± standard error (SE). Statistical significances were determined by Student's *t*-test.

RESULTS

Polarographic assays of cytochrome c oxidase utilize a redox mediator to facilitate transfer of reducing equivalents between the exogenous reductant ascorbate and cytochrome c. The dependence on cytochrome c concentration of cytochrome oxidase activity in heart mitochondria from young, aged and aged + acetyl-L-carnitine treated rats was studied. The results of a typical experiment (see FIGURE 1) show that the concentration dependence of cytochrome oxidase by these different preparations of mitochondria reveals hyperbolic saturation characteristics. The data fit a single K_m value (around 10 μM) for cytochrome c for all three types of mitochondria. The maximal activity of cytochrome oxidase was markedly reduced (around 30%) in mitochondria from aged rats when compared with that obtained in mitochondria from young rats. The lower activity of this enzymatic system observed in mitochondria from aged rats was restored to the level of young rats by following treatment of aged rats with acetyl-L-carnitine. This compound had no effect on the activity of cytochrome oxidase in mitochondria isolated from young rats (results not shown).

The statistical analysis of the kinetic parameters of cytochrome oxidase in heart mitochondria from young, aged, and aged + acetyl-L-carnitine treated rats obtained from four experiments is presented in TABLE 1.

The lower activity of cytochrome oxidase in mitochondria from aged rats could be due, in principle, to a change in enzyme mass. To assess this, the cytochrome oxidase content of mitochondrial preparations from young and aged rats was measured. For these studies, chemical reduction by dithyonite was used to obtain reduced-minus oxidized difference spectra. The data reported in TABLE 2 show that the heme aa_3 content was practically the same in mitochondria from both young and aged rats. When the kinetic data of cytochrome oxidase are expressed on a per heme aa_3 basis, it is clear that young and aged mitochondrial preparations exhibit different molecular activity (see also TABLE 2). These results indicate that the catalytic efficiency of the active oxidase molecules is changed with aging.

Changes in cytochrome oxidase activity may affect the rates of mitochondrial respiration and phosphorylation. Respiratory activities of cardiac mitochondria from young, aged, and aged + acetyl-L-carnitine treated rats are reported in TABLE 3. Mitochondria from aged rats exhibited a significant decline (around 25%) in state 3 respiration compared to mitochondria from young animals. There was also a slight decline in state 4 respiration. Treatment of aged rats with acetyl-L-carnitine restored these decreased rates of respiration to the level observed in mitochondria from young rats.

In healthy mitochondria, respiration is tightly coupled to the production of ATP which, in turn, is translocated across the inner mitochondrial membrane from the matrix of these organelles to the cytosol by a stoichiometric exchange with cytosolic

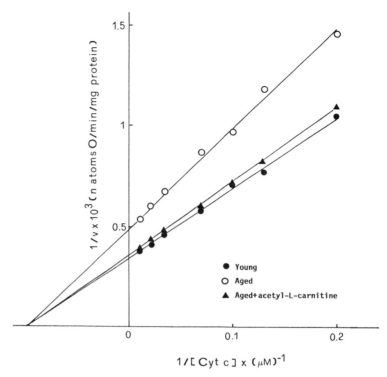

FIGURE 1. Double reciprocal plots of cytochrome c oxidase activity in heart mitochondria isolated from young, aged, and aged + acetyl-L-carnitine treated rats. The rate of oxidation of ascorbate (10 mM) in the presence of TMPD (1 mM) and various concentrations of cytochrome c was measured with mitochondria from young, aged, and aged + acetyl-L-carnitine rats as described in Materials and Methods. The experiment shown is representative of five different experiments that gave similar results.

ADP. This exchange is carried out by a membrane bound transport protein, the adenine nucleotide translocase. There are numerous reports in the literature that the rate of mitochondrial ATP production when supported by NAD linked substrates declines with aging (see Reference 1 for a review with relevant references),

TABLE 1. Kinetic Parameters of the Cytochrome Oxidase in Heart Mitochondria from Young, Aged, and Aged + Acetyl-L-carnitine Treated Rats[a]

| Animals | Cytochrome Oxidase | | Decrement |
	K_m (μM)	V_{max} (natoms O/min/mg prot.)	
Young	10.5 ± 0.7	3180 ± 352	
Aged	11.3 ± 0.8	2290 ± 285	28%
Aged + ac. carn.	11.0 ± 0.8	3090 ± 341	

[a]Note: The K_m and V_{max} values were calculated from double reciprocal plots similar to those reported in FIGURE 1. Results are expressed as mean $\pm$ SE for four separate experiments.

TABLE 2. Cytochrome Oxidase Content in Heart Mitochondria from Young and Aged Rats[a]

Animals	Cytochrome Oxidase (nmol heme aa₃/mg prot.)	Turnover Number (nmol e⁻/sec/nmol aa₃)
Young	0.412 ± 0.04	258 ± 25
Aged	0.406 ± 0.05	188 ± 19

[a]Note: Results are expressed as mean $\pm$ SE for four separate experiments.

and this effect has been attributed by several investigators to changes in the composition and in the phisical properties of the mitochondrial membrane.[3–24]

It has been shown that the activity of the ADP carrier is decreased in rat heart mitochondria from aged rats.[4,5] This decrease was ascribed to an altered membrane lipid environment of this carrier protein. The effect of pretreatment of aged rats with acetyl-L-carnitine on the activity of the ADP carrier was studied. The results reported in FIGURE 2 confirm that the activity of the ADP carrier in rat heart mitochondria is reduced (by more than 30%) with aging. Pretreatment of aged rats with acetyl-L-carnitine restores the activity of this carrier system to the level of young rats.

Acetyl-L-carnitine may restore the activity of the ADP carrier either by increasing the amount of the carrier molecules or by restoring the correct lipid composition of the mitochondrial membrane, altered by aging. The first possibility was tested by measuring the content of ADP carrier in mitochondria from young, aged, and aged + acetyl-L-carnitine treated rats. The content of ADP carrier was measured by titrating the ADP carrier activity with carboxyatractiloside (CAT). CAT is a very specific, noncompetitive tight-binding inhibitor which is bound by a 1:1 stoichiometry to the translocator.[25] Thus the content of the active adenine nucleotide translocator can be determined by the amount of CAT sufficient to completely inhibit ADP transport. The titration of ADP transport by increasing concentrations of CAT in mitochondria from young, aged, and aged + acetyl-L-carnitine treated rats is reported in FIGURE 3. The inhibition plots are biphasic with all these three types of mitochondria. Maximal inhibition of ADP transport was achieved by approximately the same concentration of CAT in all three populations of mitochondria. This indicates that the amount of ADP carrier is the same in mitochondria from young, aged, and aged + acetyl-L-carnitine treated rats.

The activity of cytochrome oxidase is known to be dependent on the phospholipid composition of the mitochondrial membranes. To examine the possible role of changes in bulk membrane lipids in affecting oxidase function, the temperature dependence of the oxidase activity in mitochondria isolated from young, aged, and

TABLE 3. Respiratory Activities of Cardiac Mitochondria from Young, Aged, and Aged + Acetyl-L-carnitine Treated Rats[a]

Animals	Respiratory Activity (natom O/min/mg protein)		RCR	ADP/O
	State 3	State 4		
Young	320 ± 33	38 ± 4.1	8.4	2.78
Aged	240 ± 26	30 ± 3.5	8.0	2.71
Aged + ac. carn.	312 ± 29	37 ± 3.7	8.4	2.74

[a]Note: Rates of mitochondrial respiration were measured polarographically using pyruvate + malate as substrates. Results are expressed as means $\pm$ SE for four separate experiments.

aged + acetyl-L-carnitine treated rats was examined. The Arrhenius plots of a typical experiment of cytochrome oxidase activity in mitochondria from these three types of mitochondria are reported in FIGURE 4. Mitochondrial preparation from young rats exhibited a biphasic plot of log respiration rate versus reciprocal temperature, with change in the slope at 29.5 ± 3.1°C. With heart mitochondria preparation from aged rats, the Arrhenius plot for cytochrome oxidase activity was also biphasic, but the position of the break point was shifted to a higher temperature, 32 ± 3.4°C. This difference in temperature dependence of cytochrome oxidase activity suggests a different lipid environment of the active enzyme molecules in mitochondrial membrane from young and aged rats. Treatment of aged rats with acetyl-L-carnitine restored the altered Arrhenius plot profile for mitochondrial cytochrome c oxidase to that observed in mitochondria from young rats.

To ascertain the possible involvement of membrane lipids in affecting the cytochrome oxidase activity, the phospholipid composition of mitochondrial preparation from young, aged, and aged + acetyl-L-carnitine was analyzed. TABLE 4 compares the phospholipid patterns of mitochondrial membrane from these three types of rats. No appreciable variation in mitochondrial phospholipid composition of either of these three types of rats occurred, except for negatively charged phospholipid cardiolipin, the level of which was markedly reduced in aged animals and brought back to the level of young rats by pretreatment of aged rats with acetyl-L-carnitine.

Chemical changes in the mitochondrial cardiolipin were further investigated by analyzing the fatty acyl profiles of this phospholipid. The fatty acid patterns of the mitochondrial cardiolipin of young, aged, and aged + acetyl-L-carnitine treated rats

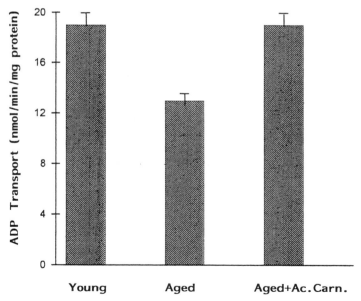

FIGURE 2. ADP transport in heart mitochondria isolated from young, aged, and aged + acetyl-L-carnitine treated rats. The transport of ADP in mitochondria was measured as described in Reference 21. The results are expressed as mean ± SE for four different experiments.

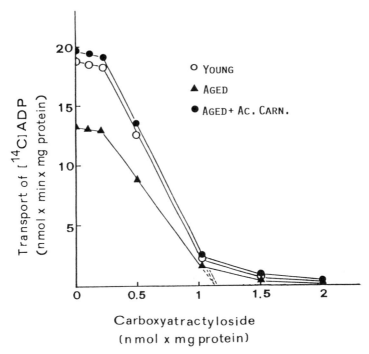

FIGURE 3. Inhibition of ADP transport by carboxyatractyloside in heart mitochondria isolated from young, aged, and aged + acetyl-L-carnitine treated rats. The inhibition of ADP transport by carboxyatractyloside was studied as described in Reference 21. The experiment shown is representative of four different experiments that gave similar results.

are shown in TABLE 5. No apreciable alteration of cardiolipin fatty acyl distribution was observed in any of these three populations of mitochondrial membranes. There was also no alteration of fatty acid composition of phosphatidylcholine, phosphatidylethanolamine, phosphatidylserine, and phosphatidylinositol in mitochondrial membranes isolated from these different types of animals (results not shown).

DISCUSSION

The present study demonstrates that aging affects the kinetic characteristics of cytochrome oxidase in rat heart mitochondria. While the apparent K_m value for cytochrome c is similar in mitochondrial preparations from young and aged rats, the maximal activity of this enzyme complex is markedly reduced in mitochondria from aged rats. These results can be interpreted to indicate that while the nature of the cytochrome oxidase appears unaffected, the mass of this enzymatic system is lowered in mitochondria from aged rats. However, the content of cytochrome oxidase, determined as heme aa_3 level, appears to be the same in mitochondria from young and aged rats. Thus, the lower cytochrome oxidase activity observed in mitochondria from aged rats does not appear to be dependent on a decrease in the mass of this

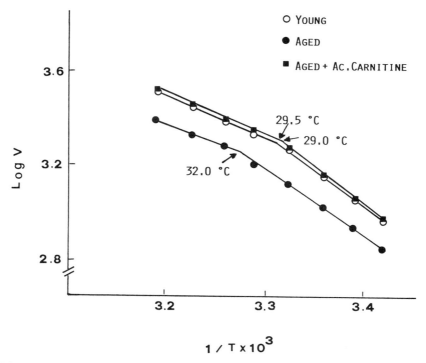

FIGURE 4. Temperature dependence of cytochrome c oxidase activity in heart mitochondria from young, aged, and aged + acetyl-L-carnitine treated rats. The rate of oxidation of ascorbate (10 mM) in the presence of TMPD (1 mM) and cytochrome c (50 μM) was determined at various temperatures, in the medium described in Materials and Methods. The experiment shown is representative of four different experiments that gave similar results.

enzyme complex. However, age-related changes in the amount and in the conformation of specific subunits of this enzyme complex cannot be excluded.

Cytochrome oxidase is considered, together with adenine nucleotide translocase, an important factor in the regulation of mitochondrial respiration.[26,27] A decrease in

TABLE 4. The Effect of Aging and Acetyl-L-carnitine Treatment on Phospholipid Composition in Rat Heart Mitochondria[a]

Phospholipid	Distribution (mol%)			
	Young	Treated Young	Aged	Treated Aged
DPG	14.1 ± 1.1	15.2 ± 1.3	9.8 ± 1.0	14.6 ± 1.2
PE	35.0 ± 1.7	34.8 ± 1.5	32.4 ± 1.7	32.8 ± 1.8
PI	1.4 ± 0.4	1.6 ± 0.3	1.5 ± 0.3	1.8 ± 0.5
PS	2.4 ± 0.4	2.5 ± 0.5	3.1 ± 0.7	2.6 ± 0.5
PC	47.1 ± 1.5	45.9 ± 1.4	53.2 ± 1.6	48.2 ± 1.7

[a]Note: DPG = cardiolipin; PE = phosphatidylethanolamine; PI = phosphatidylinositol; PS = phosphatidylserine; PC = phosphatidylcholine. Results are expressed as mean ± SE for four experiments.

the mitochondrial cytochrome oxidase activity, as observed in aged rats, should be associated with a decrease in mitochondrial state 3 respiration. The results reported in TABLE 3 clearly demonstrate that mitochondria from aged rats exhibit a lower rates of state 3 respiration compared to those obtained with young rats. There is also a good correlation between the degree of decline of mitochondrial state 3 respiration and that of cytochrome oxidase in aged animals. The decrease in adenine nucleotide translocase activity, as observed in aged rats, may also contribute to the lower rates of state 3 respiration in mitochondria from aged rats. Treatment of aged rats with acetyl-L-carnitine restores the reduced activity of the mitochondrial cytochrome oxidase and that of adenine nucleotide translocase as well as the reduced respiratory activity to the level of young rats.

Cytochrome oxidase is an integral protein of the inner mitochondrial membrane, and its activity is tightly dependent on the lipid microenvironment. The difference in temperature dependence of cytochrome oxidase activity in mitochondria from young and aged rats (see FIGURE 4) indicates that the lipid environment of the active enzyme molecules in these two types of mitochondrial membranes is not the same. Interestingly, the difference in temperature dependence of cytochrome oxidase

TABLE 5. Cardiolipin Fatty Acid Composition in Mitochondrial Membranes Isolated from Young, Aged, and Aged + Acetyl-L-carnitine Treated Rats[a]

	Cardiolipin		
Fatty Acid	Young	Aged	Aged + Ac. Carnitine
16:0	11.3 ± 0.9	10.9 ± 0.8	10.5 ± 0.7
16:1	3.0 ± 0.5	2.4 ± 0.4	3.1 ± 0.4
18:0	2.4 ± 0.3	3.2 ± 0.3	2.9 ± 0.2
18:1	6.2 ± 0.3	8.0 ± 0.7	7.8 ± 0.4
18:2	72.0 ± 2.0	70.1 ± 1.9	70.9 ± 1.8
20:3	2.1 ± 0.2	2.0 ± 0.3	2.2 ± 0.3
20:4	1.9 ± 0.2	2.6 ± 0.3	1.4 ± 0.2
22:6	1.1 ± 0.2	0.8 ± 0.1	1.2 ± 0.1

[a]Note: Each value represents the mean ± SE obtained from four separate experiments.

activity in mitochondria from young and aged rats was abolished by following treatment of aged rats with acetyl-L-carnitine.

The mammalian inner mitochondrial membrane has a unique composition, compared to other cellular and organelles membrane. This membrane contains little cholesterol or other sterol, while it is enriched in phospholipids. Among phospholipid species, cardiolipin has interesting chemical and structural characteristics, being highly acidic and having a head group (glycerol) that is esterified to two phosphodiglyceride backbone fragments rather than one. Cardiolipin also has a highly specialized physiological distribution, being almost exclusively localized in the inner membrane of mitochondria where it is biosynthesized. Several studies have shown that tightly associated cardiolipin is required for optimal electron transport activity of heart cytochrome oxidase.[10,11,28–30] There is also evidence for specific interaction between cardiolipin and the enzyme (for review, see Reference 31), although the origin of this dependence is still unclear. Among the ways in which cardiolipin may affect the catalytic activity of cytochrome oxidase, it has been recently suggested that this phospholipid modifies the environment of the enzyme complex in such a way as to facilitate conformational changes of two forms of the cytochrome oxidase, which differ in kinetic activity.[32] The results reported in TABLE 4 document a marked and almost specific decrease (more than 30%) in the content of cardiolipin in the mitochondrial preparation from aged rats. This reduced level of cardiolipin in mitochondria from aged rats is brought back to the level of young rats by treatment of aged rats with acetyl-L-carnitine. These changes in the cardiolipin levels are accompanied by parallel changes in the mitochondrial cytochrome oxidase activity. Thus, the most obvious explanation of the effect of acetyl-L-carnitine on cytochrome oxidase activity is the restoration of the correct lipid microenvironment (cardiolipin level) of this enzyme system in the inner mitochondrial membrane, altered by aging. It should be noted that treatment of young rats with acetyl-L-carnitine had no effect either on the mitochondrial cytochrome oxidase activity or on the level of cardiolipin. This suggests that the observed effects of acetyl-L-carnitine are related to changes produced by aging.

Previous results in the literature have shown a decreased activity of the adenine nucleotide translocase in heart mitochondria from aged rats.[4,5] This result has been confirmed in the present investigation. This decreased translocating activity has been attributed to changes in membrane phospholipid composition. We have found that the lower activity of the adenine nucleotide translocase in heart mitochondria from aged rats is restored to the level of young rats by treating aged animals with acetyl-L-carnitine. Cardiolipin has been reported to be required for optimum activity of adenine nucleotide translocase.[4] Thus, as proposed for cytochrome oxidase activity (see above) and phosphate carrier,[17] the observed effect of acetyl-L-carnitine on the activity of the adenine nucleotide carrier in aged animals can be explained, at least in part, on the ground of a restoration of the integrity of the mitochondrial membrane lipid microenvironment (cardiolipin content) of this carrier protein.

CONCLUSIONS

The results here reported demonstrate that the activity of cytochrome oxidase and that of adenine nucleotide translocase decline with aging. The factor responsible for this decline appears to be, at least in part, a modification of the lipid composition of the mitochondrial membrane and more specifically a decrease in the level of cardiolipin, a phospholipid located at the level of the inner mitochondrial membrane and specifically required for the optimum functioning of these proteins.

Acetyl-L-carnitine is capable of restoring the integrity of the cardiac mitochondrial membrane altered by aging (specifically the cardiolipin content), thereby restoring the normal activity of cytochrome oxidase, adenine nucleotide translocase, and phosphate carrier,[17] all systems that require cardiolipin for their optimal activity. This, in turn, should allow more efficient oxidative phosphorylation, thereby improving cardiac performance in aged animals.

It remains for us to ascertain the molecular mechanism by which acetyl-L-carnitine restores the normal level of cardiolipin in cardiac mitochondrial inner membrane of aged animals.

ACKNOWLEDGMENTS

The authors would like to thank Mr. L. Gargano and F. Fracasso for excellent technical assistance.

REFERENCES

1. HANSFORD, R. G. 1983. Biochim. Biophys. Acta **726:** 41–80.
2. LEWIN, M. B. & P. S. TIMIRAS. 1984. Mech. Ageing Dev. **24:** 343–351.
3. NOHL, H. 1982. Gerontology **28:** 354–359.
4. NOHL, H. & R. KRAMER. 1980. Mech. Ageing Dev. **14:** 137–144.
5. KIM, J. H., E. SHRAGO & E. ELSON. 1988. Mech. Ageing Dev. **46:** 279–290.
6. HANSFORD, R. G. 1978. Biochem. J. **170:** 285–295.
7. PARADIES, G. & F. M. RUGGIERO. 1990. Biochim. Biophys. Acta **1016:** 207–212.
8. PARADIES, G. & F. M. RUGGIERO. 1991. Arch. Biochem. Biophys. **284:** 332–337.
9. PARADIES, G., F. M. RUGGIERO & P. DINOI. 1992. Int. J. Biochem. **24:** 783–787.
10. ROBINSON, N. C., F. STREY & L. TALBERT. 1980. Biochemistry **19:** 3656–3661.
11. FRY, M., G. A. BLONDIN & D. E. GREEN. 1980. J. Biol. Chem. **255:** 9967–9970.
12. SILIPRANDI, N., D. SILIPRANDI & M. CIMAN. 1965. Biochem. J. **96:** 777–780.
13. GADALETA, M. N., V. PETRUZZELLA, M. RENIS, F. FRACASSO & P. CANTATORE. 1990. Eur. J. Biochem. **187:** 501–506.
14. RUGGIERO, F. M., F. CAFAGNA, M. N. GADALETA & E. QUAGLIARIELLO. 1990. Biochem. Biophys. Res. Commun. **170:** 621–626.
15. CURTI, D., F. DAGANI, M. R. GALMOZZI & F. MARZATICO. 1989. Mech. Ageing Dev. **47:** 39–45.
16. PETRUZZELLA, V., L. G. BAGGETTO, F. PENIN, F. CAFAGNA, F. M. RUGGIERO, P. CANTATORE & M. N. GADALETA. 1992. Arch. Gerontol. Geriatr. **14:** 131–144.
17. PARADIES, G., F. M. RUGGIERO, M. N. GADALETA & E. QUAGLIARIELLO. 1992. Biochim. Biophys. Acta **1103:** 324–326.
18. PARADIES, G. & F. M. RUGGIERO. 1988. Biochim. Biophys. Acta **935:** 79–86.
19. TAYER, W. S. & E. RUBIN. 1981. J. Biol. Chem. **256:** 6090–6097.
20. KUBOYAMA, M., F. C. YONG & T. E. KING. 1972. J. Biol. Chem. **247:** 6375–6383.
21. DOUSSIERE, J., E. LIGETI, G. BRANDOLIN & P. V. VIGNAIS. 1984. Biochim. Biophys. Acta **766:** 492–500.
22. BLIGH, E. G. & W. J. DYER. 1959. Can. J. Biochem. Physiol. **37:** 911–917.
23. RUGGIERO, F. M., C. LANDRISCINA, G. V. GNONI & E. QUAGLIARIELLO. 1984. Lipids **19:** 171–178.
24. CLANDININ, M. T. & S. M. INNIS. 1983. Mech. Ageing Dev. **22:** 205–208.
25. KLINGEMBERG, M. 1980. J. Membr. Biol. **56:** 97–105.
26. ERECINSKA, M. & D. F. WILSON. 1982. J. Membr. Biol. **70:** 1–14.
27. KADENBACH, B. 1986. J. Bioenerg. Biomembr. **18:** 39–54.
28. MARSH, D. & G. L. POWELL. 1988. Bioelectrochem. Bioenerg. **20:** 73–82.
29. POWELL, G. L., P. F. KNOWLES & D. MARSH. 1987. Biochemistry **26:** 8138–8145.
30. HOCH, F. L. 1992. Biochim. Biophys. Acta **1113:** 71–133.
31. DAUM, G. 1985. Bichim. Biophys. Acta **822:** 1–42.
32. ABRAMOVITCH, D. A., D. MARSH & G. L. POWELL. 1990. Biochim. Biophys. Acta **1020:** 34–42.

Cysteine Restores the Activity of ATP-Sensitive Potassium Channels of Skeletal Muscle Fibers of Aged Rats[a]

D. TRICARICO, R. WAGNER, R. MALLAMACI, AND
D. CONTE CAMERINO[b]

Unit of Pharmacology
Department of Pharmacobiology
Faculty of Pharmacy
University of Bari
Via Orabona no. 4I-70125
Bari, Italy

INTRODUCTION

Several studies have documented a decrease in muscle performance with senescence in both human and animals.[1,2] Age-related changes in the contractile proteins may at least in part be responsible for the decrease of muscle contraction.[3] Other factors have been proposed to contribute to the alterations of muscle functionality in aged rats. Properties of the sarcolemma change with age, the membrane potential declines,[4] intracellular Na^+ rises, and the intracellular K^+ concentration decreases.[4] The loss of K^+ from the fibers and the accumulation of extracellular K^+ ion in muscle T-tubules may depress the amplitude and slow down the conduction of action potential.[4]

There are numerous reports documenting changes in the biophysical and pharmacological properties of ion channels expressed during various stages of development in excitable tissues, including skeletal muscle. For example, the sodium current becomes sensitive to nanomolar concentrations of tetrodotoxin as the muscle matures.[5] Calcium currents with different kinetics ("transient" and "sustained" current types) have been observed in muscles from neonatal mice.[6] The transient-type current, which is insensitive to the dihydropyridine class of calcium channel inhibitors, disappears during postnatal development, while the sustained current increases. Both the channel density and conductance of ATP-sensitive potassium channels (K^+_{ATP}) of neonatal myocytes are significantly smaller than in adult cells, as determined by single channel patch clamp analysis.[7,8] Apamin-sensitive K^+ channels are expressed in fetal rat skeletal muscle, then disappear during development; they will reappear after denervation of adult muscle.[9]

Not much is known about changes in ion channel properties that may occur in skeletal muscle during aging, as opposed to development. Macroscopic recordings have shown that the resting K^+ conductance of skeletal muscle fibers in aged rats increases with age, while chloride conductance decreases.[10] The excitability characteristics of skeletal muscle fibers also change during aging; the duration of action potential increases and the firing capability decreases.[10]

[a]This work was supported by CNR P. F. "Invecchiamento" cod. no. 931338.
[b]Author to whom correspondence should be addressed.

To assess whether the macroscopic changes in K^+ conductance that occur during aging in skeletal muscle are due to alterations of single K^+ channel properties or to the appearance of a novel K^+ channel population (or both), we used the patch clamp technique to survey the K^+ channels present on the surface membrane of resting skeletal muscle fibers from 7–11 ("adult"), 20–23, and 25 month old ("aged") rats. Most of our studies focused on K^+_{ATP}, the most frequently observed K^+ channel type in our experiments. In particular, experiments were performed to evaluate differences in gating behavior and sensitivity to ATP and cysteine between K^+_{ATP} channels of adult and aged fibers.

METHODS

Single muscle fibers were prepared from muscles (flexor digitorum brevis) from the hind feet of adult and aged rats using a modification of the method of Bekoff and Betz[11] (1987). In particular, adult and aged rats were sacrificed by CO_2 atmosphere replacement, after which both hind limbs were removed, skinned, and immersed in Ringer solution. The feet were then pinned dorsal side up in a Sylgard-coated dish filled with Ringer solution. The Ringer in the dish was then replaced with 2 ml of enzyme solution containing 3 mg/ml collagenase (3.3 U/mg, Type XI-S, Sigma Chemical Co., St., Louis, Mo.) dissolved in Ringer. The muscle was incubated for 1.5–2 hours at 30°C under 95% O_2/5% CO_2 atmosphere in a Dubnoff rocker (rpm 0.8). Dissociated cells were washed several times with fresh Ringer solution and transferred to a Ringer-filled recording chamber.

Patch pipettes were pulled in two stages from Corning 7052 glass (Garner Glass Co., Calif.) on a patch electrode puller (DMZ-Universal Puller, Zeitz-Instrumente, Germany). Electrodes typically had "bubble numbers" of around 6–7 before fire polishing.[12] Pipettes were then coated with Sylgard to within 150 μm–50 μm of the pipette tip and fire polished (MF-83 Pipette microforge, Narishighe, Japan) to give bubble numbers of 3–4 and resistances of 8–9 MΩ when filled with our usual pipette solution. With most cell preparations, high-resistance seals of 20 to 70 GΩ readily formed after pressing the patch pipette lightly against the membrane, releasing the positive pressure in the pipette, and applying a small amount of suction to the electrode by syringe (1 ml capacity).

Solutions (Concentrations in mM)

Pipette: 150 KCl, 2 $CaCl_2$, 10 MOPS, pH 7.2.

Bath: 145 NaCl, 5 KCl, 1 $MgCl_2$, 0.5 $CaCl_2$, 5 glucose, 10 MOPS (3-[N-morpholino] propanesulfonic acid), pH 7.2 ("normal Ringer"). 150 KCl, 2 $CaCl_2$, 10 MOPS, pH 7.2 ("pipette solution"). 150 KCl, 5 EGTA, 10 MOPS, pH 7.2 ("symmetrical potassium"). 400 KCl, 5 EGTA, 10 MOPS, pH 7.2 ("high potassium").

Cysteine and Na_2ATP (Sigma Chemical Co., St. Louis, Mo.) were dissolved in symmetrical potassium solution.

Hardware and Software

Isolated muscle fibers were patch clamped in an RC-13 recording chamber (Warner instrument Corp. Hamden, Conn.).

Single channel activity was recorded using an Axopatch 1D patch amplifier with a CV-3 headstage. Single channel currents were recorded under constant voltage ("steady state") at 20°C. Currents were filtered at 2 kHz (4 pole bessel, -3 dB) and sampled at 20 kHz and 12 bit resolution and stored on the hard disk of an 80386/33 personal computer. The data acquisition hardware (TL-1 Interface, AXON Instruments) was driven by the Fetchex data acquisition program (pClamp software package, AXON Instruments). Data were analyzed using pClamp and our own custom software.

Experiments were performed using standard single channel patch clamp technique.[13] In the *cell-attached* configuration, the bath contained "symmetrical potassium" solution. *Inside-out* patches were rapidly formed by withdrawing the patch electrode from the cell while in the cell-attached configuration.[13]

Direct inspection of the recorded current records was used to measure the single channel current at various voltages, using the cursor method provided by the program Fetchan (pClamp, AXON Instrument). The single channel conductance was then calculated as the slope of the voltage-current relationship of the channel. Other analysis methods are described in the appropriate sections of this paper.

Open Probability Analysis

Software was developed by one of us (R. Wagner) to analyze Fetchex data files containing multiple channels or subconductance levels of identical amplitude. This software determines the fraction of an "episode" spent at every conductance level, for each episode in the file, and outputs these data to a tab-delimited ASCII file for further analysis. Channel (or sublevel) independence and the number of channels (or subconductance states) present in the record can be determined by summing the fraction of time at each conductance level and fitting the data to an appropriate binomial distribution. If the data indicate that the channels are gating independently, the open probability (P_{open}) of a single channel (or subconductance state) is obtained as one of the parameters of the fit. Further insight into the gating process may be obtained by examining graphs of the output data in various forms. Details about the program are available directly from the authors.

RESULTS

ATP-sensitive K$^+$ channels (K$^+_{ATP}$) were encountered during steady-state patch clamp recording from the surface membrane of adult and aged rat skeletal muscle fibers.

The K$^+_{ATP}$ Channel of Adult and Aged Rat Muscle Fibers

Under our recording conditions, the K$^+_{ATP}$ channel was the most commonly observed K$^+$ channel on the surface membrane of both adult and aged rat skeletal muscle fibers. *Cell-attached* recordings made at positive pipette potential with 150 mM KCl in the pipette and 150 mM KCl and 5 mM EGTA in the bath ("symmetrical potassium") revealed inward currents flowing through single channels. The reversal potentials of the observed single channels currents were around 0 mV, as expected for currents carried by K$^+$ ions. Analysis of the gating behavior of K$^+_{ATP}$ channels in

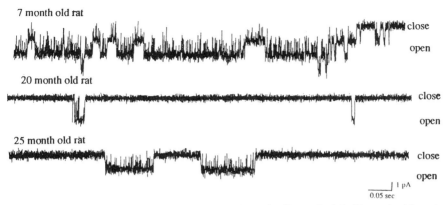

FIGURE 1. ATP-sensitive K$^+$ channel of skeletal muscle fibers of adult (7-month-old) and aged (20- and 25-month-old) rats. The recordings were performed in steady-state condition at −60 mV voltage membrane in inside-out configuration, at 20°C. Acquisition rate 20 kHz, filter 2 kHz. 820 msec of traces are shown. The direction of ionic currents follows the standard convention: downward deflection on the current records indicate the movement of positively charged ions from the extracellular side of the membrane to the intracellular side (inward current). The traces showed are referred to patch no. 14, 18, and 27 respectively of 7-, 20-, and 25-month-old rats.

three patches from 7-month-old rat fibers held at −60 mV ΔV_m identified 10.2 ± 1 transitions/sec ($n = 3$ patches) between open and closed conductance levels during 30.512 seconds of recording. The number of transitions/sec increased to 97 ± 2 ($n = 3$ patches) and 96 ± 3 ($n = 4$ patches) respectively for the 20- and 25-month-old rat fibers, thus indicating, in the cell-attached configuration, a slight increase of channel gating activity with aging. As was expected for K$^+_{ATP}$ channels, the excision of cell-attached patches from fibers of 7-month-old rats into the *inside-out configuration* dramatically increased channel activity. In contrast, when patches were excised from fibers from aged rats, no increase of channel activity was detected (FIGURE 1). Open probability analysis revealed that the P_{open} of the channels from aged fibers was about 10 times lower as compared to the P_{open} of channels from adult rats in the range of potentials going from −80 mV to +60 mV (TABLE 1). Increasing the concentration of K$^+$ in the bath solution shifted the reversal potential from 0 mV to the left, confirming that the channel under study was K$^+$/selective.

TABLE 1. Effects of Aging on the Open Probability of Isolated Patches Containing ATP-Sensitive Potassium Channels from Rat Skeletal Muscle Fibers[a]

Age (months)	Open Probability (P_{open})	Number of Patches
7–11	0.196 ± 0.034	9
20–23	0.057 ± 0.016	10
25–26	0.041 ± 0.013	4

[a]The probability of a channel being open was determined under steady-state recording conditions at a transmembrane potential of −70 mV in the inside-out patch configuration in the absence of ATP. The values are expressed as mean ± standard error.

The application of 100 μM ATP to the cytoplasmic face of patches from muscle fibers of both adult and aged rats reduced the P_{open} of the channels, indicating that the channels are indeed ATP sensitive. The frequency of occurrence of K^+_{ATP} channels in patches decreased with the age of the rats, from 56% in 7-month-old rat fibers to 39% and 30%, respectively, in fibers from 20–23 and 25-month-old rats. A minimum of 3 and a maximum of 8 simultaneously open channels were observed in the fibers from adult (7–11 month old) rat muscle. In contrast, no more than 2 simultaneously open channels were observed in fibers from aged rats.

No significant difference in the single channel conductance was observed between adult and aged rat channels. The amplitude of the current through K^+_{ATP} channels at -70 mV was -4.71 ± 0.09 pA ($n = 10$ channels) in 7-month-old rat fibers and -4.80 ± 0.12 pA ($n = 10$ channels) in 20-month-old rat fibers. The current-voltage relationships of channels from both adult and aged fibers showed weak inward rectification (FIGURE 2). In symmetrical K^+, the slope conductance was 60.06 ± 1.57 pS ($n = 10$ channels), 60.06 ± 2.32 pS ($n = 8$ channels), and 56.5 ± 2.4 pS ($n = 4$ channels), respectively, for channels from 7–11, 20–23, and 25-month-old rat fibers.

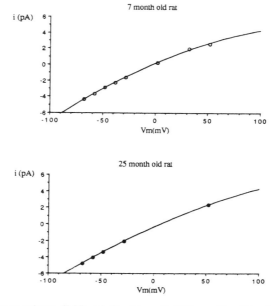

FIGURE 2. Current-voltage (I-V) relationships of ATP-sensitive K^+ channel of skeletal muscle fibers of adult (7-month-old) and aged (25-month-old) rats. Single channel currents were recorded in steady-state condition and inside-out configuration at 20°C. The amplitude of the current records has been measured by direct inspection of the traces by cursor method. The single channel conductance has been calculated by linear regression analysis as slope of the I-V relationships. The equations that best fitted the data points were: $y = -0.23099 + 0.059036x$ with correlation coefficent of 0.993 and $y = -0.15386 + 0.058204x$ with correlation coefficent of 0.997 respectively for 7- and 25-month-old rat I-V relationships. Either the pipette solution and the solution bathing the cytoplasmic face of the channel contained 150 mM KCl. The I-V relationships reported are referred to patches no. 42 and 43 respectively of 7- and 25-month-old rats.

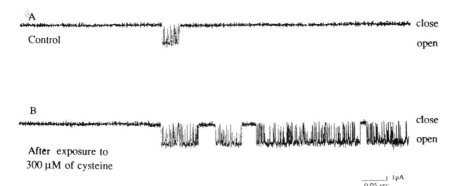

FIGURE 3. ATP-sensitive K$^+$ channel of skeletal muscle fibers of 20-month-old rat before (trace A) and after application to the cytoplasmic face of the channel of cysteine (trace B). The recordings were performed in steady-state condition at -70 mV voltage membrane in inside-out configuration, at 20°C. Acquisition rate 20 kHz, filter 2 kHz. 700 msec of traces are showed. The direction of ionic currents follows the standard convention: downward deflection on the current records indicates the movement of positively charged ions from the extracellular side of the membrane to the intracellular side (inward current). The traces showed are referred to patch no. 21 of 20-month-old rat.

Effect of Cysteine on K$^+_{ATP}$ Channels of 7- and 20-Month-Old Rat Fibers

The application of cysteine (100 μM and 300 μM) to the cytoplasmic face of patches from aged rat fibers containing K$^+_{ATP}$ channels produced an increase in channel openings (FIGURE 3). The P_{open} of the K$^+_{ATP}$ channels was 0.055 under control conditions and 0.081 and 0.099 after 100 μM and 300 μM cysteine, respectively. Cysteine applied at a concentration of 300 μM to the cytoplasmic surface of patches containing K$^+_{ATP}$ channels from 7-month-old rat fibers did not alter the single channel current or the P_{open} of the channels, indicating that the effect of cysteine is specific for K$^+_{ATP}$ channels from aged muscle.

Effect of ATP on K$^+_{ATP}$ Channels from Adult and Aged Rat Fibers

To assess whether differences exist in the sensitivity of adult and aged rat skeletal muscle K$^+_{ATP}$ channels to the inhibitory effect of ATP, we compared the effects of different concentrations of this nucleotide on K$^+_{ATP}$ channels from 7–11 and 20- to 23-month-old rat fibers.

The concentration of ATP required to produce a 50% decrease of the P_{open} of K$^+_{ATP}$ channels in inside-out patches was 28.5 ± 2.03 μM for channels from adult muscle and 20.53 ± 2.93 μM for channels from aged muscle (FIGURE 4). Hill plots of the concentration-dependent inhibition of P_{open} had slopes of 0.82 and 1.3 for K$^+_{ATP}$ channels from adult and aged fibers, respectively.

SUMMARY AND DISCUSSION

We have found that both the frequency of occurrence and the gating properties of K$^+_{ATP}$ channels are altered during aging in rats. The reduced density observed of

K^+_{ATP} channels in aged muscle fibers as compared to adult fibers may be due to either a change in the number of functional channels in the surface membrane or a change in the localization of channels. We found an average of 6.4 ± 1 ($n = 9$ patches) and 1.1 ± 0.2 ($n = 10$ patches) channels per isolated patch respectively, for the 7–11 and 20–23 month old rat fibers. It is possible that the K^+_{ATP} channels of adult fibers may be organized as clusters of channels, while the K^+_{ATP} channels of aged fibers may not have this type of organization and thus appear as a single units spread out over the membrane surface. A high density of K^+_{ATP} channels has been also observed in mouse and frog skeletal muscle fibers and in pancreatic β cells, where it is possible to recognize regions (so-called hot spot areas) where the channel density is extraordinarily high.[14] In addition, the observed lowering of the P_{open} of the channel with aging could have also affected the number of active channel in the patch

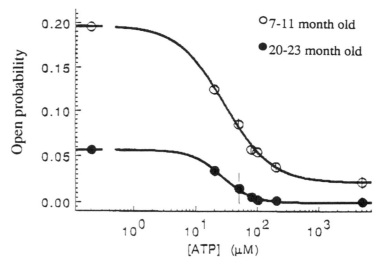

FIGURE 4. Dose-response relationships of the open probability of ATP sensitive K^+ channel of 7–11 month old rats and 20–23 month old rats versus ATP concentrations. Curves were drawn according to equation: $P_{open} = (Max - Min)/(1 + ([ATP]/EC_{50})^n)$ Each point represents mean of a minimum of 3 and a maximum of 10 experiments $\pm$ standard error.

of membrane, reducing the probability of overlapping of openings. An analysis of steady-state channel gating indicated that the P_{open} of the K^+_{ATP} channel (in the absence of ATP) was reduced in muscle from aged rats. Two major mechanisms may explain the reduced probability of the channel to be in an open state. The first involves an alteration of the oxidation state of the channel protein. Many ion channel proteins contain critical cysteine residues; the function of the channel often depends on the oxidation state of these groups.[15] For example, oxidation of sulfhydryl groups leads to prolonged openings of Ca^{2+} channels. In contrast, similar treatment of K^+_{ATP} channels in mouse skeletal muscle fibers and pancreatic β cells reduces the open probability of the channels.[15,16] In our experiments, it is possible that oxidation of thiol groups of K^+_{ATP} channels in aged fibers could have been the basis for the reduced probability of the channel being in an open state. The fact that application of cysteine to the cytoplasmic face of patches from aged muscle increased the P_{open} of K^+_{ATP} channels supports this hypothesis.

Another possible mechanism to explain the decreased number of K^+_{ATP} channels observed in patches from aged fibers may involve an inhibitory effect of Ca^{2+} on the K^+_{ATP} channel. This mechanism was recently proposed by Krippeit-Drews and Lonnendonker (1992), who claim that Ca^{2+} may irreversibly close the K^+_{ATP} channel.[17] In light of this observation, an increase in the intracellular Ca^{2+} concentration during the aging process of muscle fibers of aged rats used in our experiments may have irreversibly inhibited channel activity, and thus reduced the number of functional channels.

Finally the dose-response relationships between ATP concentrations and the reduction of P_{open} of K^+_{ATP} channels of 7–11 and 20–23 month old rat fibers showed that the channels from aged muscle are more sensitive to the inhibitory effect of ATP than are channels from adult muscle. We do not know if the different open channel probability between adult and aged channels could have influenced the access of ATP to the receptor, or if the ATP binding site has been modified. However, in agreement with previous reports,[16,18] the Hill coefficients we determined indicated the presence of one binding site for ATP per channel protein for channels from both adult and aged muscle, suggesting that no change occurs with aging in the molecularity of the reaction between ATP and the channel.

We find it interesting that the apparent density and open probability of K^+_{ATP} channels *decrease* in aged muscle, contrary to the overall *increase* in macroscopic K^+ conductance observed by De Luca *et al.* (1990).[10] It is possible that the K^+ conductance responsible for the increase in macroscopic K^+ conductance observed during aging may reside in membranes, such as T-tubule, not accessible with patch clamp electrodes.

REFERENCES

1. LARSSON, L., G. GRIMBY & J. CARLSSON. 1979. Muscle strength and speed of movement in relation to age and muscle morphology. J. Appl. Physiol. **46:** 451–456.
2. SYROVY, I. & E. GUTMANN. 1977. Changes in speed of contraction and ATPase activity in striated muscle during old age. Exp. Gerontol. **5:** 31–35.
3. CARLSEN, R. C. & D. A. WALSH. 1987. Decrease in force potentiation and appearance of α-adrenergic mediated contracture in aging rat skeletal muscle. Pflügers Arch. **408:** 224–230.
4. JONES, D. A. 1981. Muscle fatigue due to changes beyond the neuromuscular junction. *In* Human Muscle Fatigue: Physiological Mechanism. Ciba Foundation **82:** 178–191. Pitman Medical. London, England.
5. FRELIN, C., H. P. M. VIJVERBERG, G. ROMEY, P. VIGNE & M. LAZDUNSKI. 1984. Different functional states of tetrodotoxin sensitive and tetrodotoxin resistant Na^+ channels occur during the in vitro development of rat skeletal muscle. Pflügers Arch. **402:** 121–128.
6. BEAM, K. G. & C. N. KNUDSON. 1988. Calcium currents in embryonic and neonatal mammalian skeletal muscle. J. Gen. Physiol. **91:** 781–798.
7. CHEN, F., G. T. WETZEL, W. F. FRIEDMAN & T. S. KLITZNER. 1992. ATP-sensitive potassium channels in neonatal and adult rabbit ventricular myocytes. Pediatr. Res. **32/2:** 230–235.
8. WAHLER, G. M. 1992. Developmental increases in the inward rectifying potassium current rat ventricular myocytes. Am. J. Physiol. (Cell-Physiol.) **262/5,1:** C1266–1272.
9. SCHMID-ANTOMARCHI, H., J. F. RENAUD, G. ROMEY, M. HUGUES, A. SMID & M. LAZDUNSKI. 1985. The all-or-none role of innervation in expression of apamin receptor and apamin-sensitive Ca^{2+}-activated K^+ channel in mammalian skeletal muscle. Proc. Natl. Acad. Sci. USA **82:** 2188–2191.

10. DE LUCA, A., M. MAMBRINI & D. CONTE CAMERINO. 1990. Changes in membrane ionic conductances and excitability characteristics of rat skeletal muscle during aging. Pflügers Arch. **415:** 642– 644.
11. BEKOFF, A. & W. J. BETZ. 1977. Physiological properties of dissociated muscle fibers obtained from innervated and denervated adult rat muscle. J. Physiol. Lond. **271:** 25– 40.
12. COREY, D. P. & C. F. STEVENS. 1983. Science and technology of patch-recording electrodes. *In* Single-Channel Recording. B. Sakmann & E. Neher, eds. **3:** 53–68. Plenum press. New York & London.
13. HAMILL, O. P., E. MARTY, E. NEHER, B. SAKMANN & F. J. SIGWORTH. 1981. Improved patch-clamp techniques for high-resolution current recording from cells and cell-free membrane patches. Nature **391:** 85–100.
14. DUNNE, M. J. & O. H. PETERSEN. 1991. Potassium selective ion channels in insulin-secreting cells: physiology, pharmacology and their role in stimulus-secretion coupling. Biochim. Biophys. Acta **1071:** 67–82.
15. SHAHIDUL, I., P. BERGGREN & O. LARSSON. 1993. Sulfhydryl oxidation induces rapid and reversible closure of the ATP-regulated K^+ channel in the pancreatic β-cell. FEBS **319**(1/2): 128–132.
16. WEIK, R. & B. NEUMCKE. 1989. ATP-sensitive potassium channels in adult mouse skeletal muscle: characterization of the ATP-binding site. J. Membr. Biol. **110:** 217–226.
17. KRIPPEIT-DREWS, P. & U. LONNENDONKER. 1992. Dual effects of calcium on ATP-sensitive potassium channels of frog skeletal muscle. Biochim. Biophys. Acta **1108:** 119– 122.
18. SPRUCE, A. E., N. B. STANDEN & P. R. STANFIELD. 1987. Studies of the unitary properties of adenosine-5'-triphosphate regulated potassium channels of frog skeletal muscle. J. Physiol. Lond. **382:** 213–236.

α-Glycerophosphocholine in the Mental Recovery of Cerebral Ischemic Attacks

An Italian Multicenter Clinical Trial

GIUSEPPE BARBAGALLO SANGIORGI,
MARIO BARBAGALLO, MARCELLO GIORDANO,
MARIA MELI, AND RITA PANZARASA

Institute of Internal Medicine and Geriatrics
University of Palermo
Via Del Vespro 141
90127 Palermo, Italy

INTRODUCTION

Patients affected by acute ischemic cerebral event (TIA, p-TIA, stroke) may develop a syndrome characterized by sensitive-motor and, often, cognitive deficit, depending on the type of occlusion and individual response.[1,2]

Cerebrovascular disease is commonly considered to be the second cause of dementia, and stroke in particular accounts for 20–25%.[3] The term "dementia" implies a change in the mental state, from one level of mental functioning to a lower one over time. The explanation of the elevated risk of dementia following stroke is not yet fully understood: injury of different and multiple brain regions, each specific for certain cognitive functions, might lead to dementia simply on an additive basis, or a multiplicative mechanism may apply with the cumulative effect of several lesions. Many drugs, have been clinically tested in order to assess their role in the functional recovery of these patients.

Among these, α-glycerophosphocholine (α-GPC), a new molecule belonging to a class of choline donors, has shown a very promising profile on the basis of pharmacokinetics and pharmacological studies: in animals it has shown to exert an integrated neuronal function[4] and to facilitate learning and memory in a dose-related way.[5,6] Once α-GPC crosses the blood-brain barrier, it directly increases the synthesis and the release of acetylcholine, and serves as a precursor for membrane phospholipids, improving the functionality of neuronal membranes.[7–9] In healthy human volunteers, it has been possible to prevent the memory deficit produced by scopolamine.[10] And both in open and controlled clinical studies[11–14] on a substantial number of patients,[15] it has shown a good therapeutic effect on the outcome of dementia regardless of its etiology.

The aim of the present study was to assess α-GPC efficacy and tolerability in the treatment of neuropsychic symptoms following acute stroke.

MATERIAL AND METHODS

Experimental Design

The present study was an open multicenter uncontrolled trial involving 176 centers of internal medicine, geriatrics, and neurology spread all over Italy.

TABLE 1. Clinical Assessment and Evaluation Time

	First Part		Second Part	
	Baseline	1st Month	3rd Month	6th Month
Demography and run-in assessment	X			
SYS/DIAS BP and HR	X	X	X	X
Mathew Scale	X	X		
MMSE		X	X	X
GDS		X	X	X
Crichton Rat. Scale		X	X	X
Blood Analyses	X		X	X
α-GPC therapy	1000 mg/day im		3 × 400 mg/day orally	

The study was carried out in two phases that lasted 6 months altogether: during the first part (which lasted from day 1 to day 28, generally in hospital), the patients were treated parenterally with α-GPC at the dosage of 1000 mg/day, and in the second part (which lasted from day 29 to the end of the 6th month), the patients were treated orally with α-GPC at a dosage of 1200 mg/day, at a regimen of 400 mg three times a day.

The clinical assessments were made at the admission visit (baseline), at the end of the first part, and after 3 and 6 months from the beginning.

TABLE 1 reports the list of the clinical assessments and the checking times.

First part (baseline, 28th day): the clinical assessments consisted of patient's medical history (only at baseline), physical and neurological examination, arterial blood pressure and heart rate control, Mathew Scale and blood analyses.

Second part (28th day or secondary baseline, 3rd month, 6th month): the clinical assessments consisted of physical and neurological examination, Minimental State Test, Crichton Rating Scale, Global Deterioration Scale, arterial blood pressure and heart rate control, blood analyses (only at the 6th month).

Experimental Sample

The study population consisted of 2058 patients 45–85 years of age, with diagnosis of cerebral ischemic attacks (stroke or TIA), within the previous 10 days.

The exclusion criteria were patients with a baseline Mathew score < 35, or presenting consciousness deficit such that no cooperation was possible in performing the assessment tools requested by the protocol, or those receiving pharmacological therapy with psychotropic or nootropic drugs, or with short life expectancy, or with previous psychiatric and neurologic diseases, or with severe renal, liver, or heart diseases and neoplasms. Furthermore those patients with hemorragic infarction, head injury, or intracerebral or subarachnoid hemorrage, as well as alcohol and/or drug addictions, were not considered eligible for the study.

Concomitant Treatments

Conventional treatment for stroke was accepted; concomitant treatments with other brain-related drugs were excluded. Possible concomitant treatments for other diseases had to be kept as stable as possible during the six months of the study. The short half-life anxiolitics were accepted only at doses already stabilized for 30 days, and they had to be recorded on the patients' case report forms.

Treatment Discontinuation and Adverse Effects

Investigators could discontinue the treatment at any time, and were asked to report this information on the patient's form, especially if the discontinuation was due to an adverse effect reported by the patient or detected by the investigator that could be related to the drug in study.

Statistical Analysis

Data were expressed as mean ± standard deviation (SD). The statistical analyses were performed by Medical Statistics Service (Castellanza, VA, Italy); for the analysis of continuous variables parametric tests were used, and nonparametric tests were used to assess the efficacy of the drug (Friedman test, χ^2 approximation).

RESULTS

Demographic Characteristics

A total of 2058 patients with diagnosis of ischemic attacks were recruited. Inclusion and exclusion criteria were not fulfilled by 14 patients, who were not considered in the statistical analysis for efficacy. The 14 patients were excluded on the grounds of age limits (2 patients), different diagnosis (2 patients), inappropriate dosage of the drug in study (1 patient), and for low scoring at the Mathew Scale (9 patients). Features of the 2044 remaining patients are reported in TABLE 2.

TABLE 2. Demographic Characteristics

Patients enrolled	2058	
Patients evaluated	2044	[a]
Gender:		
Males	1132	55.5%
Females	908	44.5%
Missing	4	
Mean age	70.3	±8.65
Patients aged 45–65	485	23.7%
Patients aged >65	1559	76.3%
Years of schooling:		
1–5	429	21.0%
5–8	965	47.2%
>8	397	19.4%
Missing	253	12.4%
Family history of cerebrovascular events	761	37.2%
Diagnosis: ischemic stroke	1152	56.4%
TIA	892	43.6%

[a]14 drop out.

Males and females were equally represented, accounting for 55.5 and 44.5% respectively. The mean age was 70.3 years (485 patients, 23.7%, aged 45–65; 1559 patients, 76.3%, aged 66–85 years); nearly 50% of patients had 5–8 years schooling, and around 20% each had elementary or high school diplomas; 1152 patients (56.4%) suffered from an ischemic stroke, and 892 (43.9%) from transient ischemic attack (TIA).

Most of the patients enrolled had concomitant diseases, as shown in TABLE 3. In fact, 1781 patients (87.1%) had concurrent diseases, mainly related to the cardiovascular apparatus (72.4%) and metabolic disturbances (31.5%).

In parallel, concurrent therapies were recorded for 78.3% cases, and, likewise, drugs for the cardiovascular therapy were the majority (82.5%).

Efficacy

First Part of the Study (Days 1–28)

In order to assess the efficacy of α-GPC administered intramuscularly (im) during the 28 days of the first part of the study, which took place mainly in hospital, the Mathew Scale assessment was used; this scale scores 0 (clinical death) to 100

TABLE 3. Concomitant Diseases and Drugs

Patients with concomitant diseases	1721	87.1%
Patients without concomitant diseases	263	12.9%
Concomitant Disease:		
Cardiovascular	1290	72.4%
Metabolic/diabetes	561	31.5%
Concomitant drugs:		
Cardiac therapy	1470	82.5%
Antithrombotics	588	37.5%
Drugs for diabetes	308	19.5%

(patient with perfect consciousness).[16] A minimum score = 35 was chosen for enrollment, in order to have patients with a sufficient level of consciousness to cooperate in performing the psychometric tests.

FIGURE 1 and TABLE 4 show the trends and the mean values of the scoring to this scale at baseline and on the 28th day of treatment. The mean Mathew scale value increases from 58.7 to 74.6 corresponding to 15.9 points ($p < 0.001$).

In agreement with Gelmers,[17,18] the patients were furthermore divided into two classes: "more deteriorated" (score 35–65) and "less deteriorated" (score >65). A high percentage of patients improved their conditions at the end of the first phase of the trial, moving to the "less deteriorated" class. These changes were statistically significant ($p < 0.001$).

Second Part of the Study (Days 29–180)

In order to assess the efficacy of α-GPC during the second part of the study, in which 400 mg tid were administered orally to patients mainly discharged from hospital, the Crichton Rating Scale (CRS) and the Mini Mental State Test (MMST)

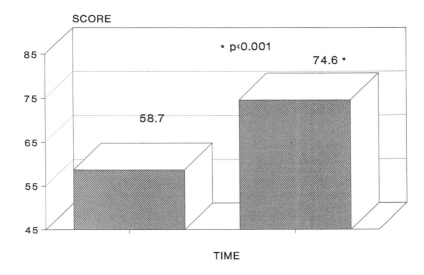

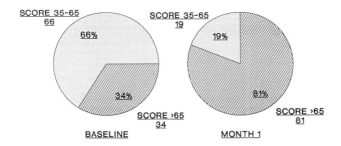

NUMBER OF PATIENTS IN TWO CLASSES
OF MATHEW SCORE

FIGURE 1. Top: Mean values of Mathew Scale in time. **Bottom:** Number and percentage in time of patients in the two classes of Mathew Scale score according to Gelmers.

TABLE 4. Mathew Scale (0–100) (First Part of the Study)

(m ± SD)	Basal (58.7 ± 12.7)	28th Day (74.6 ± 10.3)
		$p < 0.001$
Number of patients with		
score 35–65	1348 (66%)	370 (18.5%)
score > 65	696 (34%)	1635 (81.5%)

were administered to the patients on the day in which the therapy route of administration was changed (28th day) and on the 3rd and 6th month. The Crichton Geriatric Rating Scale[19] score 1–10 is considered "normal," the score 11–20 "mild deterioration," 21–30 "moderate deterioration," and > 30 "severe deterioration."

TABLE 5 and FIGURE 2 show the trend of the mean score value for the patients treated: they achieved a significant decrease (improvement) of 4.3 points, from 20.2 to 15.9, between the 28th day and the final visit. The lower part of FIGURE 2 shows the number of patients with the score corresponding to "mild deterioration": their number grows with time, increasing from 72.7% at the 3rd month to the 83.7% at the final visit (6th month).

Cognitive functions were assessed by the Mini Mental State Test in which score 0–23 is commonly considered as "abnormal deterioration" and score > 23 as "normal."[20] The mean score values increased in time, showing an improvement of 2.2 points at the 3rd month ($p < 0.001$) and above the score of normality, and a further 1.1 points at the 6th month, up to 24.3. The trend of the mean values is reported in TABLE 6 and in FIGURE 3.

Moreover, the lower part of FIGURE 3 shows the percentage of patients who recovered from an abnormal to a normal score: it increases in time, moving from 40% at the 28th day to 55.8% at the 3rd month and to 65% at the 6th month.

TABLE 5. Crichton Geriatric Rating Scale (Second Part of the Study)

(m ± SD)	28th Day (20.2 ± 7.2)	3rd Month (17.8 ± 6.05)	6th Month (15.9 ± 5.35)
		$p < 0.001$	$p < 0.001$
Number of patients with deterioration			
Mild (< 20)	1205 (59.8%)	1405 (72.7%)	1588 (83.7%)
Moderate (21–30)	613 (30.4%)	450 (23.3%)	271 (14.3%)
Severe (> 30)	197 (9.8%)	77 (4%)	38 (2%)

The degree of global deterioration was assessed with the Global Deterioration Score (GDS),[21] in which the value 0 means normality and 7 means severe deterioration. TABLE 7 and FIGURE 4 report the trend of the mean values of GDS. The mean values decreased from 2.72 at the beginning of the second phase to 2.16 at the end of the trial; the difference between the mean scores was statistically significant ($p < 0.01$).

At the end of both parts of the study, investigators were requested to report their subjective opinions about the overall clinical efficacy and tolerability of α-GPC. FIGURE 5 shows the different percentages of the investigators' opinion at the end of each one of the two parts of the study.

A "very good"/"good" efficacy was reported by 68.9% (first part) and 77.6% (second part) of the investigators; a "moderate" efficacy was reported by 24.8% (first part) and 17.5% (second part) of investigators, and a "poor"/"none" efficacy was reported by 6.3% (first part) and 4.9% (second part) of the investigators.

Tolerability

Of the 2044 patients considered for the study, 140 (6.8%) withdrew from the treatment: 101 during the first part and 38 during the second part. The reasons for

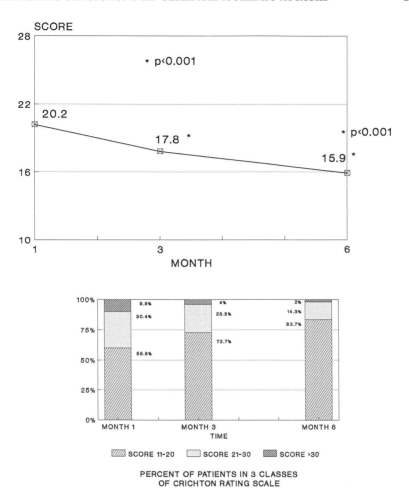

FIGURE 2. Top: Mean values of Crichton Geriatric Rating Scale in time. **Bottom:** Number and percentage in time of patients in the deterioration classes of Crichton Geriatric Rating Scale.

TABLE 6. Minimental State Test (Second Part of the Study)

(m ± SD)	28th Day (21.0 ± 6.1)	3rd Month (23.2 ± 5.4)	6th Month (24.3 ± 5.1)
		$p < 0.001$	$p < 0.001$
Number of patients with score			
0–23	1204 (60%)	851 (44.2%)	665 (35%)
>23	803 (40%)	1074 (55.8%)	1234 (65%)

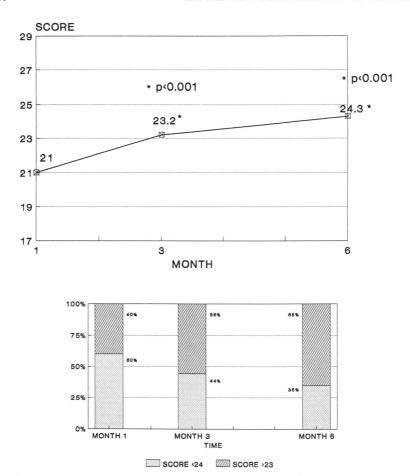

FIGURE 3. Top: Mean values of Mini Mental State Test in time. **Bottom:** Number and percentage in time of patients in the two deterioration classes of the Mini Mental State Test.

TABLE 7. Global Deterioration Scale (Second Part of the Study)

	28th Day	6th Month
m ± SD	2.72 ± 1.3	2.16 ± 1.1 $p < 0.01$

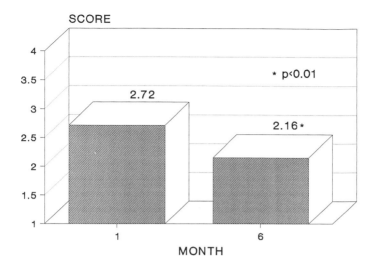

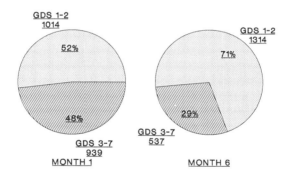

NUMBER OF PATIENTS IN TWO CLASSES
OF GDS SCORE

FIGURE 4. Top: Mean values of Global Deterioration Scale in time. **Bottom:** Number and percentage in time of patients in the classes of Global Deterioration Scale.

withdrawal are reported in TABLE 8; 41 patients died; the investigator related all the deaths to a worsening of the underlying pathology; none to the drug treatment.

Systemic tolerability was also controlled by monitoring arterial blood pressure, heart rate and blood analyses (full blood count and renal, liver functionality).

The patients were also observed for adverse events which were recorded at each control visit. TABLE 9 shows the mean values of blood pressure and heart rate: no changes occurred during all the treatment period.

No abnormal values were observed in the blood analyses as well as in the other monitoring records during the trial.

Unwanted Events

In total, 51 unwanted effects were reported by 44 out of the 2058 enrolled patients (2.14%). TABLE 10 lists all the unwanted effects complained of by the patients enrolled into the trial. Of the 2058 treated patients, 14 (0.68%) had to withdraw from the therapy with α-GPC for concomitant events: 10 in part I and 4 in part II. The reason for withdrawal were: 4 heartburn (3 in part I and 1 in part II), 2 nausea/vomit (in part I), 2 excitation/insomnia (in part I), 2 diarrhea (1 in part I, 1 in part II), 1 dizziness, 1 skin rash (in part II), 1 confusion, 1 repeated drop attacks (in part I). All the other events complained of did not result in a therapy withdrawal, and were of light or mild severity.

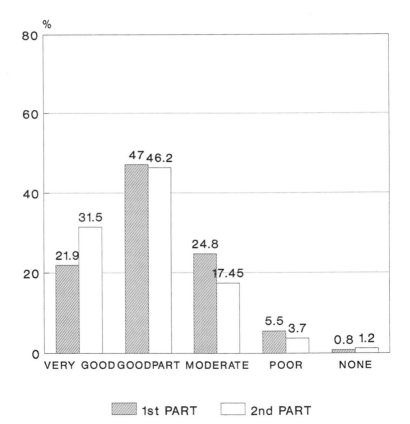

FIGURE 5. Overall clinical impression of efficacy reported by the investigators at the end of each of the two parts of the study.

TABLE 8. Discontinuation of the Trial

Reason	First Part	Second Part	Total
Drop out	52	21	73 (3.55%)
Exitus	30	11	41 (1.99%)
Unwanted events	10	4	14 (0.68%)
Improved	5	2	7 (0.34%)
Inefficacy	4	1	5 (0.24%)
	101	39	140 (6.8%)

The most frequent reported side effects were: heartburn (14), excitation-insomnia (9), nausea (8) and headache (4).

CONCLUSIONS

The present results collected from a large patient population diagnosed for acute ischemic cerebral attacks confirm the efficacy of α-GPC on the mental recovery after stroke.

At the end of the first part of the study, after 1 month of parenteral therapy with α-GPC, the results were very good both in tolerability and in efficacy: Mathew Scale reached a mean score equivalent to a less deteriorated neurological condition (> 65) and the tolerability was good: 34 events (1.66%) and 10 withdrawals (0.49%).

The improvement was maintained in time during the following 5 months of oral therapy, and a further improvement in cognitive functions (by the Minimental State Test), in behavioral functions (by the Crichton Geriatric Rating Scale), and in medical conditions related to cognitive decline (by the GDS) was statistically evaluable.

Tolerability was very good also in the second part: 17 events (0.33%) and 4 withdrawals (0.2%).

These data confirm in a large patient population the efficacy and the therapeutic role of α-GPC on the cognitive enhancement of patients with an acute cerebrovascular attacks (stroke and/or TIA): the very low incidence of adverse events confirms that α-GPC can be safely administered also for a long period after the occurrence of stroke.

TABLE 9. Arterial Blood Pressure and Heart Rate (Mean, Standard Deviation, Range)

	First Part		Second Part	
	Basal	28th Day	3rd Month	6th Month
Systolic (mean ± SD)	159 ± 23	149 ± 17	149.5 ± 15	149 ± 14.6
Range	100–240	100–200	100–200	100–205
Diastolic (mean ± SD)	90 ± 12	85 ± 9	85 ± 8	85 ± 8
Range	50–140	50–170	60–150	60–150
Heart rate (mean ± SD)	81.5 ± 12	78.5 ± 8.5	78.7 ± 8	78.6 ± 7
Range	45–152	50–120	45–165	56–110

TABLE 10. List of the 51 Adverse Events[a]

	Total	First Part	Second Part
Heartburn	14	10 (3)	4 (1)
Nausea-vomit	10	9 (2)	1
Excitation-insomnia	9	5 (2)	4
Headache	4	3	1
Diarrhea	3	2 (1)	1 (1)
Dizziness	2		2 (1)
Skin rash	2	1	1 (1)
Gastric bleeding	1		1
Increased γ-GT	1		1
Increased ALAT/ASAT	1		1
Confusion	1	1 (1)	
Anemia and low vit. B12	1	1	
Supraventricular arrhythmia	1	1	
Repeated drop attacks	1	1 (1)	

[a]The number in parenthesis indicates number of drop-out patients.

SUMMARY

The clinical efficacy and the tolerability of α-glycerophosphocholine (α-GPC), a drug able to provide high levels of choline for the nervous cells of the brain and to protect their cell walls, have been tested in a clinical open multicenter trial on 2044 patients suffering from recent stroke or transient ischemic attacks. α-GPC was administered after the attack at the daily dose of 1000 mg im for 28 days and orally at the dose of 400 mg tid during the following 5 months after the first phase.

The evaluation of the efficacy on the psychic recovery was done by the Mathew Scale (MS) during the period of im drug administration, and using the Mini Mental State Test (MMST), the Crichton Rating Scale (CRS), and the Global Deterioration Scale (GDS) during the following period of oral administration.

The MS mean increased 15.9 points in 28 days in a statistically significant way ($p < 0.001$) from 58.7 to 74.6. At the end of the 5 month oral administration, the CRS mean significantly decreased 4.3 points, from 20.2 to 15.9 ($p < 0.001$); the MMST mean significantly increased ($p < 0.001$) from 21 to 24.3 at the end of the trial, reaching the "normality" score at the 3rd month assessment. The GDS score at the end of the trial corresponded to "no cognitive decline" or "forgetfulness" in 71% of the patients. Adverse events were complained of by 44 patients (2.14%); in 14 (0.7%) the investigator preferred to discontinue therapy.

The most frequent complaints were heartburn (0.7%), nausea-vomit (0.5%), insomnia-excitation (0.4%), and headache (0.2%).

The trial confirms the therapeutic role of α-GPC on the cognitive recovery of patients with acute stroke or TIA, and the low percentage of adverse events confirms its excellent tolerability.

REFERENCES

1. LOEB, C. 1986. La diagnosi di attacco ischemico transitorio: una diagnosi facile? Aggiornamento del medico **10**(2): 86–89.

2. STAZI, C., F. CARPINTERI & F. STAZI. 1986. Ictus cerebrale: dall'etiologia alla terapia. Clin. Ter. **118**: 433–447.
3. TATEMICHI, T. K., M. A. FOULKES, J. P. MOHR, J. R. HEWITT, D. B. HIER, T. R. PRICE & P. A. WOLF. 1990. Dementia in stroke survivors in the stroke data bank cohort. Stroke **21**(6): 858–866.
4. SCHETTINI, G., C. VENTRA, T. FLORIO, M. GRIMALDI, *et al.* 1992. Molecular mechanisms mediating the effect of α-glycerylphosphorylcholine, a new cognition-enhancing drug, on behavioral and biochemical parameters in young and aged rats. Pharmacol. Biochem. Behavior **43**: 139–151.
5. GOVONI, S., C. LOPEZ, F. BATTAINI, *et al.* 1990. Effetti di alfa-GFC sul comportamento di evitamento passivo del ratto e sui livelli di acetilcolina. Basi Raz. Ter. **20**(1): 55–60.
6. DRAGO, F., L. NARDO, V. FRENI, *et al.* 1990. Effetti comportamentali di α-GFC in modelli di invecchiamento cerebrale patologico. Basi Raz. Ter. **20**(1): 65–68.
7. SPANO, P. F. & M. TRABUCCHI. 1990. Farmacocinetica e metabolismo di 14^C colina alfoscerato nel ratto. Basi Raz. Ter. **20**(1).
8. MISSALE, C., S. SIGALA & P. F. SPANO. 1990. Effetto modulatore di α-GFC sulla trasmissione colinergica nell'ippocampo di ratto. Basi Raz. Ter. **20**(1): 13–15.
9. AMENTA, F., E. BRONZETTI, M. DEL VALLE, *et al.* 1990. Neuroanatomia dell'invecchiamento cerebrale nell'animale da esperimento: effetto del trattamento con α-GFC. Basi Raz. Ter. **20**(1): 31–38.
10. CANAL, N., M. FRANCESCHI, M. ALBERONI, *et al.* 1990. Effetto di α-GFC sulla amnesia causata da scopolamina. Basi Raz. Ter. **20**(1): 75–78.
11. MOGLIA, A., S. BERGONZOLI & P. DE MOLINER. 1990. Effetto di α-GFC nel modificare il brain mapping in pazienti con Age Associated Memory Impairment (AAMI). Basi Raz. Ter. **20**(1): 83–89.
12. BASSI, S., M. G. ALBIZZATI, R. PIOLTI & L. FRATTOLA. 1990. Esperienza clinica con colina alfoscerato in pazienti affetti da demenza degenerativa primaria e multiinfartuale. Gnosis **5**: 55–62.
13. DI PERRI, R., G. COPPOLA, L. A. AMBROSIO, A. GRASSO, F. M. PUCA & M. RIZZO. 1991. A multicentre trial to evaluate the efficacy and tolerability of α-glycerylphosphoryocholine versus cytidine diphosphocholine in patients with vascular dementia. J. Int. Med. Res. **19**: 330–341.
14. FRATTOLA, L., R. PIOLTI, S. BASSI, M. G. ALBIZZATI, G. GALETTI, B. GRUMELLI, N. CANAL, *et al.* 1991. Multicenter clinical comparison of the effects of choline alphoscerate and cytidine diphosphocholine in the treatment of multiinfarct dementia. Curr. Ther. Res. **49**(4): 683–693.
15. BAN, T. A., R. PANZARASA, S. BORRA, D. DEL DUCHETTO & O. FJETLAND. 1991. Choline alphoscerate in elderly patients with cognitive decline due to dementing illness. New trends Clin. Neuropharmacol. **5**(3/4): 1–35.
16. MATHEW, N. T., J. S. MEYER, V. M. RIVERA, J. Z. CHARNEY & D. HARTMANN. 1972. Double blind evaluation of glycerol therapy in acute cerebral infarction. Lancet **7791** (Dec. 23).
17. GELMERS, H. J., K. GORTER, C. J. DE WEERDT & H. J. A. WIEZER. 1988. A controlled trial of nimodipine in acute ischemic stroke. N. Engl. J. Med. **318**(4): 203–207.
18. GELMERS, H. J., K. GORTER, C. J. DE WEERDT & H. J. A. WIEZER. 1988. Assessment of intraobserver variability in a Dutch multicenter study on acute ischemic stroke. Stroke **19**(6): 709–711.
19. GUY, W. 1976. ECDEU Assessment Manual for Psychopharmacology. Revised 1976. Department of Health, Education and Welfare Publication (ADM) 76–338. Bethesda, Md.
20. FOLSTEIN, M. F. 1983. The Mini Mental State Examination. *In* Assessment in Geriatric Psychopharmacology. T. Crook, S. Ferris & R. Barbus, Eds. Mark Powley Ass., Inc. New Canaan, Conn.
21. REISBERG, B., S. H. FERRIS, M. J. DE LEON & T. CROOK. 1982. The Global Deterioration Scale (GDS). An instrument for the assessment of primary degenerative dementia (PDD). Am. J. Psych. **139**: 1136–1139.

APPENDIX

For contributing and assessing the patients, thanks are due to following investigators:

Addis L.	Ospedale Dettori Tempio Pausania (SS)
Aguggia M.	Ospedale S. Luigi Gonzaga Orbassano (TO)
Ambrosio L.A.	Ospedale Dell'Annunziata Cosenza
Amedoro G.	Ospedale Civile Rieti
Amodio E.	Ospedale Umberto I Frosinone
Andreotti M.	Presidio Ospedaliero Varallo Sesia (VC)
Angeletti R.	Ospedale Civile Tarquinia (VT)
Ansaldi E.	Ospedale Civile SS. Antonio e Biagio Alessandria
Appiotti A.	Ospedale Mauriziano Torino
Arcara A.	Casa Di Cura Sant'Anna Palermo
Bagnato F.	Ospedale Civile G. Ciaccio Catanzaro
Barba V.R.	Ospedale S.Giuseppe Da Copertino Copertino (LE)
Barbi G.	Ospedale S. Anna Como
Bargnani C.	Ospedale Di Chiari (BS)
Belfiore A.	Ospedale Civile Ostuni (BA)
Bendandi P.	Casa Di Cura S. Francesco Ravenna
Bernacchi G.	Ospedale S. Leonardo Castellammare Di Stabia (NA)
Bernadi A.	Ospedale Di Rovereto (TN)
Bertuzzi A. Pascal G.C.	Istituti Ospedalieri Carlo Poma Mantova
Bettini R.	Ospedale Del Ponte Varese
Bonaduce V.	Ospedale Consorziale Bari
Bonasera N.	Ospedale Civico e Benfratelli Palermo
Bonincontro C.	Ospedale Civile Vasto (CH)
Bosi L.	Arcispedale S. Anna Ferrara
Cafagna D.	Ospedale Cattinara Trieste
Calcara G.	Ospedale S. Marta e. S. Venera Acireale (CT)
Camardella G.	Ospedale Civile Rieti
Cassani P.	Ospedale S. Biagio Domodossola (NO)
Castiglione R.	Ospedale Villa Sofia Palermo
Cataliotti C.	Ospedale S. Giovanni Di Dio e Isidoro Giarre (CT)
Cella L.	Ospedale S. Francesco Barga (LU)
Cerini G.	Ospedale M. Sarcone Terlizzi (BA)
Cerri C.	Ospedale Trabattoni Ronzoni Seregno (MI)
Cesareo E.	Ospedale A. Tortora Pagani (SA)
Ciannella L.	Ospedale G. Rummo Benevento
Clivati A.	Ospedale Citta' Di Sesto S. Giovanni (MI)
Codeluppi P.	Ospedale Civile I. Caffi Poggiorusco (MN)
Conti A.	Ospedale San Luca Firenze
Cortesi P.P.	Ospedale Pierantoni Forli'
Curti A.	Ospedale S. Giovanni Decoll. Andosilla Civitacastellana (VT)
Cusumano V.	Ospedale Civile Vittorio Emanuele III Monselice (PD)
D'Agnolo B.	Ospedale Cattinara Trieste
D'Angelo D.	Ospedale Generale Provinciale Giulianova (TE)
D'Auria N.	Fond. Praxis S. Maria a Vico (CE)
D'Avanzo A.	Ospedale Civile Avellino
De Angelis A.	Fond. Praxis S. Maria a Vico (CE)
De Falco F.A.	Ospedale Loreto Mare (NA)
Del Papa M.	Ospedale Civile Civitanova Marche (MC)
Di Taranto A.	Ospedale F. Lastaria Lucera (FG)
Fabriani P. Favilla A.	Ospedale F. Lotti Pontedera (PI)
Fabrizi De Biani G.	Ospedale Serristori Figline Valdarno (FI)
Fabrizi G.	Ospedale P. Burresi Poggibonsi (SI)
Facchini G.	Ospedale Del Comprensorio Lugo (RA)

Faggi L. Aimone G.	Ospedale Maggiore Lodi
Ferrari E.	Ospedale S. Margherita Pavia
Ferrari L.	Ospedale Civile Umberto I Enna
Ferrini L.	Ospedale Della Misericordia Montegranaro (AP)
Finocchiaro S.	Presidio Ospedaliero Ferrarotto Alessi Catania
Fiorina L.	Ospedale Civile Castellamonte (TO)
Galanti F.	Ospedale San Giovanni Roma
Galbiati G. Galli G.C.	Ospedale Di Lecco (CO)
Galeone F.	Ospedale Della Val Di Nievole Pescia (PT)
Galvanini G.T.	Presidio Ospedaliero Di Villafranca e Verona (VR)
Galzio R.	Ospedali Ed Istituti Riuniti Teramo
Ganga A.	Universita' Degli Studi Sassari
Gelarda G.	Ospedale Civico e Benfratelli Palermo
Gentile M.	Policlinico Umberto I Roma
Giamundo A.	II Policlinico Napoli
Giorgetti C.	Ospedale S. Chiara Pisa
Gorgone G.	Ospedale M. Raimondi S. Cataldo (CL)
Guerrieri G.	Ospedale Maggiore Modica (RG)
Gugliucci N.	Ospedale Civile Oliveto Citra (SA)
Guideri R.	Ospedale S. Andrea Massa Marittima (SI)
Guizzardi G.	Casa Di Cura De Cesaris Spoltore (PE)
Guizzaro A.	I Policlinico Napoli
Gurioli L. Desiderato P.	Ospedale Civile Cuorgne' (TO)
Gusmaroli V.	Ospedale Agnelli Pinerolo (TO)
Jorini G.M. Bazzani M.	Ospedale Civile Asola (MN)
Italiano F.	Ospedale Martini Nuovo Torino
La Rosa G.	Ospedale Regina Margherita Messina
Lagana' G.	Ospedale Morelli Reggio Calabria
Lai M.	Casa Di Cura Tomasini Ierzu (NU)
Laperuta A.	Ospedale A.Tortora Pagani (SA)
Lavitola G.	Ospedale Dell'Annunziata Cosenza
Leo F.	Ospedale G. Panico Tricase (LE)
Lipizer A.	Stabilimento Ospedaliero Gorizia
Loni G.	Ospedali Riuniti Livorno
Losi F.	Casa Di Cura S. Antonino Piacenza
Maffei R.	Ospedale S. Maria Della Pieta' Nola (NA)
Maffini S.	Ospedale Civile Cortemaggiore Piacenza
Maggi S.	Ospedale Civile Modugno (BA)
Magoni M.	Universita' Degli Studi Brescia
Manca P.	Ospedale Civile Sondrio
Mancini M. Bompani R.	Ospedale G. Stuard Parma
Mandarini A.	Ospedale Cardarelli Napoli
Mansoldo G.	Centro Ospedaliero S. Chiara Trento
Marangolo M.	Ospedale G. Garibaldi Catania
Marano R.	Policlinico Bari
Marchesi D.	Ospedale Domus Salutis Brescia
Mariella F.	Ospedale Civile Martina Franca (TA)
Marinangeli B.	Casa Di Cura Stella Maris S. Benedetto D. Tronto (AP)
Mengoli M.	Ospedale Civile S. Sebastiano Correggio (RE)
Molinari E.	Policlinico San Matteo Pavia
Morbelli E.	Casa Di Cura Societa' Esercizio Cesano Boscone (MI)
Morino U	Ospedale Martini Nuovo Torino
Munari L.	Ospedale Civile Padova
Murgia B.	Ospedale S. Francesco Nuoro
Musco A.	Ospedale Basso Ragusa Militello In Val Di Catania (CT)
Napoli S.	Ospedali Riuniti Sanremo e Bussana Sanremo (IM)

Neviani V.	Casa Di Cura Hesperia Modena
Nevola C.	Ospedale Civile Avellino
Nicolino A.	Fondaz. Clinica Del Lavoro Campoli Del Monte Taburno (BN)
Orefice G.	II Policlinico Napoli
Pacifici P.	Ospedale Civile S. Maria Dei Laici Amelia (TR)
Pagano S.	Casa Di Cura Orestano Palermo
Pagliano F.	Ospedale Generale Carate Brianza (MI)
Palermo F.	Ospedali Riuniti G. Melacrino e F. Bianchi Reggio Calabria
Papuzzo M.	Clinica S. Marco Latina
Pascalis L.	Ospedale S. Giovanni Di Dio Cagliari
Pedace C.	Ospedale S. Foiano Arezzo
Petroni A.	Clinica Di Lorenzo Avezzano (AQ)
Pipicelli G.	Ospedale Civile Soverato (CZ)
Pisani L.	Pio Albergo Trivulzio Milano
Pittera A.	Ospedale SS. Salvatore Paterno' (CT)
Platania S. Tringale G.	Ospedale Civile E Muscatello Augusta (SR)
Polizzi C.	Ospedale S. Biagio Marsala (TP)
Pomante P.	Clinica S. Anna Pomezia (ROMA)
Ponseveroni A.	Ospedale Misericordia e Dolce Prato (FI)
Porcellati C.	Ospedale Civile R. Silvestrini Perugia
Pozzuoli L.	Ospedale Civile Caserta
Principe M.	Ospedale S. Camillo De Lellis Manfredonia (FG)
Princi R.	Ospedale Civile Locri (RC)
Pumilia G.	Ospedale Civico e Benfratelli Palermo
Puoti F. Cotrufo R.	I Policlinico Napoli
Raganato G.	Ospedale S. Giuseppe Da Copertino Copertino (LE)
Rampino A.	Casa Di Cura Citta' Di Udine
Rapex G.	Ospedale M. Montessori Chiaravalle (AN)
Rascio L.	Ospedale S. Camillo Roma
Rastelli G.	Ospedale Civile Fidenza (PR)
Renzi D. Artese D.	Ospedale SS. Trinita' Popoli (PE)
Ricca M.	Ospedale Di Camerata Firenze
Rizzo D.	Ospedale Cardarelli Napoli
Rocchi G.	Stabilimento Ospedaliero Sacile (PN)
Rodari T.	Ospedali Riuniti Verbania e Pallanza Verbania (NO)
Rollandi M.	Ospedale Civile S. Andrea La Spezia
Rossini P.M.	Ospedale Fatebenefratelli Roma
Salvi P.	Ospedale Quarenghi S. Pellegrino (BG)
Sarapo G.	Ospedale Civile Villa D'Agri (PZ)
Sardi A.	Ospedale Civile Chivasso (TO)
Sarno A.	Ospedale Villa Camaldoli Napoli
Scarda G. Neri A.	Ospedale S. Filippo Neri Roma
Schioppa M.	Ospedale Vecchio Pellegrini Napoli
Schisano G.	Ospedale Nuovo Pellegrini Napoli
Sechi F. Molinu M. Testoni M.	Ospedale Presidente A. Segni Ozieri (SS)
Sesti A.G.	Casa Di Cura Villa Kraus Firenze
Sgro G.	Ospedale Dell'Annunziata Sulmona (AQ)
Simone P.	Casa Sollievo Della Sofferenza S. Giovanni Rotondo (FG)
Solinas F.	Ospedale Presidente A. Segni Ozieri (SS)
Spedo A.	Ospedale Civile Migliorini e Balzan Badia Polesine (RO)
Stella L.	Ospedale Cardarelli Napoli
Tagliabue P. Balbis E.	Ospedale S. Andrea Vercelli
Tavormina F.	Ospedale S. Antonio Abate Trapani

Tessitore A.	Ospedale Cardarelli Napoli
Timpanaro S.	Presidio Ospedaliero Vittorio Emanuele II Catania
Trampetti P.	Ospedale Civile Montefalco (PG)
Travaglini A.	Ospedale Civile S. Maria Terni
Tridico N.	Ospedale Civile Rossano (CS)
Venco A. Serena G.	Ospedale Di Circolo Varese
Vicari E.	Ospedale V. Cervello Palermo
Viglierchio P.	Ospedale San Paolo Savona
Vigna L.	Ospedale G. Ferrari Castrovillari (CS)
Vivalda L.	Ospedale Martini Nuovo Torino
Voglini C.	Ospedale S. Ambrogio Mortara (PV)
Volpe D.	Ospedale S. Raffaele Arcangelo e Fatebenefratelli Venezia
Zanardi M. Morena M. Rossi M.	Ospedale Civile Ge-Sampierdarena
Zito F.	Ospedale SS. Annunziata Taranto

Screening an Elderly Population for Verifiable Adverse Drug Reactions

Methodological Approach and Initial Data of the Berlin Aging Study (BASE)[a]

MARKUS BORCHELT AND ANN L. HORGAS

Freie Universität Berlin
Universitätsklinikum Rudolf Virchow (Charlottenburg)
Forschungsgruppe Geriatrie
Haus 9, Spandauer Damm 130
14050 Berlin, Germany

INTRODUCTION

Elderly subjects are generally considered to be at high risk for adverse drug reactions (ADR).[1–3] Though chronological age per se has been frequently implicated in this phenomenon,[4,5] increasing evidence suggests multimorbidity, concomittant polypharmacy,[6–9] and physiological changes in the pharmacodynamics and pharmacokinetics of drugs[10,11] as the principal phenomena underlying the age-related increase in the incidence of ADR.

The evidence, however, is not conclusive, and discussion of the role of age as an independent risk factor in ADR remains controversial.[12,13] This controversy may in part arise from the methodological difficulties associated with studies of ADR in the aged. Although a substantial number of investigations have been undertaken, the precise prevalence rate of adverse drug reactions among elderly adults is still unclear.[14] Different sampling procedures and assessment strategies account for some of the discrepancies in ADR rates across different studies. To date, most studies have focused on clinical samples,[15] especially on patients hospitalized due to adverse reactions to drugs,[5,8,16,17] and on patients who develop adverse reactions during a hospital stay.[13,18] However, reported prevalence rates differ remarkably, ranging from 10% to 31% and from 2% to 44%, respectively. Relatively few studies have focused on community-dwelling older adults.[19–21] Within these studies, reported rates of ADR also vary substantially between 8% and 42%.[10]

With regard to the assessment of ADRs, many studies have relied on voluntary physician reporting,[12,22] retrospective chart review, or patients' self-reports.[21] Spontaneous reporting, however, is likely to underestimate the actual rate of ADR.[12] This is especially true for elderly populations since multimorbidity, which is prevalent in old

[a]The Berlin Aging Study (BASE) is financially supported by two German Federal Departments: the Department of Research and Technology (13 TA 011: 1988–1991) and the Department of Family and Senior Citizens (1991 to present). The institutions involved are the Free University of Berlin and the Max-Planck-Institute for Human Development and Education, Berlin, where the study is housed. The Steering Committee is cochaired by Paul B. Baltes and Karl Ulrich Mayer, and it consists of the directors of the four cooperating research units (Paul B. Baltes, psychology; Karl Ulrich Mayer, sociology; Elisabeth Steinhagen-Thiessen, internal medicine and geriatrics; Hanfried Helmchen, psychiatry) and the field research coordinator, Reinhard Nuthmann.

age, is often considered first as a potential cause for any new symptom. In addition, concomittant polypharmacy adds substantially to the methodological problems of assessing specific drug etiologies among elderly patients.[23]

Accurate estimation of ADR prevalence among older adults is also hampered by the lack of standardization in both the definition of adverse drug reactions and the screening procedures used to assess them. The World Health Organization defined an adverse reaction as any response to a drug "which is noxious and unintended and which occurs at doses used in man for prophylaxis, diagnosis, or therapy."[24] Though this definition seems clear, it does not help in defining a specific event as the result of a specific drug course. At a more fundamental level, definitions of specific drugs and drug groups that are considered causal agents of ADR are often arbitrary or inexplicit. Diuretics, for instance, may or may not be considered antihypertensive agents, an ambiguity that will influence detection and reporting of adverse effects involving this drug class. However, in an attempt to standardize the process of determining whether or not a clinical manifestation (e.g., symptom, laboratory alteration) is the result of a specific drug, detailed algorithms have been developed that can be used to estimate the likelihood that a specific event is an ADR.[15,25] Though an important contribution in the field, considerable interrater variability[26,27] and intermethod variability[28] persist, due to the role of individual judgment in evaluating risk as well as due to the lack of method sensitivity, specificity, and predictive validity.[26-28] In each of these studies and published algorithms, screening for ADR begins with presentation of a specific clinical sign or symptom and proceeds backwards to evaluate the potential source. This reliance on presenting clinical manifestations contributes (a) to the underestimation of the prevalence of ADR in elderly subjects, especially since it has been documented that elders underreport symptoms,[21] and (b) to the unclear definition of ADR since it is rarely, if ever with regard to relatively "minor" events (e.g., headache, GI upset, rash), specified which clinical manifestations warrant further investigation as potential ADR.

Thus, using an alternative assessment methodology, the purpose of the present study is to evaluate explicitly defined ADR risks in a representative sample of old and very old adults based on screening of their drug regimens, and to evaluate the cooccurrence of corresponding verifiable laboratory manifestations. Specifically, the objectives of this investigation are (1) to examine the overall prevalence of drug-related risks for fluid/electrolyte imbalance and renal dysfunction, (2) to estimate the cooccurrence of corresponding alterations in nine commonly used laboratory screening parameters, (3) to identify all potentially involved drug etiologies, and (4) to evaluate the magnitude of age effects relative to drug effects on variation in laboratory parameters.

SAMPLE

The data reported here represent a subset of the intensive 14-session data collection protocol of the ongoing multidisciplinary Berlin Aging Study, comprised of assessments from four different disciplines (e.g., internal medicine, psychiatry, sociology, and psychology). The BASE sample is designed to be representative of the western part of the city of Berlin and to oversample the very old and the male population. Specifically, it is a probability sample of community-dwelling and institutionalized individuals aged 70 to 100+ years which is drawn from the city registration office (in the Federal Republic of Germany, every citizen is registered). The present subsample ($n = 336$) was stratified by age and sex by randomly selecting, within each cell of the original study design, 28 individuals from the larger parent sample of

TABLE 1. Sample Description

Demographic Characteristics	Percent		χ^2 (df)[b]
	Current Sample ($n = 336$)	First-wave Sample[a] ($n = 156$)	
Age (yrs)			
70–84	50.0	50.0	—
85–100+	50.0	50.0	—
Sex			
Women	50.0	50.0	—
Men	50.0	50.0	—
Martial status			
Married	30.7	25.0	4.2 (3)
Widowed	54.2	58.3	
Divorced	6.5	5.1	
Never married	8.6	11.5	
Housing types			
Institutionalized	15.5	17.3	0.4 (1)
Education			
Primary	67.5	69.5	1.4 (2)
Lower secondary	25.1	24.0	
Matriculation/university	7.4	6.5	
Vocational training	57.4	59.6	0.3 (1)
Income (DM)			
< 1,000	3.8	4.5	2.4 (4)
1000– < 1400	20.0	16.7	
1400– < 1800	28.0	25.6	
1800– < 2200	16.4	19.2	
> 2200	33.8	34.0	

[a]Subjects contacted before August 24, 1991.[29]
[b]All chi-square statistics not significant ($p > 0.10$).

individuals who completed the intensive protocol. This intermediary sample reflects the stratification strategy of the BASE study and is comparable to both the initial stratified sample ($n = 156$) and the final sample ($n = 516$) which is not yet available for analysis. TABLE 1 summarizes demographic characteristics of the current sample as well as those obtained for the first wave of BASE participants ($n = 156$) who were contacted before August 24, 1991. In comparison, the current sample's characteristics were within statistical boundaries of the initial sample. As previously reported,[29] no major selection effects were observed for this initial sample when a variety of demographic and basic functioning variables were considered. One exception was 12-month mortality rate following initial contact for BASE participants: elderly volunteers who completed the entire 14-session protocol had a lower mortality rate than those who refused participation or dropped out of the study.

LABORATORY SCREENING

Venipuncture was made by examining physicians at the end of the second medical session. A blood sample was obtained from all but eight participants (2.4%) who refused venipuncture. Thirty-one blood samples (9.2%) were obtained from nonfasting subjects or had a delay between venipuncture and laboratory testing longer than 8 hours and were subsequently excluded from analyses. Standard biochemical procedures were used to quantify nine parameters: serum creatinine, blood urea nitrogen (BUN), potassium, calcium, sodium, and chloride, and urine protein and hemoglobin. Twelve specific alterations were identified by comparison with standard normal ranges (TABLE 2) which were not adjusted for age.

SCREENING PROCEDURES FOR VERIFIABLE ADR

Currently used medications, prescription as well as nonprescription drugs, were assessed during the BASE data collection protocol by standardized physician interviews at the participant's place of residence. For ascertaining assessment of drug use as completely as possible, two different questionnaires were administered to all participants. The first asked directly for all drugs currently used; the second was guided by symptoms and disorders and asked for related drug use consecutively. During both these interviews, original drug containers were inspected for each reported medication. Additional validating information was gathered by telephone interviews with participants' family physicians. Therefore, accidental inconsistencies were identified instantaneously and were traced and corrected by reassessment of the questioned drugs. The questionnaires were administered in a two- to three-week interval. Within this period, newly started drugs were disregarded since laboratory testing was completed before the date of the second interview.

All reported drugs were screened for potential fluid, electrolyte, and renal ADR using computer algorithms. The reference database contained complete drug information from the German Physician's Desk Reference[30] and is comprised of 10,672 preparations from 416 different manufacturers and includes 6270 chemically defined drugs. This reference was chosen for three reasons: (1) it is the most frequently used drug reference in German clinical medicine, (2) for each preparation, a five-digit code reflecting 87 primary indication classes is provided, and (3) most importantly, a semistandardized, hierarchical system of coded ADR descriptions is presented that first combines substances with similar ADR patterns, and then specifies ADR consecutively according to the affected organ systems based on the WHO classification system.[31]

The computerized search algorithms were designed not only to check the codings of ADR descriptions for verifiable effects (i.e., alteration of laboratory parameters) but also to identify unclassified text entries for the appearance of the following keywords: renal failure, renal dysfunction, nephropathy, nephritis, hematuria, nephrotic syndrome, proteinuria, fluid imbalance, fluid retention, dehydration, electro-

TABLE 2. Normal Ranges of Laboratory Parameters in Serum

Parameter	Unit		Range
Sodium	mmol/l		134–145
Chloride	mmol/l		95–112
Potassium	mmol/l		3.4–5.2
Calcium	mmol/l		2.1–2.6
Hematocrit	%	Women	37–47
		Men	40–54
BUN[a]	mg/dl		14–46
Creatinine	mg/dl		<1.3

[a]BUN = blood urea nitrogen.

lyte imbalance, hypo-/hyperkalemia, hypo-/hypercalcemia, hyponatremia, or hypochloremia. However, no attempt was made to identify inconsistencies within the Desk Reference itself, e.g., citation of a specific ADR for one preparation but not for another containing the same ingredient(s). The drugs that were identified by the algorithms as potential causes for the 12 selected laboratory alterations are summa-

TABLE 3. Drugs Implicated in Causing Laboratory Alterations Based on Information in the Rote Liste$^{(R)}$, by Potential Effect

Renal Function			
Elevated Creatinine	Elevated BUN	Proteinuria	Hematuria
ACE-inhibitors	Cephalosporins	Griseofulvin	H$_2$-blockers
Acetaminophen	Levodopa	Laxatives	Indomethacin
Allopurinol	Loop diuretics	NSAID	Laxatives
Aminoglycosides	Nimodipine	Pyritinol	Paraldehyde
Cytostatics	Retinoids		Phenolphthalein
Diclofenac	Spironolactone		Phenylbutazone
Gold salts	Thiazides		Salicylates
Indomethacin	Triamterene		Vitamin D
Loop diuretics	Trimethoprim		
Methotrexate			
Penicilline			
Phenylbutazone			
Salicylates			
Spironolactone			
Thiazides			
Triamterene			

Electrolyte Balance			
Hypokalemia	Hyperkalemia	Hypocalcemia	Hypercalcemia
Cisplatin	ACE-inhibitors	Cisplatin	Antacids
Corticosteroids	Amiloride	Laxatives	Calcium
Laxatives	Diclofenac	Loop diuretics	Tamoxifen
Loop diuretics	Indomethacin		Thiazides
Thiazides	Spironolactone		Vitamin D
	Triamterene		

Fluid Homeostasis			
Hypernatremia	Hyponatremia	Hypochloremia	Dehydration
Corticosteroids	Carbamazepine	Thiazides	Loop diuretics
Estrogens	Cisplatin		
Guanethidine	Loop diuretics		
Methyldopa	Spironolactone		
NSAID	Thiazides		

rized in TABLE 3. This table also illustrates the uniqueness of this approach, since many references contain tables of potential ADR grouped for different drugs but only a few provide tables of drugs grouped for potential clinical manifestations of adverse effects.[32]

DEFINITION OF AT-RISK AND CONTROL GROUPS

Using the ADR screening procedure described above, subjects at specific risk for ADR were identified by their reported use of at least one drug implicated in the selected laboratory alterations. Review of the ADR descriptions for the identified drugs revealed that regular long-term treatment was an important factor in many of them. Therefore, definite risk for a specific adverse reaction was coded only if a drug was used on a regular basis for at least one year. Subjects using at least one such drug were considered at risk.

In addition, for each of the three domains assessed (i.e., renal function, electrolyte balance, and fluid homeostasis), separate control groups were defined. These consisted of subjects who used either no drugs or only drugs without any known adverse effects on the domain-specific laboratory parameters. Therefore, comparisons of drug-ADR associations were based on three relative risk groups: (1) subjects at definite risk for specific ADR, (2) subjects not at risk for these or comparable ADR (i.e., adverse effects on other parameters within the same domain), and (3) subjects at risk for comparable ADR or at questionable risk due to irregular or short-term use of implicated drugs. For example, the group at risk for drug-related hyponatremia was compared (a) to those not at risk for hyponatremia and (b) to those at risk for other fluid homeostatic alterations (e.g., dehydration) or who did not use these causal drugs in the defined manner. Therefore, all analyses were based on the entire sample excluding only subjects with missing laboratory values.

AGE-DEPENDENT ADR SUSCEPTIBILITY

With regard to the question of increasing ADR susceptibility with age, regression analyses were conducted using age, ADR risk group, and a risk-by-age interaction term as predictors. To avoid leverage points, the interaction term was defined by the product of ADR risk group and the difference between actual age and the mean age of 85 years (denoted as "age_Z"). Laboratory values that were significantly related to drug use in chi-square analyses were defined as the dependent variables Y in the overall regression equation denoted as:

$$Y = b_1 * age_Z + b_2 * risk + b_3 * (age_Z * risk) + c \qquad \text{(F1)}$$

These regression models indicated only one ADR risk group by combining the two groups at any specific or comparable/questionable risk. This combined group was contrasted against those not at risk in order to maximize statistical power for the detection of even small contributions of age to ADR susceptibility. Since "ADR risk" is coded as an indicator variable (i.e., "0" for no risk and "1" for at risk), this regression equation can be interpreted as a combination of two separate equations, one for each group as seen below.

Not at risk:

$$Y_0 = b_1 * age_Z + c \qquad \text{(F2)}$$

and at risk:

$$Y_1 = b_1 * age_Z + b_2 + b_3 * age_Z + c \qquad \text{(F3)}$$

which can be reduced to

$$Y_1 = Y_0 + b_2 + b_3 * \text{age}_Z \tag{F4}$$

Hence, coefficient b_2 in Equation F1 indicated the mean difference between both groups regardless of age whereas coefficient b_3 reflected the age-dependent change of this mean difference. An increasing difference with age would be indicated by identical signs for both b_2 and b_3 and a decrease if the signs were different. Thus, the partial F value associated with b_3 in Equation F1 was used as a test for changing ADR susceptibility with age.

RESULTS

The mean number of concurrently used drugs was 5.9 [standard deviation (SD) = 3.2] in this sample of very old adults. Evaluation of the associated ADR profiles revealed high rates of risk for potential adverse effects on renal function, electrolyte balance, and fluid homeostasis. The most common risks (TABLE 4) were due to the use of drugs with known potential for hypokalemia ($n = 110$ subjects at definite specific risk), creatinine increase ($n = 104$ subjects), BUN increase ($n = 103$),

TABLE 4. Frequencies of Laboratory Alterations by ADR Risk Group

Domain/ Alteration	ADR Risk Group						Chi-Square
	Neither Specific nor Comparable Risks		Comparable or Questionable Risks		Definite Specific Risks		
	%	$n_a/n_t{}^a$	%	$n_a/n_t{}^a$	%	$n_a/n_t{}^a$	
Renal function							
Incr. BUN	28.7	(43/150)	40.9	(18/44)	43.7	(45/103)	6.6^c
Incr. crea.	12.3	(19/155)	23.9	(11/46)	28.8	(30/104)	11.5^d
Proteinuria	12.8	(16/125)	29.2	(26/89)	23.7	(9/38)	9.0^c
Hematuria	9.6	(12/125)	9.5	(10/105)	4.8	(1/21)	0.5
Any alteration	46.4	(58/125)	62.2 (79/127)				6.3^c
Electrolyte balance							
Hypokalemia	1.3	(2/153)	5.9	(2/34)	10.9	(12/110)	11.6^e
Hyperkalemia	2.0	(3/153)	2.5	(2/81)	3.2	(2/63)	0.3
Hypocalcemia	5.2	(8/153)	3.8	(4/106)	2.6	(1/38)	0.6
Hypercalcemia	0.7	(1/153)	—	(0/89)	3.6	(2/55)	4.9^b
Any alteration	9.2	(14/153)	16.7 (24/144)				3.8^b
Fluid homeostasis							
Hypernatremia	11.6	(22/190)	6.6	(5/76)	16.7	(5/30)	2.6
Hyponatremia	1.1	(2/190)	—	(0/25)	2.4	(2/82)	1.2
Hypochloremia	0.5	(1/190)	—	(0/60)	4.3	(2/47)	6.0^c
Dehydration	4.2	(8/190)	2.9	(2/69)	5.3	(2/38)	0.4
Any alteration	16.8	(32/190)	15.0 (16/107)				0.2

$^a n_a$, number of subjects with alteration; n_t, total number of subjects per group.
$^b p < 0.10$.
$^c p < 0.05$.
$^d p < 0.01$.
$^e p < 0.001$.

TABLE 5. Possible Drug Etiologies for Laboratory Alterations that Were Significantly Associated with ADR Risk

Alteration	Cases	Possible Drug Etiologies[a]
Hypochloremia	2	Loop diuretics (2), thiazides (2)
Hypokalemia	12	Thiazides (8), loop diuretics (4), laxatives (1)
Hypercalcemia	2	Thiazides (2)
BUN increase	45	Thiazides (26), triamterene (14), loop diuretics (17), spironolactone (5), levodopa (1), trimethoprim (1)
Creatinine increase	30	Thiazides (17), loop diuretics (14), triamterene (9), ACE-inhibitors (4), allopurinol (4), acetaminophen (2), spironolactone (2), aminoglycosides (1), NSAID (1)
Proteinuria	9	Laxatives (6), NSAID (3)

[a]The total of possible etiologies per alteration did not equal the number of cases due to multiple drug use.

hyponatremia ($n = 82$), and hypercalcemia ($n = 55$). Overall, 48.1% of all subjects in the sample were at risk for at least one of the 12 potential effects studied in association with long-term regular drug use.

Alterations of laboratory parameters were also frequently observed. Signs of renal failure predominated with elevated blood urea nitrogen (BUN) in 35.7% of subjects, proteinuria in 20.2%, and elevated creatinine in 19.7%. With regard to electrolytes, hypokalemia was the most prevalent finding (5.4%), followed by hypocalcemia (4.4%). Clinical manifestation of hypochloremia was least common (1.0%).

Chi-square analyses on the frequencies of altered lab values by ADR-risk group revealed significant differences in the rates of occurrence for six of the 12 investigated alterations (TABLE 4). Compared to subjects at no risk for domain-related adverse effects, laboratory alterations specifically corresponding to ADR exposure were significantly more frequent in elderly subjects at definite risk for elevated BUN (43.7% vs. 28.7%), elevated creatinine (28.8% vs. 12.3%), proteinuria (23.7% vs. 12.8%), hypokalemia (10.9% vs. 1.3%), hypochloremia (4.3% vs. 0.5%), and hypercalcemia (3.6% vs. 0.7%). Overall, 25.8% of all subjects in the sample were identified with at least one cooccurence of a definite and specific ADR risk and the corresponding laboratory alteration.

Specific drugs that were potentially associated with these alterations are summarized in TABLE 5. Subjects with creatinine and/or BUN increase ($n = 53$) were predominantly receiving diuretic treatment due to congestive heart failure or hypertension. Only 7 of these elders (13.2%) had a preexisting diagnosis of renal failure. All elders with both manifest proteinuria and a related ADR risk ($n = 9$) were either users of laxatives or NSAIDs. None had a previously diagnosed nephrotic syndrome, though one had a preexisting nephrolithiasis. Nearly all elders with manifest hypokalemia, hypercalcemia, or hypochloremia ($n = 22$) had a long-term prescription of either thiazides or loop diuretics ($n = 17; 77.3\%$). In comparison, among subjects with no such alterations ($n = 314$), use of diuretic drugs was found in only 31.8%.

Multivariate regression analyses confirmed these results by using the original laboratory values as dependent variables (TABLE 6). Proportions of variance in laboratory values attributable to age and ADR risk were evaluated by testing the effect of removing each of the variables from the equations separately. As indicated by the change in R square on removal, proportions of variance attributable to ADR risk varied between 1.0% for variation in calcium levels and 7.3% in serum chloride levels. Variance attributable to age effects varied between 0.0% for serum chloride and 5.1% for serum calcium variability. In comparison, drug effects accounted for larger proportions of variability in serum potassium (5.7% vs. 1.9%), chloride (7.3% vs. 0.0%), and creatinine (2.7% vs. 1.9%).

By using the previously described overall regression Equation F1, the coefficient for the risk-by-age interaction term (b_3) was estimated for potassium, calcium, chloride, creatinine, and BUN as dependent variables (TABLE 6). All estimations of the coefficient for this term, which was used as an indicator of age-dependent ADR susceptibility, revealed only small values that did not reach any statistical significance. Hence, the regression models indicated that the observed adverse drug effects on the selected laboratory parameters were all independent of the subjects' ages.

TABLE 6. Multiple Regression Analyses: Estimated Coefficients for Age (b_1), ADR Risk (b_2), and Risk-by-Age Interactions (b_3) and Attributable Proportions of Variance

Dependent Variable (Y)	Estimates for Coefficients[a] (% variance)			Const.	F
	b_1	b_2	b_3		
Potassium	$+0.010^c$	-0.209^c	-0.004	$+4.222$	7.1^e
	(1.9)	(5.7)	(0.2)		
Calcium	-0.004^e	$+0.023^b$	$+0.001$	$+2.282$	8.5^e
	(5.1)	(1.0)	(0.0)		
Chloride	$+0.002$	-2.145^e	-0.030	$+105.113$	12.7^e
	(0.0)	(7.3)	(0.1)		
Creatinine	$+0.009^c$	$+0.127^d$	-0.001	$+1.000$	6.8^e
	(1.9)	(2.7)	(0.0)		
BUN	$+0.497^d$	$+5.194^c$	-0.022	$+41.596$	7.0^e
	(2.5)	(1.8)	(0.0)		

[a]Equations were denoted for each dependent variable Y as $Y = b_1 * \text{age}_z + b_2 * \text{ADR risk} + b_3 * \text{age}_z * \text{ADR risk} + \text{const.}$ with binary coding of ADR risk ($0 = \text{no}/1 = \text{yes}$ for both the groups at primary and secondary or questionable risk) and $\text{age}_z = \text{age} - 85$.
[b]$p < 0.10$.
[c]$p < 0.05$.
[d]$p < 0.01$.
[e]$p < 0.001$.

DISCUSSION

The analyses reported here used a methodologically different approach to the assessment of ADR in elderly subjects. This method first assessed all drugs reported by the participants for specific potential ADR, rather than beginning with a clinical manifestation and inferring an ADR. In a second step, evidence of laboratory alterations consistent with adverse effects of the identified drugs were assessed and the congruence between drug use and laboratory manifestation evaluated. This method provides valuable contributions towards more reliable estimates of the prevalence of ADR since it evaluates all of the medications used by elderly subjects, rather than evaluating one drug in relation to a specific, presenting clinical manifestation. In addition, these analyses rely on objective laboratory parameters rather than subjective symptom reports, thus providing more reliable evidence for verifiable ADR.

In addition, the present investigation is based on explicitly defined groups at ADR risk and tested the occurence of specific potential ADRs against a control group. It should be noted, however, that subjects in the control groups were also using drugs, though not necessarily those being implicated in the specific adverse effects under investigation. Therefore, assignment of subjects to the control groups is heavily dependent on complete identification of all potential adverse outcomes of drug regimen by the screening procedure used. Exclusion of a drug from the list of potential ADR-inducing agents in the German Physician's Desk Reference[30] does not automatically imply concensus on its safety, since ADR reference sources vary markedly in the ADRs that they identify.[33] Misclassification errors of this type, however, can be assumed to increase the likelihood of accepting the null hypothesis of no statistical relationship between drug and effect, thereby underestimating rather than overestimating the magnitude of verifiable ADR in this sample.

It is important to note that six of the nine laboratory parameters investigated in this study were significantly influenced by drug use. In particular, long-term use of diuretics has been identified as presenting serious risks for electrolyte imbalance and renal impairment in elderly patients. It should be mentioned, however, that these relationships were analyzed without controlling for additive effects (e.g., simultaneous risks for hypokalemia due to concommitant treatment with loop diuretics and laxatives), or counterbalancing effects (e.g., simultaneous hydrochlorothiazide and triamterene treatment with both the risk for hypo- and hyperkalemia).

Further, the statement of "verifiable" ADR should be interpreted cautiously. Due to the cross-sectional design of this study, dechallenge and rechallenge of the potentially offending drugs and controlling for individual differences in disease course was not possible. Therefore, the congruence between use of drugs with potential ADR risk and observed laboratory alterations reflects probable, but not definite, ADR.

Finally, initial analyses of age as a factor that potentially increased susceptibility for adverse drug effects on laboratory parameters suggest little, if any, effect. In order to examine this question more definitively, however, additional analyses are needed. Though beyond the scope of the present paper, multivariate regression models must be used that control for the existence and severity of medical conditions and the total number of drugs taken in order to examine the independent effect of age more carefully.

In conclusion, a different approach to assessing ADR, one that screens all currently used medications for potential effects, provides an alternative view of the prevalence of ADR in elderly subjects. Though restricted to estimates of ADR in a limited number of domains rather than global prevalence rates, this approach indicates that elderly subjects are at considerable risk for ADR that influence fluid, electrolyte, and renal parameters. Thus, monitoring of medications for these effects is highly recommended, especially in elderly patients on long-term drug therapy. In addition, use of the implicated drugs, especially long-term diuretic treatment, must be taken into account when interpreting laboratory findings in patients of advanced old age.

SUMMARY

Older adults are known to carry the largest risk for potential adverse drug reactions (ADR) due to the increased number of diseases and concurrent drug therapies. Prevalence rates of the most frequently used drugs in this population have already been evaluated, but the actual rates of specific drug-related risks (e.g., renal dysfunction) have not. Precise estimates of specific ADR risks rely on careful evaluation of the complete drug regimen for potential adverse effects, especially for elderly subjects. In addition, evaluations of manifest ADR have generally been based on reviews of individual medical records or self-reported symptoms. Systematic screening of a representative sample of elders for verifiable potential ADR has not been performed to date and is methodologically challenging. However, the present study attempts to assess both the prevalence of explicitly defined risks for known ADR and the corresponding cooccurrence of laboratory parameter alterations using a new approach. Initial findings are reported for a nearly-representative, age and sex stratified sample of 70 to 100+ year old subjects ($n = 336$) who participated in the Berlin Aging Study (BASE). Analyses focused on adverse drug effects on fluid and electrolyte balance and renal function. The results indicated an overall prevalence rate of 50% for selected ADR risks and a rate of 26% for the cooccurence of corresponding laboratory alterations. By taking age into account, preliminary multivariate analyses did not support the hypothesis of increasing ADR susceptibility with advancing age.

REFERENCES

1. HARTSHORN, E. A. & D. S. TATRO. 1991. Principles of drug interactions. *In* Drug Interaction Facts. D. S. Tatro, Ed.: xix–xxvi. J. B. Lippincott. St. Louis, Mo.
2. TANNER, L. A., C. BAUM, C. PRELA & D. L. KENNEDY. 1986. Spontaneous adverse reaction reporting in the elderly for 1986. J. Geriatr. Drug Ther. **3:** 31–54.
3. ZUCKERMAN, I. H. & L. H. ODERDA. 1986. Drug therapy in the elderly patient-1986. Consultant Pharmacist **5:** 191–195.
4. KLEIN, U., M. KLEIN, H. STURM, M. ROTHENBÜHLER, R. HUBER, P. STUCKI, I. GIKALOV, M. KELLER & R. HOIGNE. 1976. The frequency of adverse drug reactions as dependend upon age, sex, and duration of hospitalization. Int. J. Clin. Pharmacol. **13:** 187–195.
5. WILLIAMSON, J. & J. M. CHOPIN. 1980. Adverse reactions to prescribed drugs in the elderly: a multicentre investigation. Age Ageing. **9:** 73–80.
6. BORCHELT, M., M. LINDEN, J. P. FISCHER & B. GEISELMANN. 1991. Impact of multimedication on health status of the very old. Paper presented at the 44th Annual Scientific Meeting of the Gerontological Society of America, San Francisco. Gerontologist **31.**
7. CARBONI, P., M. PAHOR, R. BERNABEI & A. SGADARI. 1991. Is age an independent risk factor of adverse drug reactions in hospitalized medical patients? J. Am. Geriatr. Soc. **39:** 1093–1099.
8. GRYMONPRE, R. E., P. A. MITENKO, D. S. SITAR, F. Y. AOKI & P. R. MONTGOMERY. 1988. Drug-associated hospital admissions in older medical patients. J. Am. Geriatr. Soc. **36:** 1092–1098.
9. SMUCKER, W. D. & J. R. KONTAK. 1990. Adverse drug reactions causing hospital admission in an elderly population: experience with a decision algorithm. J. Am. Board Family Practitioners **3:** 105–109.
10. DENHAM, M. J. 1990. Adverse drug reactions. Br. Med. Bull. **46:** 53–62.
11. VESTAL, R. E. & G. W. DAWSON. 1985. Pharmacology and aging. *In* Handbook of the Biology of Aging. C. E. Finch & E. L. Schneider, Eds.: 744–819. Van Nostrand Reinhold. New York, N.Y.
12. BURKE, L. B., H. M. JOLSON, R. A. GOETSCH & J. C. AHRONHEIM. 1993. Geriatric drug use and adverse drug event reporting in 1990: a descriptive analysis of two national data bases. In Annual Review of Gerontology and Geriatrics: Focus on Medications and the Elderly. J. W. Rowe & J. C. Ahronheim, Eds. **12:** 1–28. Springer. New York, N.Y.
13. NOLAN, L. & K. O'MALLEY. 1988. Prescribing for the elderly. I. Sensitivity of the elderly to adverse drug reactions. J. Am. Geriatr. Soc. **36:** 143–149.

14. AVORN, J. 1990. Reporting drug side effects: signals and noise. (Editorial.) JAMA. **263:** 1823.
15. KARCH, F. E. & L. LASAGNA. 1975. Adverse drug reactions: a critical review. JAMA **234:** 1236–1241.
16. HURWITZ, N. 1969. Predisposing factors in adverse reactions to drugs. B. Med. J. **1:** 536–539.
17. LEVY, M., W. KEWITZ, J. HILLEBRAND & M. ELIAKIM. 1980. Hospital admissions due to adverse drug reactions: a comparative study from Jurusalem and Berlin. Eur. J. Clin. Pharmacol. **17:** 25–31.
18. SEIDL, L. G., G. F. THORNTON, J. W. SMITH & L. E. CLUFF. 1966. Studies on the epidemiology of adverse drug reactions. III. Reactions in patients on a general medical service. Bull. Johns Hopkins Hosp. **119:** 299–315.
19. HUTCHINSON, T. A., K. M. FLEGEL, M. S. KRAMER, D. G. LEDUC & M. S. HOPINGKONG. 1986. Frequency, severity and risk factors for adverse reactions in adult outpatients: a prospective study. J. Chronic Dis. **39:** 533–542.
20. KELLAWAY, G. S. M. & E. MCCRAE. 1979. Intensive monitoring for adverse drug effects in patients discharged from acute medical wards. N. Zealand Med. J. **78:** 525–528.
21. KLEIN, L. E., P. S. GERMAN & D. M. LEVINE. 1984. Medication problems among outpatients. Arch. Intern. Med. **144:** 1185–1188.
22. CASTLEDEN, C. M. & H. PICKLES. 1988. Suspected adverse drug reactions in elderly patients reported to the Committee on Safety of Medications. Br. J. Clin. Pharmacol. **26:** 347–353.
23. GROHMANN, R., P. DIRSCHEDL, E. RENNIG, J. SCHERER & L. G. SCHMIDT. 1986. Methodological problems in assessment of adverse drug reactions with drug combinations. Pharmacopsychiatry **19:** 300–301.
24. 1970. International drug monitoring—the role of the hospital, World Health Organization. Drug Intelligence Clin. Pharmacol. **4:** 101.
25. KRAMER, M. S., J. M. LEVENTHAL, T. A. HUTCHINSON & A. R. FEINSTEIN. 1979. An algorithm for the operational assessment of adverse drug reactions. I. Background, description, and instructions for use. J. Am. Med. Assoc. **242:** 623–632.
26. HUTCHINSON, T. A., K. M. FLEGEL, H. HOPINGKONG, W. S. BLOOM, M. S. KRAMER & E. G. TRUMMER. 1983. Reasons for disagreement in the standardized assessment of suspected adverse drug reactions. Clin. Pharmacol. Therapeutics. **34:** 421–426.
27. LOUIK, C., P. G. LACOUTURE, A. A. MITCHELL, R. KAUFFMAN, F. H. LOVEJOY, J. Y. SUMNER & S. SHAPIRO. 1985. A study of adverse reaction algorithms in a drug surveillance program. Clin. Pharmacol. Therapeutics **38:** 183–187.
28. PERE, J. C., B. BEGAUD, F. HARAMBURU & H. ALBIN. 1986. Computerized comparison of six adverse drug reaction assessment procedures. Clin. Pharmacol. Therapeutics **40:** 451–461.
29. BALTES, P. B., K. U. MAYER, H. HELMCHEN & E. STEINHAGEN-THIESSEN. 1993. The Berlin Aging Study: Overview and Design. Ageing Society **13:** 483–515.
30. ROTE LISTE. 1990. Editio Cantor. Aulendorf.
31. 1988. International classification of diseases, injuries, and causes of death (ICD) (German version). Kohlhammer. Köln, Germany.
32. WOOD, A. J. J. & J. A. OATES. 1987. Adverse reactions to drugs. *In* Harrison's Principles of Internal Medicine. E. Braunwald, K. J. Isselbacher, R. G. Petersdorf, J. D. Wilson, J. B. Martin & A. S. Fauci, Eds.: 352–358. McGraw-Hill. New York, N.Y.
33. HORGAS, A. L. & M. A. SMYER. 1992. Prescription drug use and drug-drug interactions in nursing home residents: relationships to health outcomes. Paper presented at the 45th Annual Scientific Meeting of the Gerontological Society of America, Washington, D.C.

Aging and Vasoconstrictor Responses Mediated by α_2-Adrenoceptors and 5-HT$_1$ and 5-HT$_2$ Receptors[a]

JAMES R. DOCHERTY

Department of Physiology
Royal College of Surgeons in Ireland
123 St. Stephen's Green
Dublin 2, Ireland.

INTRODUCTION

Postural hypotension is common in the elderly, but little is known of alterations in responsiveness of peripheral veins with aging. Hence, this study examines how vasoconstrictor responsiveness is altered by aging in a human vein.

Aging is associated with a variety of changes in the cardiovascular system.[1] A large number of studies have examined how vasoconstrictor responses mediated by noradrenaline (NA) or 5-hydroxytryptamine (5-HT) are altered by aging both in experimental animals and man. Before discussing how vasoconstrictor responses to these agents are altered by aging in the human saphenous vein, it is worth reviewing available data on the effects of aging on responses involving α-adrenoceptors and 5-HT receptors.

α-Adrenoceptors

α_1-Adrenoceptors are found on most types of smooth muscle, including vascular and intestinal, as well as cardiac muscle, and mediate contraction, but for the purpose of this discussion we will look at cardiovascular receptors. In physiological studies, the majority of investigators have examined the contractile response of isolated smooth muscle and looked for alterations in either the potency of agonist or in the maximum contractile response. The results of these studies are shown in TABLE 1.

Most studies have failed to find any change with age in contractile responses mediated by α_1-adrenoceptors in human and dog arteries and rat and rabbit blood vessels. However, studies employing the rat aorta, a tissue widely used in aging research, have generally found that aging causes a decreased contractile responsiveness, or a decrease in receptor reserve. A decreased α-adrenoceptor mediated maximum inotropic response has been reported in rat heart with increasing age (TABLE 1).

Pharmacological studies of ligand binding sites have reported a decrease in the number of α_1-ligand binding sites in rabbit heart and a decrease or no change in rat heart (TABLE 1). These changes in ligand binding site number are accompanied by a decreased biochemical response in terms of phosphoinositol (PI) response in rat heart (TABLE 1).

TABLE 1. Effects of Aging on Responses Mediated by α_1-Adrenoceptors

Species and Tissue	Response	Effect of Aging	Reference
Human, dog arteries	Contraction	No change	2, 3, 4
Rat aorta	Contraction	No change	5
		Decrease	6–8
Rat blood vessels	Contraction	No change	9, 10
		Decrease	11
Rat heart	Inotropic response	Decrease	12
	PI formation	Decrease	13, 14
	mRNA	Decrease	12
	Ligand binding	No change	15
		Decrease	14
Rabbit heart	Ligand binding	Decrease	16
Human systemic	Pressor	Decrease	17
		No change	18
Rabbit, rat systemic	Pressor	No change	16, 19

α_2-Adrenoceptors

α_2-Adrenoceptors are involved in two major types of response at different locations. On peripheral nerve terminals, α_2-adrenoceptors function as inhibitory prejunctional receptors and mediate an inhibition of transmitter release both as autoreceptors (on adrenergic nerves) or as heteroceptors (on other types of nerve). α_2-Adrenoceptors are also present postjunctionally on smooth muscle, where like α_1-receptors they mediate a contraction, and on glands, such as the Islets of Langerhans, where they mediate inhibition of secretion. Very few studies have looked at the effects of aging on α_2-adrenoceptor function, mainly since α_2-adrenoceptor mediated responses are generally difficult to find, but studies, such as they are, are listed in TABLE 2. In pharmacological studies of ligand binding sites, most studies have found no age-related change in affinity or number of α_2-adrenoceptors on platelets. In line with the reports of no consistent change in the number of α_2-ligand binding sites with age, there is no consistent evidence for any change in the aggregatory response mediated by these receptors on platelets, although two studies report an increased aggregation. An increased aggregatory response with age also appears to occur for other agents such as collagen and arachidonic acid.

Studies of the effects of aging on α_2-adrenoceptors mediating contractions of smooth muscle have been hindered by the lack of suitable isolated tissues containing α_2-adrenoceptors. However, the human saphenous vein is an example of a tissue in

TABLE 2. Effects of Aging on Responses Mediated by α_2-Adrenoceptors

Species and Tissue	Response	Effect of Aging	Reference
Human saphenous vein	Contraction	Decrease	20, present data
Human platelet	Ligand binding	No change	21, 22
		Decrease	23
		Increase	24
	Aggregation	No change	21
		Increase	24
Rat systemic	Pressor	Decrease	25

which contractions to noradrenaline are mediated predominantly, if not exclusively, by α_2-adrenoceptors (see Discussion). In contrast to the situation with isolated tissues, vascular α_2-adrenoceptors mediating contraction can be relatively easily identified *in vivo,* and indeed these postjunctional α_2-adrenoceptors were first identified in the pithed rat preparation. In the pithed rat preparation, the pressor potency of the α_2-adrenoceptor agonist xylazine is reduced by aging, but no such age-related difference can be seen for the α_1-adrenoceptor agonist amidephrine.[25] However, this age-related difference in the pressor potency of xylazine is abolished by the angiotensin converting enzyme inhibitor captopril, suggesting that an age-related decline in angiotensin levels (or responsiveness) causes the change in α_2-responsiveness. It is well known that, *in vitro,* the demonstration of an α_2-adrenoceptor mediated contraction can be dependent on an ongoing contraction to other vasoconstrictors such as angiotensin, and so alterations in levels of angiotensin *in vivo* may also have implications for α_2 responsiveness.

TABLE 3. Effects of Aging on Responses Mediated by 5-HT

Species and Tissue	Response	Effects of Aging	Reference
Human saph. vein	Contraction	Decrease	20, present data
Human forearm	Pressor	No change	26
Rat aorta	Contraction	Decrease	27
		Increase	28
Dog coronary artery	Contraction	No change	29
Rat coronary artery	Contraction	Increase affinity	30
		Decrease number	30
Rat carotid artery	Contraction	No change	28
Rat cerebrovasculature	Contraction	Increase	31

5-Hydroxytryptamine

5-hydroxytryptamine in the periphery, although present as a neurotransmitter in some nerves, is located mainly in platelets and chromaffin cells. Most studies looking at the effects of aging on smooth muscle contractions mediated by 5-HT have failed to examine which subtype of 5-HT was involved. However, since the predominant 5-HT receptor mediating contractions in many tissues is the 5-HT_2 receptor, it can be assumed, except if noted otherwise, that 5-HT_2 receptors are being examined. During aging, most studies report no change in the contractile potency of 5-HT (TABLE 3), but a decreased or even increased potency has been reported in the rat aorta and the rat cerebrovasculature.

Since platelets are a major source of 5-HT, it is of interest to examine how aging affects platelet 5-HT function. 5-HT content of platelets is reported to be decreased in aged female (but not male) rats,[32] and in man.[33]

The objects of this study were to investigate the effects of aging on responses of human saphenous vein to NA and 5-HT.

METHODS

Human saphenous veins were obtained from predominantly female patients aged 32–68 years, undergoing surgical removal of varicose veins, and apparently healthy segments of side branches of the main vein were chosen for experimentation. Rings (3–5 mm length) were attached to myograph transducers under 1 g tension for isometric tension recording in organ baths at 37°C in Krebs-Henseleit solution of the following composition (mmol l^{-1}): NaCl 119, $NaHCO_3$ 25, (+)-glucose 11.1, KCl 4.7, $CaCl_2$ 2.5, KH_2PO_4 1.2, $MgSO_4$ 1.0, ascorbic acid 0.28, tetrasodium EDTA 0.03. Additionally, in experiments examining responses to noradrenaline (NA), the following were present (mmol l^{-1}): corticosterone 0.03, cocaine 0.003, propranolol 0.001. Rings were preexposed to NA or 5-HT (10 μmol l^{-1}) for 5 min, and thereafter bathing fluid was changed every 15 min except during agonist administration. After 30 min, a cumulative concentration-response curve was carried out to NA or 5-HT (0.5 log unit increments) beginning with 1 nmol l^{-1}, until a maximum response to NA or 5-HT was reached. If the maximum response obtained to NA or 5-HT was less than 0.5 g, the experiment was discarded. A second concentration-response curve to 5-HT was carried out 120 min later, following 60 min exposure to receptor antagonist or vehicle. Agonist potency was expressed as an EC_{20}, EC_{50}, or EC_{80} (concentration producing 20%, 50%, or 80% of maximum contraction) or as a pD_2 ($-\log EC_{20}$, EC_{50}, or EC_{80}).

STATISTICAL EVALUATION

Results are expressed as mean ± standard error of the mean (SEM) or mean and 95% confidence limits. The EC_{20}, EC_{50}, or EC_{80} values were calculated from the original traces. Linear regression analysis was used to evaluate the correlation between parameters, and a probability level of 0.05 or less was taken as being significant.

DRUGS

The following drugs were used: cocaine hydrochloride (Sigma); corticosterone (Sigma); 5-hydroxytryptamine hydrochloride (Sigma); ketanserin hydrochloride (gift: Janssen, Ireland); methiothepin maleate (gift: Roche, Grenzach, Germany); noradrenaline bitartrate (Sigma); (±)propranolol hydrochloride (Sigma).

Drug stocks were dissolved in distilled water and dilutions made up in distilled water, with the exceptions of corticosterone which was made up in 100% ethanol, and ketanserin which was dissolved in a small amount of HCl.

RESULTS

In human saphenous vein, NA produced isometric contractions with an EC_{50} of 0.60 μmol l^{-1} (95% confidence limits of 0.36–1.00 μmol l^{-1}, $n = 32$ veins) and a maximum contraction of 1.73 ± 0.23 g. 5-HT produced isometric contractions with an EC_{50} of 0.20 μmol l^{-1} (95% confidence limits of 0.13–0.31 μmol l^{-1}, $n = 19$ veins) and a maximum contraction of 1.26 ± 0.16 g. There was no significant correlation between maximum contraction to either agonist and age.

There was a significant negative correlation between NA potency (expressed as a pD_2: $-\log EC_{50}$) and age for veins from 32 patients aged 32–59, so that NA was less potent with increasing age ($r = 0.36$, $p < 0.05$, $n = 32$). There was a significant negative correlation between 5-HT potency and age for veins from 19 patients aged 33–68, so that 5-HT was less potent with increasing age ($r = 0.59$, $p < 0.01$, $n = 19$).

In the human saphenous vein, the 5-HT$_2$ receptor antagonist ketanserin (1 μM) produced a nonparallel shift in the concentration-response curve for 5-HT so that ketanserin produced large shifts in the response to high concentrations of 5-HT but had little effect on the response to low concentrations of 5-HT (see FIGURE 1). It can be shown that responses to low concentrations of 5-HT are mediated by 5-HT$_1$ receptors, and responses to high concentrations of 5-HT are mediated by 5-HT$_2$ receptors, based on the actions of ketanserin and since the nonselective 5-HT$_1$ and 5-HT$_2$ receptor antagonist methiothepin produced approximately parallel shifts in the 5-HT concentration response curve (FIGURE 2). Hence, the effects of aging on the 5-HT EC$_{20}$ and EC$_{80}$ values were also examined as a measure of 5-HT$_1$ and 5-HT$_2$ potency, respectively. However, 5-HT EC$_{20}$ ($r = 0.47$, $p < 0.05$, $n = 19$) and EC$_{80}$ ($r = 0.54$, $p < 0.05$, $n = 19$) values were also significantly affected by aging (FIGURE 3).

DISCUSSION

The major finding of this study is that the potencies of NA and 5-HT are reduced with age, over the age range 32–68 years, in saphenous veins obtained from varicose vein surgery. Before discussing the implications of this finding, it is necessary to identify the receptors involved and to discuss the possible causes.

α_2-ADRENOCEPTORS IN THE HUMAN SAPHENOUS VEIN

In the human saphenous vein, we have previously demonstrated that contractions to NA are mediated by the α_2-adrenoceptor subtype. The α_2-adrenoceptor subtype

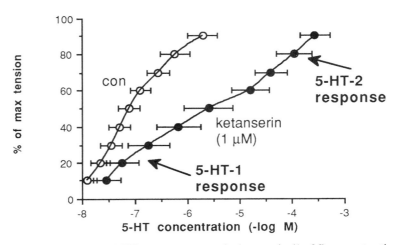

FIGURE 1. Effects of the 5-HT$_2$ receptor antagonist ketanserin (1 μM) on contractions of human saphenous vein produced by 5-HT. Note that ketanserin produced a large shift in the effects of high concentrations of 5-HT but only a small shift in the effects of low concentrations, demonstrating that the 5-HT$_2$ response requires high concentrations of 5-HT. Hence, the 5-HT EC$_{20}$ can be used as a measure of the 5-HT$_1$ component of the response and the 5-HT EC$_{80}$ can be used as a measure of the 5-HT$_2$ component of the response.

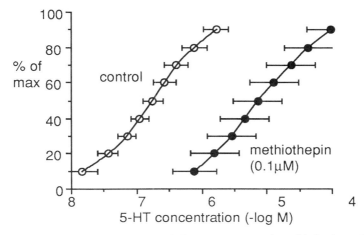

FIGURE 2. The nonselective 5-HT1 and 5-HT2 receptor antagonsit methiothepin produces an approximately parallel shift in the 5-HT concentration contractile response curve. This confirms that $5-HT_1$ receptors mediate the response to low concentrations of 5-HT.

selective antagonist yohimbine is 10 times more potent than the α_1-adrenoceptor subtype selective antagonist prazosin at inhibiting both nerve stimulation and agonist evoked contractions.[34,35] Indeed, there was a significant correlation for a series of 12 antagonists between potency at inhibiting agonist-evoked contractions in the human saphenous vein and affinity for α_2-adrenoceptor ligand binding sites.[35] Hence, the human saphenous vein is a useful model for the vascular α_2-adrenoceptor. In a previous study from this laboratory, there was an age-related decline in the potency of NA in veins from female patients.[20]

$5-HT_2$ AND $5-HT_2$ RECEPTORS IN THE HUMAN SAPHENOUS VEIN

In the human saphenous vein, we have previously demonstrated that contractions to 5-HT are mediated by 2 subtypes of receptor: a $5-HT_2$-receptor which mediates contractions to high concentrations of 5-HT, and a $5-HT_1$-like receptor which mediates contractions to low concentrations of 5-HT.[36] The potencies of ketanserin and methiothepin in the human saphenous vein (K_B values of 8.50 and 9.00) are very close to their K_i values at $5-HT_2$ ligand binding sites (8.86 and 8.76, respectively),[37] demonstrating that the vein contains a population of $5-HT_2$ receptors, mediating responses to high concentrations of 5-HT.

The receptor that mediates contractions to low concentrations of 5-HT can be clearly demonstrated to be $5-HT_1$-like: resistant to ketanserin, but antagonized by nonselective antagonists such as methiothepin. The receptor does not resemble the newly characterized $5-HT_4$ receptor since the potency of methiothepin in the present study is much higher than its potency at putative $5-HT_4$ receptors in human atria (6.84).[38]

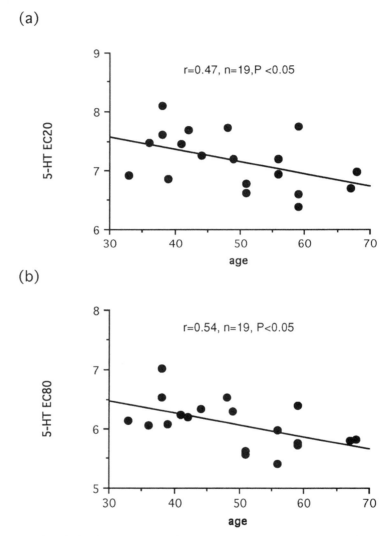

FIGURE 3. Correlation between potency (expressed as EC_{20} or EC_{80}, $-\log M$) of 5-HT at (a) 5-HT_1 receptors and (b) 5-HT_2 receptors in human saphenous veins and age. Potency at 5-HT_1 receptors was measured at the EC_{20} level and potency at 5-HT_2 receptors was measured at the EC_{80} level. Each point represents potency in an individual vein.

ALTERED AGONIST POTENCY WITH AGE

Decreased agonist potency can be caused by alteration in the affinity of the agonist for the receptor, or by alteration in the number of receptors in the case of a tissue with spare receptors. Since NA and 5-HT are physiological agonists and demonstrate relatively high potency in the human saphenous vein, it can probably be assumed that there are spare receptors for both agonists in the human saphenous vein. The decreased potency is more likely to be due to a decreased number of receptors, since alterations in affinity would need an alteration in receptor structure or environment, and since altered receptor number with aging has been reported much more frequently than altered affinity.[1] However, since responses to both NA and 5-HT declined with age, it is also possible that the age-related alteration occurs not at the receptor level, but at the level of the G-protein or beyond.

Although the increased plasma levels of NA found in the elderly (see Reference 1) might be expected to cause a reduction in the number of vascular α-adrenoceptors (down regulation), this is unlikely to explain why this effect occurs in the human saphenous vein but not in some other human blood vessels,[2,3] nor does it explain the altered response to 5-HT. Admittedly, the predominant α-adrenoceptor mediating contractions of the human saphenous vein in our studies is an α_2-adrenoceptor,[35] whereas the predominant α-adrenoceptor in vascular tissues is α_1.[39] A convenient model of α_2-adrenoceptor function is the α_2-ligand binding site on the human platelet, which has been extensively investigated in aging studies with conflicting results: a decrease,[23] no change,[21,40] or even an increase[24] in the number of α_2-ligand binding sites with age. However, a recent study comparing groups of elderly subjects found that platelet α_2-ligand binding site number was reduced in elderly subjects with postural hypotension as compared to control elderly subjects.[41] It should be noted that nerve stimulation induced contractions of human saphenous vein are also mediated mainly by α_2-adrenoceptors at least in veins from young patients, although the proportion of the response mediated by α_2-adrenoceptors declines with age.[42]

POSTURAL HYPOTENSION

Postural (orthostatic) hypotension is caused by the inability to compensate adequately for pooling of the blood in the legs on assuming an upright posture, and may result in loss of consciousness. The elderly respond to postural stress with diminished changes of heart rate and diastolic blood pressure even in the absence of postural hypotension,[43-46] and this may be a manifestation of diminished baroreflex function. Postural hypotension is common in the elderly, with reported incidences ranging from 10%,[47] to 20–30%,[43,48] rising to 30–50% in those over 75 years.[49] However, various factors can explain these wide variations in reported incidence of postural hypotension including day to day,[50] time of day, and time of measurement after standing[51] variability. Furthermore, some of the high incidences quoted may be due to the increasing prevalence of diseases such as diabetes, and to the side effects of drugs, such as tricyclic antidepressants and monoamine oxidase inhibitors, again given with increasing frequency in the elderly. In elderly subjects with postural hypotension, a failure to increase peripheral resistance sufficiently[44] or arterial rigidity[43] has been implicated. Diminished ability to constrict limb veins, due to diminished responsiveness of α_2-adrenoceptors and 5-HT$_1$ and 5-HT$_2$ receptors would result in increased pooling of blood in the legs during postural change resulting in larger falls in cardiac output and blood pressure. Coupled with this, venous valve incompetence could further increase pooling. The synthetic mineralo-corticoid fludrocortisone can be used in to increase fluid volume in postural hypotension: demonstrating the usefulness of increasing blood volume to counteract venous pooling.

In conclusion, this study demonstrates that the potencies of NA and 5-HT are reduced with increasing age in saphenous veins obtained from females undergoing varicose vein surgery.

SUMMARY

The potencies of noradrenaline (NA) at producing α_2-adrenoceptor mediated contractions, and of 5-hydroxytryptamine (5-HT) at producing 5-HT$_1$ and 5-HT$_2$ receptor mediated contractions were investigated in rings of human saphenous vein obtained from varicose vein surgery. There was a significant negative correlation between agonist potency and age for NA at α_2-adrenoceptors ($r = 0.52$, $n = 21$, $p < 0.05$) and for 5-HT at both 5-HT$_1$ ($r = 0.47$, $n = 19$, $p < 0.05$) and 5-HT$_2$ ($r = 0.54$, $n = 19$, $p < 0.05$) receptors, so that both agonists were less potent with increasing age. This demonstrates an age-related decrease in α_2-adrenoceptor and 5-HT$_1$ and 5HT$_2$ mediated contractile responsiveness in the human saphenous vein.

ACKNOWLEDGMENTS

The kind assistance of Mr. Shanik and Mr. Moore of St. James's Hospital, Dublin in supplying saphenous vein samples is gratefully acknowledged.

REFERENCES

1. DOCHERTY, J. R. 1990. Ageing and the cardiovascular system. Pharmacol. Rev. **42:** 103–125.
2. SCOTT, P. J. W. & J. L. REID. 1982. The effect of age on the responses of human isolated arteries to noradrenaline. Br. J. Clin. Pharmacol. **13:** 237–239.
3. STEVENS, M. J., S. LIPE & R. F. W. MOULDS. 1982. The effect of age on the response of human isolated arteries and veins to noradrenaline. Br. J. Clin. Pharmacol. **14:** 750–751.
4. TODA, N. & I. SHIMIZU. 1987. Neuroeffector function in mesenteric arteries isolated from beagles of different ages. J. Pharmacol. Exp. Ther. **240:** 223–227.
5. HYNES, M. R. & S. P. DUCKLES. 1987. Effect of increasing age on the endothelium-mediated relaxation of rat blood vessels in vitro. J. Pharmacol. Exp. Ther. **241:** 387–392.
6. TUTTLE, R. S. 1966. Age related changes in the sensitivity of rat aortic strips to norepinephrine and associated chemical and structural alterations. J. Gerontol. **21:** 510–516.
7. SIMPKINS, J. W., F. P. FIELD & R. J. RESS. 1983. Age-related decline in adrenergic responsiveness of the kidney, heart and aorta of male rats. Neurobiol. Aging **4:** 233–238.
8. HYLAND, L., P. WARNOCK & J. R. DOCHERTY. 1987. Age-related alterations in alpha-1 and beta-adrenoceptor mediated responsiveness of rat aorta. Naunyn-Schmiedeberg's Arch. Pharmacol. **335:** 50–53.
9. DUCKLES, S. P., B. J. CARTER & C. L. WILLIAMS. 1985. Vascular adrenergic neuroeffector function does not decline in aged rats. Circ. Res. **56:** 109–116.
10. DOHI, Y. & T. F. LUSCHER. 1990. Aging differentially affects direct and indirect actions of endothelin-1 in perfused mesenteric resistance arteries of the rat. Br. J. Pharmacol. **100:** 889–893.

11. FOUDA, A.-K. & J. ATKINSON. 1986. Sensitivity to noradrenaline andelectrical stimulation decreases with age in the rat tail artery. Naunyn-Schmiedeberg's Arch. Pharmacol. **334:** 37–39.
12. KIMBALL, K. A., L. E. CORNETT, E. SEIFEN & R. H. KENNEDY. 1991. Aging: changes in cardiac α-1 adrenoceptor responsiveness and expression. Eur. J. Pharmacol. **208:** 231–238.
13. BORST, S. E., N. NARANG, F. T. CREWS & P. J. SCARPACE. 1983. Reduced alpha-1 adrenergic receptor-mediated inositide hydrolysis in cardiac atria of senescent cycle. Clin. Pharmacol. Ther. **34:** 90–96.
14. MIYAMATO, A. & H. OHSHIKA. 1989. Age-related changes in [^{3}H]prazosin binding and phosphoinositide hydrolysis in rat ventricular myocardium. Gen. Pharmacol. **20:** 647–651.
15. SCHAEFER, W. & R. S. WILLIAMS. 1986. Age dependent changes in expression of alpha-1 adrenergic receptors in rat myocardium. Biochem. Biophys. Res. Commun. **138:** 387–391.
16. DALRIMPLE, H. W., C. A. HAMILTON & J. L. REID. 1982. The effect of age on peripheral alpha-adrenoceptors in vivo and in vitro in the rabbit. Br. J. Pharmacol. **77:** 322P.
17. ELLIOTT, H. L., D. J. SUMNER, K. MCLEAN & J. L. REID. 1982. Effect of age on the responsiveness of vascular alpha-adrenoceptors in man. J. Cardiovasc. Pharmacol. **4:** 388–392.
18. ROSENDORFF, C., B. KALLIATAKIS, H. M. RADFORD & J. PATTON. 1988. Age dependence of the pressor sensitivity to noradrenaline and angiotensin II during calcium channel blockade in hypertensive patients. J. Cardiovasc. Pharmacol. **12:** S69–S71.
19. DOCHERTY, J. R. & L. HYLAND. 1986. Alpha-adrenoceptor responsiveness in the aged rat. Eur. J. Pharmacol. **126:** 75–80.
20. DOCHERTY, J. R. 1993. Effects of aging on the vasoconstrictor responses to noradrenaline and 5-hydroxytryptamine in the human saphenous vein. Cardiol. Elderly **1:** 327–330.
21. ELLIOTT, J. M. & D. G. GRAHAME-SMITH. 1982. The binding characteristics of [^{3}H]dihydro-ergocryptine on intact platelets. Br. J. Pharmacol. **76:** 121–130.
22. BUCKLEY, C., D. CURTIN, T. WALSH & K. O'MALLEY. 1986. Ageing and platelet alpha-2 adrenoceptors. Br. J. Clin. Pharmacol. **21:** 721–722.
23. BRODDE, O.-E., M. ANLAUF, N. GRABEN & K. D. BOCK. 1982. Age dependent decrease of alpha-2 adrenergic receptor number in human platelets. Eur. J. Pharmacol. **81:** 345–347.
24. YOKOYAMA, M., K. KUSUI, S. SAKAMOTO & H. FUKAZAKI. 1984. Age-associated increments in human platelet alpha-2 adrenoceptor capacity: possible mechanism for platelet hyper-activity to epinephrine in aging man. Thromb. Res. **34:** 287–295.
25. DOCHERTY, J. R. 1988. The effects of ageing on vascular alpha-adrenoceptors in pithed rat and rat aorta. Eur. J. Pharmacol. **146:** 1–5.
26. BLAUW, G. J., P. VAN BRUMMELEN, P. C. CHANG, P. VERMEIJ & P. A. VAN ZWIETEN. 1988. Arterial dilatation and venous constriction induced by serotonin in the elderly. Drugs **36**(Suppl. 1): 74–77.
27. DOCHERTY, J. R. 1988. Changes in adrenoceptor function with age. *In* Vascular Neuroeffector Mechanisms. J. A. Bevan, H. Majewski, R. A. Maxwell & D. F. Story, Eds.: 281–287. IRL Press. Oxford, England.
28. EMMICK, J. T. & M. L. COHEN. 1986. Ageing and vasodilatation to atrial peptides. Clin. Exp. Hypertens. **A8:** 75–90.
29. TODA, N., K. BIAN & S. INOUE. 1987. Age-related changes in the response to vasoconstrictor and dilator agents in isolated beagle coronary arteries. Naunyn-Schmiedeberg's Arch. Pharmacol. **336:** 359–364.
30. NYBORG, N. C. B. 1991. Ageing is associated with increased 5-HT-2-receptor affinity and decreased receptor reserve in rat isolated coronary arteries. Br. J. Pharmacol. **102:** 282–286.
31. HAJDU, M. A., R. T. MCELMURRY, D. D. HEISTAD & G. L. BAUMBACH. 1993. Effects of aging on cerebral vascular responses to serotonin in rats. Am. J. Physiol. **264:** H2136–H2140.

32. YONEZAWA, Y., H. KONDO & T. A. NOMAGUCHI. 1989. Age-related changes in serotonin content and its release reaction of rat platelets. Mech. Ageing Dev. **47:** 65–75.
33. SHUTTLEWORTH, R. D. & J. R. O'BRIEN. 1981. Intraplatelet serotonin and plasma 5-hydroxytryptamine in health and disease. Blood **57:** 505–509.
34. DOCHERTY, J. R. & L. HYLAND. 1985. Evidence for neuro-effector transmission through postjunctional alpha-2 adrenoceptors in human saphenous vein. Br. J. Pharmacol. **84:** 573–576.
35. SMITH, K., S. CONNAUGHTON & J. R. DOCHERTY. 1992. Investigations of the subtype of α_2-adrenoceptor mediating contractions of the human saphenous vein. Br. J. Pharmacol. **106:** 447–451.
36. DOCHERTY, J. R. & L. HYLAND. 1985. An examination of 5-hydroxytryptamine receptors in human saphenous vein. Br. J. Pharmacol. **89:** 77–81.
37. ENGEL, G., M. GOTHERT, D. HOYER, E. SCHLICKER & K. HILLENBRAND. 1986. Identity of inhibitory presynaptic 5-hydroxytryptamine (5-HT) autoreceptors in the rat brain cortex with 5-HT_{1B} binding sites. Naunyn-Schmiedeberg's Arch. Pharmacol. **332:** 1–7.
38. KAUMANN, A. J., L. SANDERS, A. M. BROWN, K. J. MURRAY & M. J. BROWN. 1990. A 5-hydroxytyptamine receptor in human atrium. Br. J. Pharmacol. **100:** 879–885.
39. DOCHERTY, J. R. 1989. The pharmacology of alpha-1 and alpha-2 adrenoceptors: evidence for and against a further subdivision. Pharmacol. Ther. **44:** 241–284.
40. JONES, S. B., D. B. BYLUND, C. A. REISER, W. O. SHEKIM & G. W. CARR. 1983. Alpha-2 adrenergic receptor binding in human platelets: alterations during the menstrual cycle. Clin. Pharmacol. Ther. **34:** 90–96.
41. ROBINSON, B. J., L. I. STOWELL, R. H. JOHNSON & K. T. PALMER. 1990. Is orthostatic hypotension in the elderly due to autonomic failure. Age Ageing **19:** 288–296.
42. HYLAND, L. & J. R. DOCHERTY. 1985. An investigation of age-related changes in pre- and postjunctional alpha-adrenoceptors in human saphenous vein. Eur. J. Pharmacol. **114:** 361–364.
43. MACLENNAN, W. J., M. R. P. HALL & J. I. TIMOTHY. 1980. Postural hypotension in old age: is it a disorder of the nervous system or of blood vessels. Age Ageing **9:** 25–32.
44. WILLIAMS, B. O., F. L. CAIRD & I. M. LENNOX. 1985. Haemodynamic response to postural stress in the elderly with and without postural hypotension. Age Ageing **14:** 193–201.
45. VARGAS, E., M. LYE, E. B. FARAGHER, C. GODDARD, B. MOSER & I. DAVIES. 1986. Cardiovascular haemodynamics and the response of vasopressin, aldosterone, plasma renin activity and plasma catecholamines to head-up tilt in young and old healthy subjects. Age Ageing **15:** 17–28.
46. SMITH, J. J., C. V. HUGHES, M. J. PTACIN, J. A. BARNEY, F. E. TRISTANI & T. J. EBERT. 1987. The effect of age on haemodynamic response to graded postural stress in normal men. J. Gerontol. **42:** 406–411.
47. MADER, S. L., K. R. JOSEPHSON & L. Z. RUBENSTEIN. 1987. Low prevalence of postural hypotension among community-dwelling elderly. J. Am. Med. Soc. **258:** 1511–1514.
48. CAIRD, F. I., G. R. ANDREWS & R. D. KENNEDY. 1973. Effect of posture on blood pressure in the elderly. Br. Heart J. **35:** 527–530.
49. ROBBINS, A. S. & L. Z. RUBENSTEIN. 1984. Postural hypotension in the elderly. J. Am. Geriatr. Soc. **32:** 769–774.
50. LIPSITZ, L. A. 1989. Altered blood pressure homeostasis in advanced age: clinical and research implications. J. Gerontol. **44:** M179–M183.
51. MACRAE, A. D. & C. J. BULPITT. 1989. Assessment of postural hypotension in elderly patients. Age Ageing **18:** 110–112.

Does Any Correlation Exist between a High Plasma Digoxin Level and an Electrocardiogram in Older and Younger Patients?

ZIJAD DURAKOVIĆ

Department of Internal Medicine
Rebro
University Hospital
Medical Faculty
University of Zagreb
Zagreb, Croatia

INTRODUCTION

Observation of the effect of digitalis is important in elderly patients in whom cardiac changes are often present and renal reserve is reduced by 30 to 50%, shile the serum creatinine level may be within the normal limits,[1-7] since digoxin is mainly excreted via the kidneys.[6-9] The digitalis effect on the heart is assessed by ECG analysis. The P-R interval, Q-T segment depression, conduction disturbances, and arrhythmias are usually determined in ECGs.

The purpose of the present study was to analyze the clinical symptoms, ECG changes, plasma creatinine, and potassium level in older and younger patients with high plasma digoxin level, and to ascertain whether changes of these parameters indicate hypersaturation with digitalis more often in the elderly than in younger patients.

PATIENTS AND METHODS

From April 1978 to April 1993, a high plasma digoxin level was found in 171 patients aged 65 to 92 years, and in 58 patients aged 35 to 64 years. The etiology of congestive heart failure is presented in TABLE 1, and age groups in TABLE 2.

All patients were treated with maintenance doses of medigoxin (Lanitop-Pliva-Boehringer), usually 0.1 mg/day. All of them answered the criteria for digoxin use because of signs of congestive heart failure due to systolic or combined systolic-diastolic dysfunction verified clinically and by echocardiography before that treatment. The following clinical signs of digitalis overdose were recorded: anorexia, nausea, vomiting, and less specific signs like fatigue and headache. The plasma digoxin level was measured in all patients by radioimmunoassay "Abbott".[10] The sensitivity of the method is 0.1 μg/l. The coefficient of variation was 10%. Venous blood samples (2 ml) were taken 5 hours after the last medigoxin dose from patients in the reclining position. The blood was drawn into a test tube in which 0.2 ml of heparin had been added previously. The aim was to establish digoxin concentration in the dynamic equilibrium state, i.e., when the speed of entry into the body was the same as the speed of elimination.

TABLE 1. Etiology of Congestive Heart Failure in Older and Younger Patients

Etiology	Age (years)		
	65–92	35–64	Total
Atherosclerotic hearth disease (with atrial fibrillation)	109	29	138
Hypertensive heart disease	40	15	55
Chronic pulmonary heart disease with atrial fibrillation	16	4	20
Cardiomyopathy	4	9	13
Constrictive pericarditis	2	1	3
Total	171	58	229

The electrocardiogram was recorded when blood was taken for digoxin analysis with patients in reclining position, a three channel electrocardiography, at a paper speed of 25 mm/sec (RIZ, Zagreb, Croatia). The following leads were recorded: I-III, aVR-aVF, V_1-V_6. The following changes were analyzed: atrioventricular block of the first degree and second degree, apart from Möbitz II, frequent premature beats, atrial tachycardia, junctional rhythm. The following parameters were examined in particular: atrioventricular conduction disturbances, i.e., prolonged P-R interval with regard to heart frequency, and corrected Q-T interval. The latter was analyzed in two ways: according to the formula of Bazzet[11,12] where the finding was considered to be normal if it measured between 0.396–0432 sec in women, and in men between 0.396–0.422 sec, while it was considered shortened if it amounted to 0.370 sec or less (lead II):

$$\text{I corrected Q-T interval} = \frac{\text{measured Q-T interval}_s}{\sqrt{\text{R-R interval}_s}}$$

The Q-T interval was also analyzed according to Staniforth's formula:[13]

$$\text{II corrected Q-T interval} = \frac{\text{measured Q-T interval}_s}{\sqrt[3]{\text{R-R interval}_s}}$$

The P-T-Q index was calculated according to the formula of Joubert;[14,15] the condition for this analysis was the existence of P-wave (II or V_1 lead), i.e., sinus

TABLE 2. The Number of Patients with a High Plasma Digoxin Level According to Age and Sex

Age	Sex		Total
	Males	Females	
35–44	3	4	7
45–54	11	6	17
55–64	13	21	34
65–74	35	59	94
75–84	22	40	62
85–92	7	8	15
Total	91 (39.7%)	138 (60.3%)	229 (100%)

rhythm:

$$\text{P-T-Q index} = \text{P-R interval}_s \times \frac{\text{negative T-wave}_{mm}}{\text{I corrected Q-T interval}_s}$$

The statistical analysis was carried out by means of the correlation coefficient.[16] Creatinine and potassium levels in the serum were recorded in all patients on admission to the hospital and during the treatment. ECGs were performed and used for this analysis after correction of serum electrolytes.

RESULTS

Among the 171 elderly patients with a high plasma digoxin level, the majority were between 65 and 74 years of age, while 58 younger patients were aged 55 to 64 years. There were more women than men (60.3:39.7%), as shown in TABLE 2.

TABLE 3. Conduction Disturbances and Arrhythmias in the Electrocardiogram in Older and Younger Patients with a High Plasma Digoxin Level

Plasma Digoxin Level (nmol/l)	Conduction Disturbances		Arrhythmias		Without These Changes		Total	
	Older	Younger	Older	Younger	Older	Younger	Older	Younger
2.5–3.0	16	4	19	8	15	11	57	23
3.1–3.5	33	3	19	1	1	6	52	10
3.6–4.0	9	1	11	2	6	2	27	6
4.1–4.5	9	2	12	4	3	5	22	11
4.6–5.0	4	2	3	0	2	4	6	5
5.1–6.2	3	0	5	2	1	1	7	3
Total	74 (43.2%)	12 (20.6%)	69 (40.3%)	17 (29.3%)	28 (16.3%)	29 (50.1%)	171 (100%)	58 (100%)

Clinical symptoms of hypersaturation with digitalis occurred in 83 older (54.6%) and 19 younger patients (35.2%). Conduction disturbances were present in 43.2% of elderly and 20.6% of younger patients, while 40.3% of elderly and 29.3% younger patients presented with arrhythmias. Both changes were present in a group of rhythm disturbances, whereas 16.3% of elderly and 50.1% of younger patients were without these changes. This is shown in TABLE 3.

In 74 of the 152 elderly patients (47.4%), sinus rhythm appeared in the ECG, and in 18 (39.6%) of the younger patients. A correlation between the P-R interval and high plasma digoxin level in elderly group ($p < 0.01$), and in younger patients ($p < 0.05$) was found. Thirty-seven elderly patients (21.6%) and 15 of the 58 younger patients (25.8%) had a shortened I corrected Q-T interval. No correlation was found between the elevated plasma digoxin concentration and this parameter. Sixty-three of the 171 elderly patients (36.8%) and 17 of the 54 younger patients (32.7%) had negative T wave in the ECG (with sinus rhythm and calculated P-T-Q index). A correlation between these parameters ($p < 0.01$) was noted in elderly patients, and no correlation was found in younger ones.

In 84 elderly patients (49.1%) and in 17 of the younger patients (29.3%), elevated values of serum creatinine level were found; 13 elderly patients had a value from 375 to 750 μmol/l (two in the younger group), while this value amounted to 750–1500 μmol/l) in 16 elderly patients (4 in the younger group). There was no correlation between serum creatinine level and high plasma digoxin level. A lowered value of serum potassium level was found in 7 elderly patients (5.2%) and 3 younger ones (5.2%), while increased values were found in 25 elderly (14.6%) and in three younger patients (5.1%). In 3 patients it reached the value of 6.0 mmol/l, while in one 6 mmol/l. Those data are presented in TABLE 4.

DISCUSSION

In a group of 171 elderly and 58 younger patients treated with digitalis glycosides in whom the plasma digoxin level reached 2.5 to 6.2 nmol/L, no correlation was found between the I corrected Q-T interval (when the second root from the heart frequency was calculated), or the II corrected Q-T interval (when the third root of the heart frequency was calculated) and plasma digoxin levels. A shortened, cor-

TABLE 4. The Correlation between the Electrocardiogram, Serum Potassium and Creatinine Values, and High Plasma Digoxin Level in Elderly and Young Patients

		Correlation Coefficient		Statistical
	Parameters	Older Patients	Younger Patients	Difference
High plasma digoxin level	P-R interval	+0.212*	+0.308**	*p < 0.01 **p < 0.05
	I corrected Q-T interval	+0.092	+0.144	NS
	II corrected Q-T interval	+0.096	+0.135	NS
	P-T-Q index	+0.393*	+0.265	*p < 0.01
	Serum potassium level	+0.046	+0.058	NS
	Serum creatinine level	+0.099	+0.083	NS

rected Q-T interval was found in 23.3% of the elderly and in 25.8% of the younger patients analyzed by the first method, and in 32.2% calculated by the second method. Although the corrected Q-T interval analyzed by the second method was often somewhat shorter than it had been when analyzed by the first method, no significant difference was found. There was a correlation between the P-R interval and high plasma digoxin level in elderly (p) and in younger patients ($p < 0.01$) and between the P-T-Q index and high plasma digoxin level in the elderly. This partly agrees with the results obtained in our earlier study in which we found a slight correlation between the P-R interval and high plasma digoxin level ($r = +0.34$ in all age groups) and slight correlation between the I corrected Q-T interval and high plasma digoxin level.

Some authors reported a high correlation between the plasma digoxin level and P-T-Q index[14,15] when values were within the therapeutic range. However, our results are not in agreement with the results reached by others. In those studies, healthy volunteers were included and different plasma digoxin concentrations used. Although 49% of the elderly patients and 29% of the younger ones had chronic renal failure, no correlation between high plasma digoxin levels and creatinine or serum potassium was found. This was probably due to careful adjustment of the dose of digitalis in renal insufficiency. It is known that in chronic renal failure, false positive plasma digoxin levels can be measured,[17] and even with this constatation we were not able to find a correlation between these two parameters.

According to some authors, arrhythmias were very frequent in patients hypersaturated with digitalis,[18] and this is contrary to our results. On the other hand, some authors[19] found a high correlation between changes in the ECG and plasma digoxin level.

In our earlier study among patients with high plasma digoxin level of all age groups,[14,20] more than half of the elderly and one-third of the younger patients had clinical signs of hypersaturation with digitalis, and also almost half of the elderly and one-fifth to one-third of the younger ones had arrhythmia or conduction disturbances. In our present study, the frequency of clinical hypersaturation with digitalis in elderly patients was higher than in the quoted study.[1,4] Arrhythmias and conduction disturbances as well as correlation coefficient of high plasma digoxin level, P-R interval, and P-T-Q index were also more frequently observed (82.5%). The corrected Q-T interval measured in two ways did not show any higher clinical values during the analysis of hypersaturation with digitalis.

It can be concluded that the effect of digitalis is not a cause of specific changes in the ECG either in the elderly or in younger patients. However, the association between prolonged P-R interval as well as changes in the P-T-Q index and high plasma digoxin level has been found more often in the elderly than in younger patients.

SUMMARY

In a group of 171 patients aged 65 to 92 years and 58 patients aged 35 to 64 years, plasma digoxin level measuring 2.5–6.2 nmol/l correlated with the clinical symptoms and the electrocardiogram. Conduction disturbances and arrhythmias as well as the P-R interval, P-T-Q index, and corrected Q-T interval in the ECG were analyzed. Clinical symptoms of hypersaturation with digitalis were present in 55.5% of the elderly and 34.4% of the younger patients. Conduction disturbances were found in 43.2% of the elderly and 20.6% of the younger patients, while arrhythmias appeared in 40.3% of the elderly and 29.3% of the younger patients: 16.3% of the elderly and 50.1% of the younger patients were without these changes. A correlation between the P-R interval and high plasma digoxin level in the elderly ($p < 0.01$) and younger patients ($p < 0.05$), as well as between the P-T-Q index and high plasma digoxin level in the elderly ($p < 0.01$), was found. There was no correlation between the corrected Q-T interval and high plasma digoxin level in both groups. No correlation was found between the high plasma digoxin level and serum creatinine level in both groups, or between the high plasma digoxin level and serum potassium level in both groups, although many patients had chronic renal failure. The effect of digitalis has not been shown to be a cause of specific changes in an electrocardiogram either in the elderly or in younger patients. However, the association between prolonged P-R interval, as well as changes in the P-T-Q index, and high plasma digoxin level has been found more often in the elderly than in younger patients.

REFERENCES

1. DURAKOVIĆ, Z., B. VRHOVAC & F. PLAVŠIĆ. 1984. Electrocardiogram and high plasma digoxin concentration. Int. J. Clin. Pharm. Ther. Toxicol. **22:** 45–47.

2. PACKER, M. 1989. Does digitalis work in chronic heart failure? The end of a 200-year old controversy. Cardiovascular Drugs Ther. **2:** 743–746.
3. LAMBERT, C. & J. L. ROULEAU. 1989. How to digitalize and to maintain optimal digoxin levels in congestive heart failure. Cardiovascular Drugs Ther. **2:** 717–725.
4. DURAKOVIĆ, Z., A. ŠMALCELJ, M. KVARANTAN, F. PLAVŠIĆ, I. BOGDAN, V. GRGIĆ & R. RADONIĆ. 1990. Is there any correlation between electrocardiographic changes and the high serum digoxin concentration in the elderly. Liječ vjesn **112:** 208–211.
5. DURAKOVIĆ, Z. 1992. Does correlation exist between the electrocardiogram and a high plasma digoxin level in the elderly? Geriatr. Forsch. **2:** 163–168.
6. SUNDAR, S., D. P. BURMA & S. K. VAISH. 1983. Digoxin toxicity and electrolytes: a correlative study. Acta Cardiol. **38:** 115–123.
7. SCHAPEL, G. J., T. E. JONES, T. C. DRAYSEY, J. M. CROCKER, G. T. DAVIES, M. A. ROBINSON, T. R. C. READ & P. E. STANLEY. 1981. The predictive value of the serum digoxin concentration in the management of hospitalized patients. Ther. Drug Monitor **3:** 137–142.
8. INGELFINGER, J. A. & P. GOLDMAN. 1976. The serum digitalis concentration—does it diagnose digitalis toxicity. N. Engl. J. Med. **294:** 867–870.
9. JOGESTRAND, T. & R. NORDLANDER. 1983. Serum digoxin determination in outpatients— need for standardization. Br. J. Clin. Pharmacol. **15:** 55–58.
10. PLAVŠIĆ, F., B. VRHOVAC, I. BAKRAN JR., M. GJURAŠIN & V. GOLDNER. 1978. Direct measurement of digoxin in serum, saliva and urine by radioimmunoassay. Liječ vjesn **100:** 510–513.
11. BAZETT, H. C. 1920. An analysis of the time relationship of the electrocardiogram. Heart **7:** 353–370.
12. KISSIN, M., M. M. SCHWARZSCHILD & H. BAKST. 1948. A nomogram for rate correction of the Q-T interval in the electrocardiogram. Am. Heart J. **35:** 990–992.
13. STANIFORTH, D. H. 1983. The Q-T interval and cycle length: the influence of atropine, hyoscine and exercise. Br. J. Clin. Pharmacol. **16:** 625–631.
14. JOUBER, P., B. KROENING & M. WEINTRAUB. 1975. Serial digoxin concentration and quantitative ECG changes. Clin. Pharmacol. Ther. **18:** 757–760.
15. JOUBER, P. H., B. N. AUCAMP & F. O. MÜLLER. 1976. Digoxin concentration in serum and saliva: relationship to ECG changes and dosage in healthy volunteers. Br. J. Clin. Pharmacol. **3:** 1053–1056.
16. MORTON, R. F. & R. J. HABEL. 1980. A Study Guide to Epidemiology and Biostatistics. University Park Press. Baltimore, Md.
17. DURAKOVIĆ, Z., D. IVANOVIĆ & A. DURAKOVIĆ. 1989. Digoxin-like substance in the serum of uremic patients before and after hemodialysis. Cardiovascular Drugs Ther. **2:** 757–760.
18. DANON, A., J. HOROWITZ, Z. BEN-ZVI, J. KAPLINSKI & S. GLICK. 1977. An outbreak of digoxin concentration. Clin. Pharmacol. Ther. **21:** 643–646.
19. AHLMARK, G. 1976. Extreme digitalis intoxication. Acta Med. Scand. **200:** 423–425.
20. DURAKOVIĆ, Z. 1992. The high plasma digoxin level: comparison with clinical symptoms and an electrocardiogram in the elderly and younger patients. Coll. Antropol. **2:** 371–376.

Neuroendocrine Immune Modulation Induced by Zinc in a Progeroid Disease—Down's Syndrome[a]

FEDERICO LICASTRO, MARIA CRISTINA MORINI,
AND LIZABETH JANE DAVIS[b]

Dipartimento di Patologia Sperimentale
Università di Bologna
Via S. Giacomo 14
40126 Bologna, I-Italy

[b]*Dipartimento di Biochimica*
Università di Bologna
Via Irnerio 48
40126 Bologna, I-Italy

INTRODUCTION

It is still unknown whether a specific set of genes controlling the velocity of the aging process exists. However, a survey of mortality curves in humans shows that the rate of aging among individuals of our species is quite different and suggests a high genetic heterogeneity of antisenescence mechanisms.[1] Moreover, if such genes are present in our genome, it would be of invaluable interest to comprehend the mechanisms regulating their expression.

On the other hand, it is unlikely that the aging of a complex organism is secondary to a single causal event or a unique rate-determining step. Thus, the aging phenotype, i.e., the complex series of age-related body changes, can be considered as the end result of several events that influence somatic development.[2–4]

According to this notion, the onset of each individual age-related event might arise during different stages of maturation and accelerate or decelerate the rate of body aging by affecting the developmental program.

An obvious conclusion from the above statements is that the concomitant effects of aging of different organs upon the expression of the aging phenotype and longevity are too complex to be successfully reproduced using simple experimental models.

A way to circumvent these tremendous difficulties is to increase our understanding of segmental aspects of the aging process within complex models. Human diseases characterized by accelerated aging, such as progeria[5] or Down's syndrome,[1] may be useful models to increase our knowledge of mechanisms that regulate aging and affect the senescence of organisms.

The major limitation of this approach is that these diseases also show abnormal elements that are not present in normal healthy subjects. Thus, progeroid syndromes have to be considered as appropriate partial or segmental models of aging,[6] where each disease may give useful information regarding the aging of an individual organ or homeostatic system.

[a]This work has been supported by funds from Ministero dell' Università e della Ricerca Scientifica e Tecnologica, Regione Emilia Romagna e Gazzoni 1907 S.p.a.

Down's Syndrome as a Model of Accelerated Aging

Down's syndrome (DS) is the most common form of human chromosomal aneuploidy, and is characterized by the presence of at least a portion of an extra chromosome 21.[7]

Clinically, infectious diseases, acute leukemia, and autoimmunity are often associated with the syndrome.[8–10] Immune defects appear during early life in these subjects, and some immune alterations resemble those found in normal elderly subjects.[11,12]

The analysis of survival curves of subjects with DS shows that mean and maximal life spans are reduced in these individuals.[13] In fact, average life span is approximately 57 years, females having a slightly higher survival rate than males. Maximum life span reaches 75 years of age, and no sex difference appears to be present.[13]

Institutionalization represents a factor negatively affecting both morbidity and survival. However, the life expectancy of DS persons has increased considerably over recent years as a consequence of a general improvement of social care and a different social behavior.

According to the criteria proposed by Martin,[1] DS subjects show several major phenotypic features of aging as well as the highest number of progeroid characteristics.

Patterns of survival rates and phenotypic features support the notion that DS may be considered a human disease characterized by an accelerated rate of aging.

The Immune Deficiency Associated with the Syndrome

The increased incidence of infectious diseases,[14] which are still today the major cause of mortality in children with DS, has suggested the presence of altered immune functions in these subjects.

An impairment of variable degree affects both nonspecific and specific immunity, as shown in TABLE 1. Generally, functional defects have been found in circulating granulocytes[15] and T lymphocytes.[16,17]

Moreover, most DS subjects show low plasma levels of zinc.[18] It is interesting to note that some immune defects can be normalized by dietary manipulation. In fact, low doses of zinc supplementation (1 mg/kg of body weight, per day) for short periods of time (maximum four months) restored the activity of a thymic hormone and improved mitogen responses of T lymphocytes.[16,18]

TABLE 1. Major Immune Defects Associated with DS

- Precocious histological and functional involution of the thymus.
- Impaired levels of serum immunoglobulins.
- Decreased plasma levels of thymic hormones.
- Decreased responsiveness to skin test stimulation.
- Decreased granulocyte functions.
- Decreased lymphocyte responses to *in vitro* stimulation with polyclonal mitogens.
- Decreased autologous mixed lymphocyte cultures.
- Altered representation of peripheral blood T cell subpopulations.
- Decreased lymphocyte natural killer activity.
- Altered sensitivity of lymphoid cells to IFNs.
- Impaired production of lymphokines.

TABLE 2. Neuropathological Similarities between Adults with DS and Patients with Alzheimer's Disease

- Reduction of brain glucose metabolism.
- Qualitative, quantitative, and topographic distribution of neuropathological degenerations.
- Decreased choline acetyltransferase and acetylcholinesterase.
- Decreased norepinephrine, dopamine, and serotonin.
- Cerebrovascular amyloid β-protein deposition.
- Similar structure and composition of plaque core proteins.

Thus, DS represents a condition where several defects of immune responses usually found in nontrisomic elderly are present early in life and some are positively affected by nutritional supplementation.

Senescence of the Brain in DS

Subjects with DS suffer variable degrees of mental retardation which becomes obvious during the few months after birth, and development slows down during infancy and childhood. The average developmental delay usually is of the order of two months during the first year of life. However, such a delay gradually lengthens and reaches one or two years for the more complex functions.

Mental deterioration and dementia were described to be associated with the syndrome 100 years ago,[19] and for over 50 years it has been known that the dementia of Alzheimer's type is often observed in adults with DS.[20]

A large number of reports show that the brains of adults with DS possess all the neurochemical and neuropathological hallmarks of Alzheimer's disease, and these are listed in TABLE 2.

Senescence of the Endocrine System in DS

Hormonal disorders are often found in subjects with DS, and in fact hyperthyroidism, hypothyroidism, and the presence of autoantibodies against thyroid gland have been described.[21,22]

Before the clinical manifestation of thyroid imbalance, a peculiar hormonal impairment is often present in subjects with DS, i.e., increased levels of thyroid stimulating hormone (TSH),[23–28] with normal levels of triiodothyronine (T3) and tetraiodothyronine (T4).[16,24,25,27,28]

However, decreased T3 levels have also been detected in some subjects with the syndrome, and the intellectual function of DS subjects with abnormal levels of both TSH and T3 was found significantly lower than that of DS subjects without thyroid hormonal imbalance.[24]

Recently, in a pilot study on children with DS, we have showed that elevated TSH and decreased reversal T3 (rT3) could be normalized after four months of zinc supplementation.[28] These findings indicated that thyroid imbalance in DS subjects might be secondary to an altered zinc availability and led us to hypothesize that the immune restoration observed in these subjects after zinc administration could be induced via neuroendocrine modulation.

Here we present data regarding plasma levels of TSH, rT3, granulocyte function, and peripheral blood lymphocyte populations of a large group of subjects with DS before, after zinc supplementation, and after a follow-up of 12 months.

SUBJECTS AND METHODS

Subjects

Fifty-one subjects with nontranslocated trisomy-21 were studied. The age interval of the subjects ranged from 1 to 19 years. Twenty were females, and 31 were males, and all were living at home. Informed consent was obtained from parents of DS children admitted to the immunological screening and the following clinical trial.

Zinc sulfate (1 mg of elemental Zn^{2+} per kg of body weight per day) was given orally for 4 months.

The control group consisted of 23 healthy children, 10 females and 13 males (1–11 years old).

Determination of Plasmic Zinc Levels

Plasmic zinc levels were measured by atomic absorption spectroscopy according to the method of Fernandez and Khan[29] modified as previously described.[18]

Detection of TSH and rT3 Plasmic Levels

Venous blood samples from DS children, before and after zinc supplementation, and from controls were taken in sterile test tubes containing heparin (20 U/ml). Levels of TSH and rT3 were measured by commercially available radioimmune assays (C.I.S., Italy for TSH; Bick, Italy for rT3).

Leukocyte Chemiluminescence (CL) Assay

One milliliter of heparinized venous blood from each subject was used. Neutrophil CL activity after activation by zymosan particles (Zymolite, Bouty Lab., Milan, Italy) was detected using 200 μl of autologous or heterologous normal plasma/serum as opsonizing sources[15] with the aid of an automatic and computerized bioluminometer (Berthold, LB 950, Munchen, Germany).

Statistical Analysis

Statistical comparisons were made according to two-tailed or paired Student's t-tests.

RESULTS

As shown in FIGURE 1, plasma levels of zinc were decreased ($p < 0.001$) before zinc supplementation in subjects with DS. However, circulating levels of zinc increased and reached the upper limit of normal values after dietary zinc supplement. One year after the cessation of zinc administration, zinc plasma levels were again slightly decreased ($p < 0.05$).

Levels of plasma TSH were increased ($p < 0.001$) in subjects with DS, but after zinc supplementation they reached normal values (FIGURE 2A). One year after the cessation of the nutritional therapy, TSH plasma levels were still within the normal range (FIGURE 2A).

Plasma levels of rT3 were very low ($p < 0.0001$) before zinc administration in DS subjects as compared with normal values (FIGURE 2B). After zinc therapy, serum rT3 increased and was still within the range of normality one year after the supplementation (FIGURE 2B).

Granulocyte activity assessed as chemiluminescence (CL) emission per single cell was low ($p < 0.001$) in DS subjects, but it increased after zinc supplementation (FIGURE 3). One year after the cessation of the dietary supplement, granulocyte CL was lower ($p < 0.001$) than that of controls (FIGURE 3).

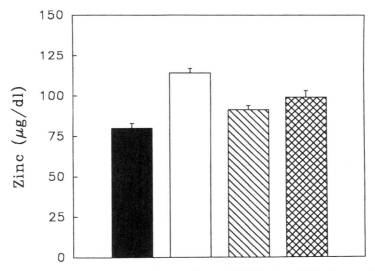

FIGURE 1. Levels of zinc in plasma from subjects with DS before (black histogram), after (white histogram), one year after the cessation of zinc supplementation (slashed histogram), and in untreated controls (cross-hatched histogram).

CONCLUSIONS

The reasons for decreased levels of zinc in subjects with DS remain unknown. In fact, low zinc plasma levels can not be simply ascribed to a gross nutritional deficit.[16,18,30] Nevertheless, low serum levels and defective intestinal absorption of vitamin A have been reported in institutionalized subjects with DS.[31,32] At present, it is unclear whether intestinal malabsorption may be responsible for zinc deficiency in these subjects, since other oligoelements such as copper[16] or magnesium[33] are usually found within normal ranges. On the other hand, a positive response to zinc supplementation[16,30] is indeed indicative of low availability of this trace element.

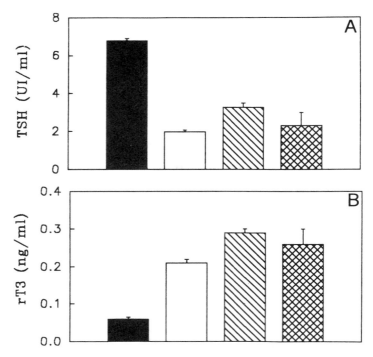

FIGURE 2. Panel A: Plasma levels of TSH in subjects with DS before (black histogram), after (white histogram), one year after the cessation of zinc supplementation (slashed histogram), and in untreated controls (cross-hatched histogram). **Panel B:** Plasma levels of rT3 in subjects with DS before (black histogram), after (white histogram), one year after the cessation of zinc supplementation (slashed histogram), and in untreated controls (cross-hatched histogram).

The reasons for abnormal levels of TSH and rT3, with a concomitant presence of normal levels of T3 and T4 (data not shown), are not of easy interpretation. Results presented here, along with other data published[28] elsewhere, suggest that in DS subjects a low zinc availability may be responsible for these biochemical alterations. Zinc deficiency might affect the metabolism of thyroid hormones and, in particular, the uptake of thyroid hormone in the peripheral tissues and/or in the hypothalamus. In fact, the receptors for thyroid hormones have been shown to belong to the steroid receptor superfamily and to have zinc fingerprints that regulate the binding of the hormones.[34,35]

The increased levels of TSH, often observed in DS subjects, might be explained as an altered steady state of the neuroendocrine axis. That is, the pituitary gland would secrete more TSH to maintain an appropriate release of T4 from the thyroid. The increased release of T4 would balance the augmented degradation of this hormone in the periphery. Such an altered thyroid steady state was normalized by dietary supplementation of zinc.

The positive effect of zinc administration upon TSH and rT3 plasma levels was still present one year after the cessation of the supplement. However, a slight increment in TSH levels was noted 12 months after the dietary supplementation.

Granulocyte CL activity was very low before zinc administration and was normalized by zinc therapy. This immune function was very sensitive as a marker of marginal zinc deficiency. In fact, one year after zinc supplementation, granulocyte activity was again impaired and paralleled the decrement of plasma zinc.

The improvement of granulocyte activity might be partially mediated by the normalization of neuroendocrine axis, pituitary-thyroid-periphery. However, a direct effect of zinc availability upon the metabolic efficiency of circulating granulocytes also seems to play a role, since their function was once again impaired one year after the cessation of the zinc therapy, when plasma zinc was also slightly decreased.

These findings suggest the presence of a hierarchical utilization of biologically available zinc in the human body. In fact, the pituitary-thyroid axis was still within the normal range 12 months after the cessation of zinc supplementation, when granulocyte CL activity was again impaired. In other words, zinc and possibly other trace elements are available first for the brain, then for the homeostatic systems such as endocrine glands, finally for other organs, i.e., the immune system.

Autoimmune thyroid disease is not uncommon in the elderly and antithyroid antibodies, along with elevated levels of TSH, are present in these subjects. Moreover, 12–15% of the elderly showed elevated levels of TSH without clinical signs of hypothyroidism and only a fraction of these subjects had elevated titers of antithyroid antibodies.[36]

It would be of interest to investigate the zinc status in elderly with elevated plasma levels of TSH, and the concomitant effect of zinc supplementation on pituitary-thyroid axis and immune responses.

In conclusion, DS appears to be a clinical condition characterized by a precocious aging of the neuroendocrine axis regulating the thyroid metabolism. Early senescence of immune responses is also present in this syndrome. Most importantly, the endocrine impairment and some deficient immune responses can be restored by dietary manipulation.

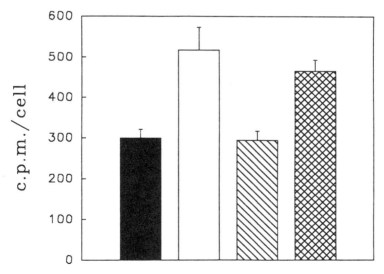

FIGURE 3. Chemiluminescence responses (cpm per single cell) of granulocytes from peripheral blood of subjects with DS before (black histogram), after (white histogram), one year after the cessation of zinc supplementation (slashed histogram), and in untreated controls (crosshatched histogram).

REFERENCES

1. MARTIN, G. M. 1979. Fed. Proc. **38:** 1962–1967.
2. MARTIN, G. M. 1988. Exp. Gerontol. **23:** 257–267.
3. MCCLEARN, G. E. 1988. Exp. Gerontol. **23:** 245–255.
4. STADMAN, E. R. 1988. Exp. Gerontol. **23:** 327–347.
5. MILLS, R. G. & A. S. WEISS. 1990. Gerontology **36:** 84–89.
6. WALFORD, R. L., F. NAEIM, K. Y. HALL, C. F. TAM, R. A. GATTI & M. A. MEDICI. 1983. In Immunoregulation. N. Fabris, E. Garaci, J. Hadden & N. A. Mitchinson, Eds.: 399–417. Plenum Publishing Corp. New York, N.Y.
7. LEJEUNE, J., M. GAUTIER & R. TURPIN. 1959. C. R. Acad. Sci. Paris **248:** 602–603.
8. HOLLAND, W. W., R. DOLL & C. O. CARTER. 1962. Br. J. Cancer **16:** 177–186.
9. ROBISON, L. L., M. E. NESBIT, H. N. SATHER, C. LEVEL, N. SHAHIDI, A. KENNEDY & D. HAMMOND. 1984. J. Pediatr. **105:** 235–242.
10. FORT, P., F. LIFSHITZ, R. BELLISARIO, J. DAVIS, R. LANES, M. PUGLIESE, R. RICHMAN, E. M. POST & R. DAVID. 1984. J. Pediatr. **104:** 545–549.
11. MARTIN, G. M. 1979. Birth Defects **14:** 5–39.
12. LICASTRO, F. 1986. Immunopathol. Immunother. Lett. **2:** 6–7.
13. DUPONT, A., M. VAETH & P. VIDEBECH. 1986. J. Ment. Defic. Res. **30:** 111–120.
14. THASE, M. E. 1982. J. Ment. Defic. Res. **26:** 177–192.
15. LICASTRO, F., C. MELOTTI, R. PARENTE, L. J. DAVIS, M. CHIRICOLO, M. ZANNOTTI & F. BARBONI. 1990. Am. J. Med. Genet. **7** (suppl.): 242–246.
16. FRANCESCHI, C., M. CHIRICOLO, F. LICASTRO, M. ZANNOTTI, M. MASI, E. MOCCHEGIANI & N. FABRIS. 1988. J. Ment. Defic. Res. **32:** 169–181.
17. LICASTRO, F., M. CHIRICOLO, E. MOCCHEGIANI, N. FABRIS, A. COSARIZZA, M. MASI, G. ARENA, M. ZANNOTTI, D. MONTI, E. BELTRANDI, R. MANCINI, M. CASADEI-MALDINI & C. FRANCESCHI. 1990. J. Immunol. Res. **2:** 95–100.
18. FABRIS, N., E. MOCCHEGIANI, L. AMADIO, M. ZANNOTTI & C. FRANCESCHI. 1984. Lancet **1:** 983–986.
19. FRASER, J. & A. MITCHELL. 1976. J. Ment. Sci. **22:** 169–175.
20. WISNIEWSKI, K. E., H. M. WISNIEWSKI & G. Y. WEN. 1985. Ann. Neurol. **17:** 278–298.
21. SARE, Z., R. H. RUVALCABA & V. C. KELLEY. 1978. Clin. Genet. **14:** 154–158.
22. LOUDON, M. M., R. E. DAY & E. M. DUKE. 1985. Arch. Dis. Child. **60:** 1149–1151.
23. MURDOCH, J. C., W. A. RATCLIFFE, D. G. MCLARTY, J. C. RODGER & J. G. RATCLIFFE. 1977. J. Clin. Endocrinol. Metab. **44:** 453–458.
24. PUESCHEL, S. M. & J. C. PEZZULLO. 1985. Am. J. Dis. Child. **139:** 636–639.
25. CUTLER, A. T., R. BENEZRA-OBEITER & S. J. BRINK. 1986. Am. J. Dis. Child. **140:** 479–483.
26. FORT, P., F. LIFSHITZ, R. BELLISARIO, J. DAVIS, R. LANES, M. PUGLIESE, R. RICHMAN, E. M. POST & R. DAVID. 1984. J. Pediatr. **104:** 545–549.
27. LEJEUNE, J., M. PEETERS, M. C. DE BLOIS, M. BERGER, A. GRILLOT, M. O. RETHORE, G. VALLEE, M. IZEMBART & J. P. DEVAUX. 1988. Ann. Genet. **31:** 137–143.
28. LICASTRO, F., E. MOCCHEGIANI, M. ZANNOTTI, G. ARENA, M. MASI & N. FABRIS. 1992. Int. J. Neurosci. **65:** 259–268.
29. FERNANDEZ, F. J. & H. KHAN. 1971. Clin. Chem. Newslett. **3:** 24–28.
30. BJORKSTEIN, B., O. BACK, H. GUSTAVSON, G. HALLMANS, B. HAGGLOF, & A. TARNVIK. 1980. Acta. Paediatr. Scand. **69:** 183–87.
31. SOBEL, A. E. 1958. Am. J. Ment. Defic. **62:** 642–656.
32. WILLIAMS, C. A., H. QUINN, E. C. WRIGHT, P. E. SYLVESTER, P. J. GOSLING & J. W. DICKERSON. 1985. J. Ment. Defic. Res. **1985:** 173–177.
33. BRUHL, H. H., J. FONI, H. LEE & A. MADOW. 1987. Am. J. Ment. Defic. **92:** 103–111.
34. WEINGERB, C., C. C. THOMPSON, E. O. ONG, R. LEBO, D. J. GRUOL & R. M. EVANS. 1986. Nature **324:** 641–646.
35. BERG, J. M. 1989. Cell **57:** 1965–1068.
36. DRINKA, P. J., W. E. NOLTEN, S. VOEKS & E. LANGER. 1991. J. Am. Geriatr. Assoc. **39:** 1000–1001.

Impaired Antibody Response to Influenza Vaccine in Institutionalized Elderly[a]

M. PROVINCIALI, G. DI STEFANO, M. MUZZIOLI,
P. SCARPAZZA,[b] D. COLOMBO,[b] M. MIGLIORINO,[b]
M. BELLANI,[b] M. COLOMBO,[c] F. DELLA CROCE,[c]
M. C. GANDOLFI,[c] L. DAGHETTA,[c] AND N. FABRIS

Immunology Center
INRCA
Gerontology Research Department
Ancona, Italy

[b]*INRCA*
Casatenovo, Italy

[c]*Camillo Golgi Geriatric Institute*
Abbiategrasso, Italy

INTRODUCTION

Epidemiological studies have demonstrated an increased occurrence of influenza epidemics in elderly people, particularly in individuals living in a high-density environment, such as nursing homes.[1,2]

The high susceptibility to outbreaks of influenza and the augmented morbility and mortality rates present in elderly population have been suggested to include such people along with other high-risk groups for annual influenza immunization.[3–5]

Conflicting data exist in the literature on the effectiveness of influenza vaccination in elderly people and, in particular, on the capacity of standard influenza vaccine to confer an adequate antibody protection.[6–9]

Although extensive vaccination procedures have been generally demonstrated to be effective in reducing the rate of broncopneumonia and mortality in vaccinated elderly nursing homes subjects, compared to unvaccinated residents,[2,8] the efficacy of influenza vaccination in elderly is by far lower than in younger persons.[10,11]

The main cause for the low effectiveness of influenza vaccination in the elderly is certainly linked to the age-related impairment in antibody response,[12] particularly for T cell–dependent antigens, such as influenza viral antigens. In fact, development of serum antiinfluenza virus antibodies appears to correlate with the degree of protection conferred by influenza vaccine. In this paper, we report the results of a survey performed in the course of 1989–90 and 1991–92 winter seasons on the effectiveness of influenza virus vaccination in inducing hemoagglutinating antibody response in institutionalized elderly. In the course of the 1989–90 study, an aggressive epidemia of influenza virus occurred with a high mortality rate that led us to measure also this parameter, in spite of the relatively modest number of subjects.

[a]This work was supported by Italian Health Ministry Targeted project: "Potenziamento della vaccinazione antiinfluenzale nell'anziano."

307

PATIENTS AND METHODS

The studies performed during the winter seasons 1989–90 and 1991–92 included 260 and 112 institutionalized elderly people respectively. The subjects enrolled in the course of winter season 1989–90 were split into two groups: one received vaccine (226 subjects), and the other was used as control (34 subjects). All subjects in the study conducted in the 1991–92 winter season were treated with vaccine. The mean age of the different groups of subjects was 81.29 ± 5.97 and 80.92 ± 8.33 years for controls and vaccinated respectively in the winter season 1989–90, and 82.00 ± 8.00 years for vaccinated in the winter season 1991–92. In all groups, age ranged from 60 to 98 years.

Subjects were vaccinated with standard influenza vaccine (Sclavo, Italy) containing A/Taiwan 1/86, A/Shangai 11/87, and B/Yamagata 16/80 in the winter season 1989–90, while the influenza vaccine used in the 1991/92 study contained B/Yamagata 16/88, A/Taiwan 1/8, and A/Bejing H3N3 (Isifluzonale, ISI, Italy). The elderly subjects were in stable and relatively fair clinical conditions. Unvaccinated and vaccinated groups were not different in critical clinical areas, mental impairment, or pharmacological therapy.

Blood withdrawals were obtained at days 0 and 30 after vaccination. Antiviral antigen antibodies were assayed by a standard hemoagglutination inhibition test.[13]

All serological titers were expressed as the reciprocal of the serum dilution starting from a 1:10 dilution. The antiinfluenza virus antibody titers were converted to log to base 2. Antibody titers under 1:40 ($5.3 \log_{-2}$) were considered unprotective.

According to general convention, seroconversion was defined as a fourfold or greater rise in serum antibody titer when compared with the prevaccination titer.

Data were analyzed for statistical significance by using ANOVA for comparing different groups; the two-tailed paired Student t-test for comparing means before and after treatment; the chi-square test for analyzing proportions among groups, and the Mc Nemar's chi-square test for comparing p values for odds ratios inside each group.

RESULTS

As shown in FIGURE 1, the antibody titer of the subjects enrolled in the winter season 1989–90 did significantly increase at the time of the second blood withdrawal in both control and vaccinated groups ($p < 0.0001$). The comparison between the antibody titer present in control and vaccinated subjects was not significantly different either before or 30 days after vaccination. In the course of the winter season 1991–92, the antibody titer of elderly subjects did not increase in a significant way after vaccination.

On the basis of the antibody titer before vaccination the subjects were divided into unprotected (antibody titer < 1:40) or protected (antibody titer ≥ 1:40). As shown in TABLE 1, an increase in antibody titer was present in both protected and unprotected subjects 30 days after vaccination. A similar rise in antibody titer was observed in elderly unvaccinated subjects. The mean antibody titer reached 30 days after vaccine administration was significantly higher in unprotected vaccinated than unvaccinated subjects ($p = 0.004$). With regard to the study performed during the winter season 1991–92, a significant increase in antibody titer was present only in the group of unprotected elderly subjects (TABLE 1).

As shown in FIGURE 2, the log increase in antibody titer observed in subjects

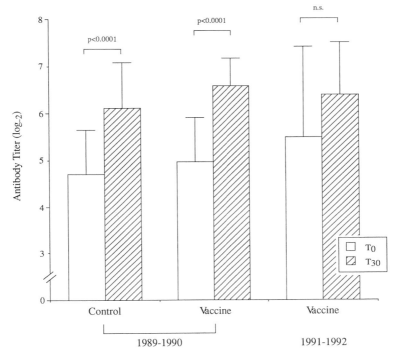

FIGURE 1. Antibody titer against influenza viral antigens in control and vaccinated elderly subjects. Blood withdrawals were done at day 0 and 30 days after vaccination.

vaccinated in the 1989–90 study was higher than the one obtained in control unvaccinated elderly considering either total or unprotected populations. The difference was statistically significant only comparing the unprotected vaccinated and control groups ($p < 0.0001$). No significant difference was present comparing the log increase in antibody titer of the protected vaccinated and control populations

TABLE 1. Evaluation of Antibody Titer to Influenza Virus before and after Vaccination in Protected and Unprotected Elderly Subjects

Winter Season	Group	Days from Vaccination	Antibody Titer ($\log_{-2}$) Unprotected	Antibody Titer ($\log_{-2}$) Protected
1989–90	Control	0	4.00 ± 0.46	5.37 ± 0.15
		30	$5.43 \pm 0.89^{a,c}$	6.80 ± 1.05^{b}
	Vaccine	0	4.29 ± 0.50	5.63 ± 0.59
		30	$6.15 \pm 1.19^{a,c}$	7.00 ± 0.93^{a}
1991–92	Vaccine	0	4.13 ± 0.37	6.85 ± 1.37
		30	5.60 ± 0.95^{a}	7.12 ± 1.62

[a] $p < 0.0001$ and [b] $p < 0.041$ when compared to the respective value at day 0.
[c] $p = 0.004$.

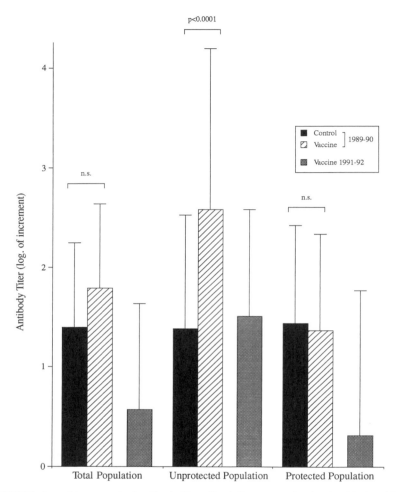

FIGURE 2. Log of increment of antibody titer after influenza vaccination in elderly subjects. Total population was split into unprotected or protected according to the antibody titer present before vaccination.

(FIGURE 2). The rise in antibody titer observed in the winter season 1991–92 in vaccinated subjects was poor and not significant.

The evaluation of the percentage of subjects who reached protective antibody titers ($\geq 1{:}40$) 30 days after vaccination revealed a significant increase in both vaccinated and control subjects in the study conducted in 1989–90 (TABLE 2). The percentage of protected subjects at the time of the second blood withdrawal was not significantly different in the two groups (80.30 vs. 65.72). The population studied in the 1991–92 winter season showed protective antibody titers before vaccination which did not increase 30 days after, as evidenced by the not significant increase in the percentage of protected subjects at time 0 and 30 (86.66 vs. 97.33, TABLE 2).

As reported in FIGURE 3, seroconversion frequencies (percentage of subjects seroconverted) were not significantly different in vaccinated and control populations studied in the winter season 1989–90. Differences were not significant even comparing unprotected vaccinated and control subjects (data not shown). The seroconversion frequency was low in the 1991–92 study and not significantly different from that of controls evaluated in the 1989–90 survey (FIGURE 3).

TABLE 3 reports the mortality rate of elderly vaccinated and unvaccinated subjects after an aggressive epidemic of influenza virus which occurred around 20 to 40 days after vaccination in the 1989–90 study. As shown, the high mortality rate observed in unvaccinated subjects was not significantly modified by vaccination procedure (7.9 vs. 10.6 percent).

DISCUSSION

Elderly persons are generally considered to be most prone to serious complications from influenza virus infection so that annual influenza vaccination is routinely used in elderly communities.[1–5]

Several observational studies have reported mixed results with regard to vaccine effectiveness in aging. In some studies, it has been reported that influenza vaccination decreases the frequency and the severity of infections in the elderly, particularly when the antigenic strains in the vaccine are closely related to the infecting virus.[1,2,10,14,15] The clinical efficacy of vaccination with viral antigens was accompanied by an adequate antibody responses only in a few cases, whereas in other studies the clinical protection conferred by influenza vaccination was much greater than expected from serological results.[10,16]

The findings of other surveys on influenza vaccination in old age have reported the poor effectiveness of standard vaccination procedures, suggesting that there may be some important differences in the ability of the elderly to respond to influenza vaccines compared with the ability of younger persons.[2,7]

The results reported in this paper on a survey performed in the course of 1989–90 and 1991–92 winter seasons demonstrate the ineffectiveness of standard influenza vaccination procedure in elderly subjects.

The increase of antibody titer found in the elderly vaccinated during the 1989–90 winter season was not significantly different from the one observed in unvaccinated subjects. The occurrence of a high aggressive influenza epidemic in the course of that survey may explain the raise in antibody titer in both populations.

The ineffectiveness of vaccination per se to ameliorate the antibody response to viral antigens was further demonstrated in the study performed in the 1991–92

TABLE 2. Evaluation of the Percentage of Protected Elderly Subjects before and after Vaccination

Winter Season	Group	Days from Vaccination		Mc Nemar test	
		0	30	χ^2	p
		Protected (%)			
1989–90	Control	15.62	65.62	15.01	<0.0001
	Vaccine	12.87	80.30	118.67	<0.0001
1991–92	Vaccine	86.66	97.33	1.50	=0.221

winter season. In this survey, the influenza virus was poorly aggressive and the only vaccination procedure was not able to increase the antibody titer.

A wide variation in seroconversion frequencies following influenza vaccination has been observed in elderly subjects. These observations have been partly explained by differences in dose and immunogenicity of the antigens used, as well as the prevaccination serum titers in the populations studied. In our study, the seroconversion frequency of vaccinated elderly was not significantly increased in comparison to unvaccinated subjects in either 1989–90 or 1991–92 studies. Even if in the latter study, the low seroconversion frequency may be explained by the high prevaccination

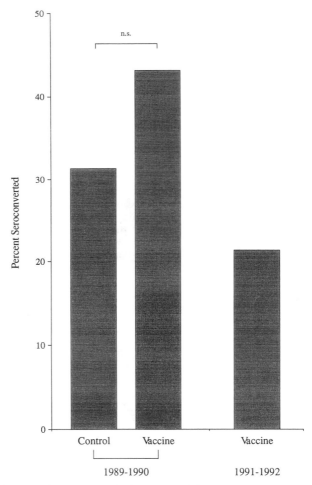

FIGURE 3. Percent of seroconverted subjects after influenza vaccination. Control and vaccinated subjects were examined for their capacity to have a fourfold or greater rise in serum antibody titer relative to the prevaccination titer.

TABLE 3. Mortality Rate of Elderly Vaccinated and Unvaccinated Subjects during 1989–90 Winter Season

	Group		
	Control	Vaccine	*p*
No. who died/total	3/38	29/273	0.815
Percent	7.9	10.6	

serum titers; in the 1989–90 survey an effective inability of influenza vaccine in increasing the percentage of seroconverted elderly may be taken into account.

The poor serological efficacy of standard influenza vaccination might explain the absence of significant differences in the mortality rate occurring during the 1989–90 winter season in the vaccinated and unvaccinated elderly population. It is questionable whether the low frequencies of seroconversion may reflect the incidence of influenza complications.

Even if our results give evidence on the ineffectiveness of influenza vaccination in elderly people, it is possible that at least a subgroup of elderly subjects might take advantage of the vaccination.

The analysis of the unprotected population of the 1989–90 survey has evidenced that even if the seroconversion frequency was not different in vaccinated and unvaccinated subjects, a significant rise in either antibody titer or log of increment of antibody titer was present in unprotected vaccinated subjects. This would suggest that vaccination does not exert its protective effect on the whole elderly population but only in a subgroup of subjects within the unprotected population.

Further studies should attempt to investigate elderly individuals with deficient responses and low antibody titers to influenza vaccine with regard to their immune status in order to evaluate the possibility of ameliorating the standard influenza vaccination by using adjuvant or immunomodulators.

ACKNOWLEDGMENTS

The authors thanks Mrs. B. Bartozzi, R. Stecconi, and Mr. M. Marcellini for their technical assistance.

REFERENCES

1. PATRIARCA, P. A., J. A. WEBER, R. A. PARKER, W. N. HALL, A. P. KENDALL, D. J. BREGMAN & L. B. SCHONBERGER. 1985. Efficacy of influenza vaccine in nursing homes. JAMA **253**(8): 1136–1139.
2. HOWELLS, C. H. L., C. K. VESSELINOVA-JENKINS, A. D. EVANS & J. JAMES. 1975. Influenza vaccination and mortality from bronchopneumonia in the elderly. Lancet **15**: 381–383.
3. BERK, L. B. & S. ALVAREZ. 1986. Vaccinating the elderly: recommendations and rationale. Geriatrics **41**(1): 79–91.
4. BARKER, W. H. & J. P. MULLOOLY. 1980. Influenza vaccination of elderly persons. JAMA **244**(22): 2547–2549.
5. GLEZEN, W. P. 1982. Serious morbidity and mortality associated with influenza epidemics. Epidemiol. Rev. **4**: 25–44.
6. LEVINE, M., B. L. BEATTIE, D. M. MCLEAN & D. CORMAN. 1987. Characterization of the immune response to trivalent influenza vaccine in elderly men. JAGS **35**: 609–615.
7. ERSHLER, W. B., A. L. MOORE & M. A. SOCINSKI. 1984. Influenza and aging: age-related

changes and the effects of thymosin on the antibody response to influenza vaccine. J. Clin. Immunol. **4:** 445–451.

8. GROSS, P. A., G. V. QUINNAN, M. RODSTEIN, J. R. LAMONTAGNE, R. A. KASLOW, A. J. SAAH, S. WALLENSTEIN, R. NEUFELD, C. DENNING & P. GAERLAN. 1988. Association of influenza immunization with reduction in mortality in a elderly population. Arch. Intern. Med. **148:** 562–565.

9. STRASSBURG, M. A., S. GREENLAND, F. J. SORVILLO, L. E. LIEB & L. A. HABEL. 1986. Influenza in the elderly: report of an outbreak and a review of vaccine effectiveness reports. Vaccine **4:** 38–44.

10. RUBEN, F. L. 1982. Prevention of influenza in the elderly. J. Am. Geriatr. Soc. **30**(9): 577–580.

11. PHAIR, J., C. A. KAUFMANN & A. BJORNSON. 1978. Failure to respond to influenza vaccine in the aged: correlation with B-cell number and function. J. Lab. Clin. Med. **92:** 822–825.

12. KISHIMOTO, S., S. TOMINO, H. MITSUYA, H. FUJIWARA & H. TSUDA. 1980. Age-related decline in the in vitro and in vitro synthesis of anti-tetanus toxoid antibody in humans. J. Immunol. **5:** 2347–2351.

13. MADORE, H. P., R. C. REICHAN & R. DOLIN. 1983. Serum antibody responses in naturally occuring influenza A virus infection determined by enzyme-linked immunoadsorbent assay, hemagglutination inhibition and complement fixation. J. Clin. Microbiol. **18:** 1345–1350.

14. BESDINE, R. W. 1986. Pneumonia and influenza: vaccination of elderly is justified. Geriatrics **41**(11): 13–16.

15. BARKER, W. H. & J. P. MULLOOLY. 1980. Influenza vaccination of elderly persons: reduction in pneumonia and influenza hospitalizations and deaths. JAMA **244:** 2547–2551.

16. ODELIN, M. F., B. POZZETTO, M. AYMARD, M. DEFAJOLLE & J. JOLLY-MILLION. 1993. Role of influenza vaccination in the elderly during an epidemic of $A \leq 1N1$ virus in 1988–1989: clinical and serological data. Gerontology **39:** 109–116.

Antagonic-Stress

A New Treatment in Gerontopsychiatry and for a Healthy Productive Life

VASILE PREDESCU,[a] DAN RIGA,[b,d] SORIN RIGA,[b]
JANINA TURLEA,[c] IOANA MOISIL BĂRBAT,[c]
AND LIVIU BOTEZAT-ANTONESCU[c]

[a] First Department of Psychiatry
"Gh. Marinescu" Clinical Hospital

[b] Institute of Neurology and Psychiatry
Berceni Road no. 10
Post Office Box 6180
RO-75622 Bucharest, Romania

[c] National Institute of Health Statistics
George Vraca Street no. 9
RO-70706 Bucharest, Romania

INTRODUCTION

The general extension of total life in the world's population determines an important growth in the number of elderly people and a continuous increase of the incidence and prevalence rates of neurological, mental, and behavioral disorders, and thus a significant decrease of active life.[1] Mental decline in normal aging and especially cognitive loss in pathological aging—organic mental disorders (OMD)—increase the limitation of activity and the need for assistance in activities of daily existence and finally the cost of social and health services.[2]

Etiopathogenic data support nondependence of the age-related brain dysfunctions only on one mechanism alone and develop a multicausal interpretation of physiopathological processes in aging.[3] Moreover, the same data advance the multimodal approach to gerontopsychopharmacotherapy[4] and promote drug combinations and multitherapies vs. monotherapies in gerontopsychiatry.[5]

The involvement of free radicals,[6] oxidative stress,[7] and deficiencies of antioxidants in brain aging, lipofuscin (age pigment) accumulation,[8] as well as in senile dementia (SD)[9] have been conducive to the study of scavengers and to the development of antioxidant therapies.[10] In the same therapeutical direction, Meclofenoxate (MF)-DCI has been proved a free radical scavenger,[11,12] a brain lipofuscinolytic agent,[13,14] a decelerator of the aging rate,[15] and an active drug in SD.[16-18] The diminution of the cerebral blood flow associated with a lower glucose and oxygen brain metabolism in normal aging as well as chronic cerebrovascular insufficiency in pathological aging and in SD[19] have been conducive to the development of antiischemic medication.[20] Therefore, cerebral vasodilators such as nicotinic acid and nicergoline (NE)-DCI, a nicotinic acid derivative esterified with ergoline, have been studied in gerontopsychopharmacotherapy.[21-22] Subsequently, NE was demonstrated as active in SD.[23-25]

---

[d] Author to whom correspondence should be addressed.

In accordance with Harman's free radical theory of aging[26] and Zs.-Nagy's membrane hypothesis of aging,[15,27] conjugated with the multimodal approach and the drug multitherapy direction in gerontopsychiatry[4,5] and starting from brain lipofuscin reduction by methionine[28] and by MF,[14] a new complex neurometabolic drug—Antagonic-Stress (AS), with nootropic, antistress, and antiaging actions—was developed and preclinically and clinically tested.[29]

Antagonic-Stress was authorized in Romania,[30,31] has successfully undergone phase III of clinical studies—being certified as such—and has recently been demonstrated as active in mild to moderate senile dementia of the Alzheimer's type (SDAT).[18,25,32]

In this paper, we present comparative and independent data, which recommend and introduce AS as a new treatment in gerontopsychiatry.

PATIENTS AND METHOD

Clinical Design and Characterization of Patients

We selected five categories of OMD (TABLE 1), using the American (DSM-III-R)[33] and international (ICD-10)[34] classifications and criteria. Double-blind, randomized, comparative, and parallel trials were performed in these diseases, in harmony with the general guidelines for clinical studies[35] and data interpretations,[36] as well as with the WHO recommendations concerning the evaluation of methods for the

TABLE 1 Multiple Studies with Antagonic-Stress (Antiaging Formula) in Gerontopsychiatry. Mental Disorders and Distribution of Comparative Groups Investigated: Placebo (PL), Meclofenoxate (MF), or Nicergoline (NE) vs. Antagonic-Stress (AS)

Diagnostic Criteria and Codes acc. to			Comparative Groups Investigated (Number of Patients)	
Classification of the Organic Mental Disorders	DSM-III-R, APA, 1987	ICD-10, Ch.V (F), WHO, 1992		
Associated with Axis III physical disorders or conditions				
• Organic amnestic disorder	294.00	F 04	PL-1 (31)	AS-1 (33)
• Organic depressive disorder	293.83	F 06.32	PL-2 (30)	AS-2 (31)
• Organic anxiety disorder	294.80	F 06.4	PL-3 (31)	AS-3 (32)
Dementias				
• Senile dementia of Alzheimer's type			MF (31)[a] NE (30)[b]	AS (32)[a,b]
• Uncomplicated	290.00	F 00.10		
• With depression	290.21	F 00.13		
• Multiinfarct dementia			PL-4 (30)	AS-4 (32)
• Uncomplicated	290.40	F 01.10		
• With depression	290.43	F 01.13		

[a]From Popa et al.[18]
[b]From Schneider et al.[25]

treatment of mental disorders.[37] AS vs. placebo (PL) investigations in OMD—amnestic (OAmD), depressive (ODeD), anxiety (OAxD), and in multiinfarct dementia (MID)—were followed by AS vs. MF or NE trials in SDAT[18,25] (TABLE 1).

Informed consent was obtained from all participants after they had received the full basic information concerning the study in which they had been included. Moreover, at the close of the trials, the PL groups benefitted by conventional treatments with cerebral activators.

Clinical characteristics of groups with OMD are shown in TABLE 2 and those with dementias in TABLE 3. The final aggregate number of old people at the end of the investigation was 343: four PL groups with 122, one MF group with 31, one NE group with 30, and five AS groups with 160 patients. Total medical and nonmedical dropouts were 9.1%.

DSM-III-R and ICD-10 clinical descriptions and diagnostic guidelines were simultaneously applied. In addition, the diagnostic process (criteria for inclusion, severity, and exclusion) was structured in five steps according to the diagnostic level: I—psychogeriatric symptomatology, II—severity, III—course and duration, IV—presence of dementia, and V—etiology (antemortem classification).[38] Criteria for severity followed from predrug multiple assessments: Wechsler Memory Scale (WMS), Hamilton Depression Scale (HDS), Hamilton Anxiety Scale (HAS), and Sandoz Clinical Assessment-Geriatric (SCAG) scale (TABLES 2 and 3). In this study, specific criteria were used for inclusion—patients of both sexes; only high education level (university); and one month before trial without interfering treatments (psychotropics, nootropics, cholinergic agents, cerebral vasodilators, antihyperlipidemic agents, anabolic or lipotropic drugs, hepatoprotectants, multivitamins, and multiminerals)—as well as for exclusion—inadequate conditions for interview and assessment; and the coexistence of severe somatic diseases.

Psychogeriatric Treatments

The same AS pharmaceutical form and administration were used in all groups. Also, all treatments were prolonged (for three months), in oral administration, 3 capsules (2 blue + 1 yellow), 3 times daily (morning, noon, and afternoon), before meals, and with liquid in abundance. A double-blind and randomized procedure was utilized in the administration of treatments: PL and AS, MF and AS, NE and AS.

The complementarity of AS composition and of its pharmaceutical form (gastro- and enterosoluble capsules) ensured the controlled release and absorption of the active substances. The retardation of nicotinic acid in enterosoluble capsules ensured its prolonged delivery and vasodilatory action. The composition of a gastro-soluble (blue) capsule is: 260 mg meclofenoxate, 150 mg methionine, 90 mg aspartic acid · Mg salt, 10 mg fructose, 8 mg vitamin B-1, 11 mg vitamin B-6, 10 mg nicotinic acid with fast release, and 10.5 mg zinc sulfate. The composition of an enterosoluble (yellow) capsule is: 315 mg orotic acid, 10 mg fructose, 80 mg nicotinic acid with prolonged release, 98 mg dipotassium hydrogen phosphate, 20 mg magnesium oxide, 2.5 mg lithium carbonate, and 0.12 mg potassium iodide. The minimal AS therapeutical active dose is 2 blue + 1 yellow capsules. For OMD and SD treatments, the therapeutical dose was three times the minimal AS active dose.

For PL groups, both blue and yellow capsules were filled with lactose (pharmaceutical adjuvant), and then only yellow capsules were enterically coated by the same procedure as for AS.

For MF groups, blue gastrosoluble capsules were each processed with 260 mg MF

TABLE 2 Characteristics of Patients with Organic Mental Disorders (OMD)—Amnestic, Depressive, and Anxiety—Associated with Axis III Physical Disorders or Conditions: Placebo and Antagonic-Stress Groups[a]

	Organic Amnestic Disorder		Organic Depressive Disorder		Organic Anxiety Disorder	
	Placebo (PL-1)	Antagonic-Stress Formula (AS-1)	Placebo (PL-2)	Antagonic-Stress Formula (AS-2)	Placebo (PL-3)	Antagonic-Stress Formula (AS-3)
Age, years						
(mean ± SD)	67.1 ± 3.9	68.5 ± 4.3	67.4 ± 4.1	68.7 ± 4.4	70.0 ± 5.0	69.1 ± 4.7
(range)	60–73	60–75	60–72	60–73	60–76	60–74
Sex (F/M)	9/22	9/24	16/14	18/13	20/11	22/10
Duration of OMD years						
(mean ± SD)	4.0 ± 1.3	4.4 ± 1.0	3.8 ± 1.2	4.2 ± 1.1	4.1 ± 1.0	3.8 ± 0.9
range	2–6	2–8	2–7	2–9	2–7	2–6
Severity of psychopathology	Memory deficit (Weschler's scale) ≤ 90		Depression (Hamilton's scale) ≥ 18		Anxiety (Hamilton's scale) ≥ 15	

[a]For each disorder, the differences between groups are not significant ($p > 0.05$; ANOVA).

TABLE 3 Characteristics of Patients with Multiinfarct Dementia and Senile Dementia of Alzheimer's Type. Placebo and Treated Groups with Meclofenoxate, Nicergoline, vs. Antagonic-Stress Formula[a]

	Multiinfarct Dementia (MID)		Senile Dementia of Alzheimer's Type (SDAT)		
	Placebo (PL-4)	Antagonic-Stress Formula (AS-4)	Meclofenoxate (MF)[b]	Nicergoline (NE)[c]	Antagonic-Stress Formula (AS)[b,c]
Age, years (mean ± SD)	65.4 ± 3.9	66.8 ± 4.1	68.6 ± 4.8	68.7 ± 4.8	70.8 ± 5.9
(range)	60–68	60–70	65–85	65–81	65–87
Sex (F/M)	10/20	10/22	15/16	14/16	15/17
Duration of dementia					
Years (mean ± SD)	1.5 ± 0.3	1.6 ± 0.4	4.4 ± 0.9	4.2 ± 1.0	4.7 ± 1.1
Range	1–3	1–4	2–7	2–8	2–10
Severity of dementia					
SCAG item 19 (no. and %)					
Moderately severe	0 (0.0%)	1 (3.1%)	1 (3.2%)	1 (3%)	2 (6.3%)
Moderate	2 (6.7%)	3 (9.4%)	4 (13.0%)	3 (10%)	4 (12.5%)
Mild to moderate	18 (60.0%)	23 (71.9%)	21 (67.7%)	18 (60%)	22 (68.7%)
Mild	10 (33.3%)	5 (15.6%)	5 (16.1%)	8 (27%)	4 (12.5%)

[a]For each disease, the differences between groups are not significant ($p > 0.05$; ANOVA).
[b]From Popa et al.[18]
[c]From Schneider et al.[25]

powder (Sintofarm, Bucharest, Romania) and yellow capsules were filled with lactose and after that were enterically coated, using the same method as for AS.

For NE groups, blue gastrosoluble capsules were each processed with 10 mg NE powder (Biofarm, Bucharest, Romania), while yellow capsules were filled with lactose and then enterically coated by the same procedure as for AS.

Psychopathological Assessments and Statistics

Complex evaluations, both pre- and posttreatments, were made with acknowledged uni- and multidimensional rating instruments: psychogeriatric assessment by SCAG scale,[39,40] Self-Assessment Scale-Geriatric (SASG)[41] and their five subscales;[42] psychopathologic rating by HDS[43] and HAS;[43] psychometric testing by digit symbol (coding) of WAIS,[44] WMS[45] and Wechsler Adult Intelligence Scale (WAIS).[44]

In OMD investigated, these instruments were applied as follows: in OAmD—digit symbol of WAIS and WMS; in ODeD—HDS; in OAxD—HAS; in MID—SCAG; and in SDAT—SCAG, SASG, digit symbol of WAIS, WMS and WAIS.

Effects of treatments resulted from comparing the total scores on digit symbol of WAIS, on HDS, HAS, SCAG, SASG, and on their five subscales; the memory quotient (MQ) on WMS; and the intelligence quotient (IQ)—full, verbal, and performance IQ—and the deterioration index on WAIS.

The statistical analysis was carried out by using an SPSS/PC+ package and an IBM PS/1 computer. Pre- vs. posttreatment comparisons were made by the analysis of variance (ANOVA). Comparing pairs of treatments (PL, MF, or NE vs. AS)—taking baseline scores as covariates—was done by the analysis of covariance (ANCOVA). Where significant F values were found, p significance level was noted. We admitted the significance level for medicine of $p < 0.05$.

RESULTS

The efficacy of AS in OMD resulted from the pre- vs. posttreatment comparisons and especially from AS vs. PL comparisons (TABLE 4). In OAmD, AS improved the visual-motor processing, attention-concentration, and short-term memory (digit symbol of WAIS) by (+)5.3—from weak (4.0–7.9) baseline to the medium superior limit (8.0–11.9) final level. In addition, an important restoration of memory-learning processes (MQ of WMS) with (+)29.9 was associated—from moderate deficit (71–80) baseline to the medium memory (91–110) final level. In ODeD, AS diminished the depression symptomatology (HDS total score) by (−)16.4, from baseline—superior limit of moderate depression (24.9–18.0) to final—inferior level of mild depression (17.9–7.0). In OAxD, AS reduced the anxiety manifestations (HDS total score) by (−)8.1, from baseline—superior limit of moderate anxiety (21.9–15.0) to final—middle level of mild anxiety (14.9–6.0). PL treatments registered a slight improvement, only in OAmD and ODeD, with statistical significance, but without psychometric or psychopathologic significance.

The effectiveness of AS in MID resulted from the pre- vs. posttreatment comparisons and especially from AS-4 vs. PL-4 comparisons (TABLE 5). AS reduced the intensity of geriatric psychopathology assessed by SCAG (1 severity interval = 18.0) in total score by (−)27.4, from superior limit of mild to moderate (72.0–54.0) level to inferior limit of mild (54.0–36.0 interval). Also, AS decreased the scores in the factor structures of SCAG as follows:

TABLE 4 Comparative Psychometric and Psychopathologic Evaluations of Antagonic-Stress Formula vs. Placebo in Prolonged Treatment (3 Months) of Organic Mental Disorders. Test of the Cognitive and Affective Profiles: Attention-Concentration by Digit Symbol of Wechsler Adult Intelligence Scale, Memory-Learning by Wechsler Memory Scale, Depression and Anxiety by Hamilton Depression and Anxiety Scales[a]

	Placebo (PL) Groups		Antagonic-Stress (AS) Groups		Significance Level (p) AS vs. PL[e]
	Baseline	Final	Baseline	Final	
Organic amnestic disorder (PL-1 and AS-1 groups)					
• Attention-concentration (score)	6.8 ± 1.4	8.3 ± 1.4^b	6.5 ± 1.4	11.8 ± 2.4^d	<0.001
• Memory-learning (memory quotient—MQ)	78.1 ± 6.9	83.9 ± 5.5^b	76.3 ± 6.6	106.2 ± 11.1^d	<0.001
Organic depressive disorder (PL-2 and AS-2 groups)					
• Depression (total score)	23.5 ± 2.3	18.1 ± 2.9^b	24.9 ± 2.3	8.5 ± 1.6^d	<0.001
Organic anxiety disorder (PL-3 and AS-3 groups)					
• Anxiety (total score)	18.2 ± 1.9	17.5 ± 1.8^c	19.2 ± 2.3	11.1 ± 1.7^d	<0.001

[a]Scores are expressed as mean ± standard deviation (SD).
[b]$p < 0.001$, final vs. baseline PL comparisons (ANOVA) are significant in amnestic (PL-1) and depressive (PL-2) organic disorders.
[c]$p > 0.05$, are not significant in organic anxiety disorder (PL-3).
[d]$p < 0.001$, all final vs. baseline AS comparisons (ANOVA) are very significant in amnestic, depressive, and anxiety organic disorders.
[e]Final AS vs. final PL scores, taking baseline scores as covariates (ANCOVA), are very significant for AS groups ($p < 0.001$) and are shown in the last column.

TABLE 5 Comparative Psychogeriatric Assessments of Antagonic-Stress Formula vs. Placebo in Prolonged Treatment (3 Months) of Multiinfarct Dementia: Heteroevaluation (Doctor) by Sandoz Clinical Assessment-Geriatric (SCAG) Scale and Its 5 Subscales[a]

	Placebo-4 (PL-4)		Antagonic-Stress Formula-4 (AS-4)		Significance Level (p) AS-4 vs. PL-4[d]
	Baseline	Final	Baseline	Final	
SCAG total score	65.2 ± 9.2	63.5 ± 9.1[b]	69.5 ± 6.8	42.1 ± 5.4[c]	<0.001
SCAG subscales					
I. Cognitive dysfunctions	14.9 ± 2.4	14.7 ± 2.3[b]	15.0 ± 2.3	9.4 ± 1.7[c]	<0.001
II. Interpersonal relationships	14.8 ± 2.5	14.4 ± 2.3[b]	16.4 ± 2.9	9.6 ± 1.6[c]	<0.001
III. Affective disorders	11.9 ± 2.4	11.3 ± 2.0[b]	13.7 ± 2.0	7.7 ± 1.6[c]	<0.001
IV. Apathy	13.3 ± 2.5	13.1 ± 2.3[b]	13.1 ± 2.7	8.7 ± 1.6[c]	<0.001
V. Somatic dysfunctions	10.3 ± 2.7	10.0 ± 2.5[b]	11.3 ± 1.9	6.7 ± 1.4[c]	<0.001

[a]Scores are expressed as mean ± SD.
[b]$p > 0.05$, ANOVA, final vs. baseline PL-4 comparisons are not significant.
[c]$p < 0.001$, ANOVA, final vs. baseline AS-4 comparisons are very significant.
[d]Final AS-4 vs. final PL-4 scores, taking baseline scores as covariates (ANCOVA), are very significant for AS-4 ($p < 0.001$) and are shown in the last column.

($-$)5.6 in the cognitive subscale (1 interval = 4.0);
($-$)6.8 in the interpersonal subscale (1 interval = 4.0);
($-$)6.0 in the affective subscale (1 interval = 3.0);
($-$)4.4 in the apathy subscale (1 interval = 4.0); and
($-$)4.6 in the somatic subscale (1 interval = 3.0).

AS efficiency in SDAT, resulting from pre- vs. posttreatment comparisons and intertreatment comparisons, pointed out the superiority of AS vs. MF and NE (TABLES 6, 7, and 8). The intensity of geriatric psychopathology assessed by SCAG (total score) was reduced by ($-$)25.1 AS, ($-$)16.3 MF, ($-$)16.0 NE, from the superior limit of mild to moderate to mild intensity. Comparative remissions (TABLE 6) in factor structures of SCAG scores were:

- in the cognitive subscale: ($-$)5.0 AS, ($-$)4.0 MF, ($-$)3.9 NE;
- in the interpersonal subscale: ($-$)6.5 AS, ($-$)3.7 MF, ($-$)4.6 NE;
- in the affective subscale: ($-$)5.6 AS, ($-$)3.6 MF, ($-$)3.2 NE;
- in the apathy subscale: ($-$)3.5 AS, ($-$)2.4 MF, ($-$)2.2 NE; and
- in the somatic subscale: ($-$)4.4 AS, ($-$)2.6 MF, ($-$)2.1 NE.

The frequency of geriatric psychopathological symptoms autoevaluated by SASG (the same types of scores and levels in scale and subscales as SCAG) was reduced by ($-$)21.1 AS, ($-$)14.1 MF, ($-$)13.7 NE, from the superior limit of mild to moderate to mild level. Comparative remissions (TABLE 7) in factor structures of SASG scores were:

- in the cognitive subscale: ($-$)4.6 AS, ($-$)3.6 MF, ($-$)3.5 NE;
- in the interpersonal subscale: ($-$)5.6 AS, ($-$)2.8 MF, ($-$)3.3 NE;
- in the affective subscale: ($-$)4.2 AS, ($-$)3.2 MF, ($-$)2.8 NE;
- in the apathy subscale: ($-$)3.0 AS, ($-$)2.2 MF, ($-$)2.2 NE; and
- in the somatic subscale: ($-$)3.8 AS, ($-$)2.3 MF, ($-$)1.9 NE.

Improvements in visual-motor processing, attention-concentration and short-term memory, tested by digit symbol of WAIS, were ($+$)4.0 AS, ($+$)1.8 NE, and ($+$)1.6 MF (TABLE 8). AS amelioration was from weak (baseline) to medium level, superior limit (final). These improvements were associated with substantial restoration of the memory learning process, tested by MQ of WMS: ($+$)27.3 AS, ($+$)18.1 MF, and ($+$)17.2 NE (TABLE 8). AS amelioration was from inferior limit of mild memory deficit (baseline) to superior limit of medium memory (final).

Improvements in cognitive performance (general intelligence) estimated by WAIS (TABLE 8) were:

- for full IQ: ($+$)21.2 AS, ($+$)7.8 MF, ($+$)10.3 NE;
- for performance IQ: ($+$)23.2 AS, ($+$)9.3 MF, ($+$)9.4 NE; and
- for verbal IQ: ($+$)16.7 AS, ($+$)9.1 MF, ($+$)7.5 NE.

Superiority of AS amelioration was:

- in performance IQ: over 2.5 times vs. MF or NE; and
- in full IQ: over 2.7 times vs. MF and over 2.1 times vs. NE.

Moreover, decreases in the impairment of cognitive functions (deterioration index of WAIS) were noted: ($-$)8.7 AS, ($-$)5.2 NE, and ($-$)4.0 MF. All three cerebral activators reduced the cognitive impairments: from possible deterioration (19%–10% interval) in baseline to nonsignificant impairment, physiological deterioration (9%–0% level) in final. AS ameliorations were over 2.2 times higher as against MF and over 1.7 times higher as against NE.

TABLE 6 Comparative Psychogeriatric Assessments of Meclofenoxate, Nicergoline, and Antagonic-Stress Formula in Prolonged Treatment (3 Months) of SDAT: Heteroevaluation (Doctor) by Sandoz Clinical Assessment-Geriatric (SCAG) Scale and Its 5 Subscales[a]

	Meclofenoxate (MF)[c]		Nicergoline (NE)[f]		Antagonic-Stress Formula (AS)[e,f]	
	Baseline	Final	Baseline	Final	Baseline	Final
SCAG total score	68.3 ± 7.2	52.0 ± 7.6[b]	66.5 ± 11.5	50.5 ± 8.6[c]	71.2 ± 7.7	46.1 ± 6.5
SCAG subscales						
I. Cognitive dysfunctions	15.3 ± 1.9	11.3 ± 2.6[d]	14.9 ± 2.9	11.0 ± 2.1[c]	15.3 ± 2.5	10.3 ± 1.9
II. Interpersonal relationships	15.9 ± 2.3	12.2 ± 2.5[c]	16.1 ± 2.6	11.5 ± 2.4[d]	16.8 ± 3.2	10.3 ± 2.0
III. Affective disorders	12.7 ± 2.3	9.1 ± 1.6[c]	12.6 ± 2.7	9.4 ± 1.9[b]	14.0 ± 2.1	8.4 ± 1.5
IV. Apathy	13.0 ± 1.9	10.6 ± 2.0[b]	12.8 ± 2.7	10.6 ± 1.9[c]	13.1 ± 2.7	9.6 ± 1.7
V. Somatic dysfunctions	11.3 ± 2.3	8.7 ± 1.9[c]	10.1 ± 2.8	8.0 ± 1.9[c]	11.9 ± 1.8	7.5 ± 1.3

[a]Scores are expressed as mean ± SD. Final vs. baseline comparisons are significant for MF, NE as well as AS ($p < 0.001$, ANOVA). Final AS vs. final MF or vs. final NE, taking baseline scores as covariates (ANCOVA) are significant for AS (at [b]$p < 0.001$, [c]$p \leq 0.01$, and [d]$p < 0.05$ levels). Results from [e]Popa et al.[18] and from [f]Schneider et al.[25]

TABLE 7 Comparative Psychogeriatric Assessments of Meclofenoxate, Nicergoline, and Antagonic-Stress Formula in Prolonged Treatment (3 Months) of SDAT: Autoevaluation (Patient) by Self-Assessment Scale-Geriatric (SASG) and Its 5 Subscales[a]

	Meclofenoxate (MF)[d]		Nicergoline (NE)[c]		Antagonic-Stress Formula (AS)[d,e]	
	Baseline	Final	Baseline	Final	Baseline	Final
SASG total score	67.4 ± 10.6	53.3 ± 13.1[c]	65.8 ± 9.5	52.1 ± 9.4[b]	68.4 ± 8.9	47.3 ± 6.5
SASG subscales						
I. Cognitive dysfunctions	15.2 ± 3.0	11.6 ± 2.8[b]	15.6 ± 2.9	12.1 ± 2.5[c]	15.7 ± 2.5	11.1 ± 2.0
II. Interpersonal relationships	14.8 ± 2.0	12.0 ± 2.1[b]	14.7 ± 2.6	11.4 ± 2.3[b]	16.2 ± 3.3	10.6 ± 2.1
III. Affective disorders	13.1 ± 2.3	9.9 ± 2.0[b]	11.9 ± 2.4	9.1 ± 1.9[b]	12.1 ± 2.3	7.9 ± 1.6
IV. Apathy	12.8 ± 2.4	10.6 ± 2.2[b]	13.3 ± 2.5	11.1 ± 2.4[b]	13.5 ± 2.6	10.5 ± 1.7
V. Somatic dysfunctions	11.5 ± 2.5	9.2 ± 2.1[b]	10.3 ± 2.7	8.4 ± 1.9[b]	11.0 ± 2.4	7.2 ± 0.9

[a]Scores are expressed as mean ± SD. Final vs. baseline comparisons are significant (ANOVA) for MF ($p < 0.001$), NE ($p < 0.001$, and $p < 0.01$), as well as AS ($p < 0.001$). Final AS vs. final MF or vs. final NE, taking baseline scores as covariates (ANCOVA) is significant for AS (at [b]$p \leq 0.001$ and [c]$p < 0.01$ levels). Results from [d]Popa *et al.*[18] and from [e]Schneider *et al.*[25]

TABLE 8 Comparative Psychometric Evaluations of Meclofenoxate, Nicergoline, and Antagonic-Stress Formula in Prolonged Treatment (3 Months) of SDAT: Testing of the Cognitive Profile by Digit Symbol of WAIS, Wechsler Memory Scale (WMS) and Wechsler Adult Intelligence Scale (WAIS)[a]

	Meclofenoxate (MF)[e]		Nicergoline (NE)[f]		Antagonic-Stress Formula (AS)[e,f]	
	Baseline	Final	Baseline	Final	Baseline	Final
Digit symbol of WAIS (score)	8.2 ± 1.4	9.8 ± 1.6^b	7.8 ± 1.2	9.6 ± 1.6^b	7.5 ± 1.6	11.5 ± 2.4
W M S − MQ	82.0 ± 6.5	100.1 ± 11.3^d	83.2 ± 6.0	100.4 ± 7.9^b	81.3 ± 9.8	108.6 ± 11.4
WAIS						
• Verbal IQ	100.2 ± 10.6	109.3 ± 12.3^b	101.8 ± 6.4	109.3 ± 7.4^b	99.5 ± 11.3	116.2 ± 11.5
• Performance IQ	93.0 ± 10.0	102.3 ± 14.5^b	91.8 ± 12.0	101.2 ± 14.7^b	87.8 ± 7.9	111.0 ± 13.5
• Full IQ	97.1 ± 7.9	104.9 ± 12.6^b	95.8 ± 7.4	106.1 ± 10.9^b	93.0 ± 8.4	114.2 ± 11.9
• Deterioration index	13.8 ± 4.4	9.8 ± 4.1^c	14.3 ± 3.3	9.1 ± 2.8^c	15.4 ± 4.3	6.7 ± 3.9

[a]Scores are expressed as mean ± SD. Final vs. baseline comparisons are significant (ANOVA) for MF ($p < 0.001$ and $p < 0.01$), NE ($p < 0.001$ and $p < 0.01$), as well as AS ($p < 0.001$). Final AS vs. final MF or vs. final NE, taking baseline scores as covariates (ANCOVA), is significant for AS (at [b]$p \leq 0.001$, [c]$p < 0.01$, and [d]$p < 0.05$ levels). Results from [e]Popa et al.[18] and from [f]Schneider et al.[25]

DISCUSSION

The assessment instruments used in this study were selected according to WHO recommendations in evaluation of treatments in mental disorders,[37] corresponding to DSM-III syndromes[43] and to their gerontopsychopathological and psychopharmacological validity, reliability, and sensitivity.[41,44,46]

Therapeutical actions of MF, NE and AS formula in OMD have to be analyzed in terms of:

- the possibility for the therapeutical class (neurometabolic nootropics, drugs acting on neurotransmitter systems, cerebral vasodilators, and antiarteriosclerotics) to interfere with pathogenic mechanisms;[47]
- the usefulness of the current pharmacological treatment strategies (vasodilators, nootropics, neurotransmitter replacements, essential nutrients, and others) in age-related cognitive disorders, memory deficits, and cerebral insufficiency;[48]
- the necessity for prolonged treatments with cerebral activators as a component part of cerebral activation therapy.[49]

In this way, MF—a neurometabolic nootropic—besides the actions presented in the introduction, increases brain RNA and protein synthesis,[50,51] improves learning and memory processes,[52] prevents scopolamine-induced amnesia,[53] completely abolishes the memory-impairing effect of clonidine[54] and has a significant antianxiety action.[55] These antiaging and neurometabolic actions support the positive effects of MF in gerontopsychiatry:[16–18] the restoration of memory and cognitive functions, antidepressant, and anxiolytic effects.

Also, NE—a cerebral vasodilator—increases brain RNA and protein synthesis, enhances noradrenaline and dopamine turnover in the brain, and inhibits human platelet aggregation.[20] These neurometabolic and antiischemic actions support the positive effects of NE in OMD and SD:[20,23–25] the improvement of memory-cognitive performance, antidepressant, and anxiolytic effects.

AS—a multiple antiaging formula with cerebroprotective, neurometabolic and nootropic actions—is composed of[29] antioxidants, scavengers, and lipofuscinolytic agents (MF and methionine), a protein synthesis activator (orotic acid), an antihyperlipidemic and antiischemic factor (nicotinic acid with fast and prolonged release), energoactive substances (aspartate and fructose), multivitamins (B-1, B-3, and B-6), multiminerals (zinc, magnesium, potassium, lithium, phosphate, sulfate, and iodide). AS is an individual drug, a complex neurometabolic and synergetic composition. Its specific actions were previously demonstrated vs. single drugs. Preclinically, AS is more efficient than MF or nicotinic acid in acute stress (contention)[56] and than MF in aging (brain lipofuscinolysis).[57] Clinically, AS is superior to MF or NE (with nicotinic acid esterified) in SDAT (in reducing psychogeriatric scores and in increasing cognitive performances).[18,25]

Also, the superiority of the AS formula vs. MF and NE as to their effectiveness in antiaging and gerontopsychiatric treatments has to be evaluated by the superiority of multitherapy vs. monotherapy. In this way, antioxidant compositions are cerebroprotective in brain ischemia,[58] improve the cerebral blood flow, decrease the erythrocyte lipofuscin level and the psychogeriatric scores in SD,[59] and are active in aging, neurological, and mental disorders.[10] Because the brain is the principal consumer of oxygen in mammals and sensitive to oxidative stress, the complementary therapeutical approaches in decreasing free radical production[60] (by improving the cerebral blood flow or/and by increasing the levels of scavenger molecules within the brain) emphasize the neccesity for combinative therapy in OMD and SD.

Brain functions, cognitive performance, and normal behavior also depend on a well-balanced and rational diet. A therapeutical demonstration in this direction was made with an optimal multivitamin and multimineral formula by improving brain electrogenesis, IQ, and behavior.[61]

The strategy of multimodal therapy (drug combinations) as a better alternative to the current unitary drug practice was demonstrated as being more efficient in OMD and SD, using animal models and senile patients,[4] as well as in demented patients, by dynamic brain mapping investigation.[5]

In the light of these facts, the AS formula—a neurometabolic antiaging multi-therapy contained in a single complex nootropic-vasodilator drug—marks progress in gerontopsychiatric treatments.

SUMMARY

A complex antiaging formula—Antagonic-Stress—was investigated vs. placebo (PL), meclofenoxate (MF)—neurometabolic nootropic and vs. nicergoline (NE)—cerebral vasodilator by comparative multiple trials (double-blind, randomized, and parallel) in gerontopsychiatry (DSM-III-R, 1987 and ICD-10, 1992 criteria). AS vs. PL studies in organic mental disorders—amnestic, depressive, anxiety, associated with axis III physical disorders or conditions, and in multiinfarct dementia were followed by AS vs. MF or NE investigations in senile dementia of Alzheimer's type. A total of 343 old people, distributed in 4 PL groups, 1 MF group, 1 NE group, and 5 AS groups were studied.

Multiple investigations, before and after three-month treatments were made: psychometric evaluation by Sandoz Clinical Assessment-Geriatric, Self-Assessment Scale-Geriatric and their 5 subscales; psychopathological rating by Hamilton Depression and Anxiety Scales; as well as psychometric testing by digit symbol of WAIS, Wechsler Memory Scale and Wechsler Adult Intelligence Scale (WAIS).

Except PL, prolonged and large dose treatments with these cerebral activators (MF, NE and especially AS) reduced the psychogeriatric-psychopathological scores and the deterioration index, and improved cognitive performance.

The therapeutical effectiveness of AS multiple formula in gerontopsychiatry and its superiority vs. monotherapy (MF or NE) are discussed in connection with its complex neurometabolic and synergetic composition, multiple antioxidative combinations, free radical scavengers, lipofuscinolytic agents, the antiischemic action of antioxidants, multivitamin and multimineral supplementation, and with the better efficacy of multitherapy vs. monotherapy in geriatrics.

ACKNOWLEDGMENTS

The authors are grateful to Prof. Dr. I. Zs.-Nagy for the possibility to present these results at the 5th International Congress of Biomedical Gerontology in Budapest, Hungary on July 1–3, 1993, as well as to Prof. Dr. D. Harman for useful discussions.

Also, the authors thank Prof. Dr. Fr. Schneider and his collective from the University of Medicine and Pharmacy in Timişoara, Romania for the kind permission to use in this paper some of their results.

REFERENCES

1. MYERS, G. C. & S. MAGGI. 1993. Worldwide population aging: implications for health research. Aging Clin. Exp. Res. **5:** 77–79.
2. HÄFNER, H., G. MOSCHEL & N. SARTORIUS, Eds. 1986. Mental Health in the Elderly. A Review of the Present State of Research. Springer. Berlin, Germany.
3. FABRIS, N., D. HARMAN, D. L. KNOOK, E. STEINHAGEN-THIESSEN & I. ZS.-NAGY, Eds. 1992. Physiopathological Processes of Aging (Towards a Multicausal Interpretation). New York Academy of Sciences. New York, N.Y.
4. CHERKIN, A. & W. H. RIEGE. 1983. Multimodal approach to pharmacotherapy of senile amnesias. *In* Brain Aging: Neuropathology and Neuropharmacology. J. Cervós-Navarro & H. I. Sarkander, Eds.: 415–435. Raven Press. New York, N.Y.
5. FÜNFGELD, E. W. 1993. Monotherapy versus multitherapy—combined therapeutical approaches for treatment of senile dementia of Alzheimer's type (SDAT). 15th Cong. Int. Assoc. Gerontol. Budapest, Hungary. Abstr. Vol: 163.
6. HARMAN, D. 1993. Free radical involvement in aging. Pathophysiology and therapeutic implications. Drug Aging. **3:** 60–80.
7. CUTLER, R. G. 1991. Human longevity and aging: possible role of reactive oxygen species. *In* Physiological Senescence and Its Postponement: Theoretical Approaches and Rational Interventions. W. Pierpaoli & N. Fabris, Eds.: 1–28. New York Academy of Sciences. New York, N.Y.
8. BRIZZEE, K. R., T. SAMORAJSKI, D. L. BRIZZEE, J. M. ORDY, W. DUNLAP & R. SMITH. 1983. Age pigment and cell loss in the mammalian nervous system: functional implications. *In* Brain Aging: Neuropathology and Neuropharmacology. J. Cervós-Navarro & H. I. Sarkander, Eds.: 211–229. Raven Press. New York, N.Y.
9. JESBERGER, J. A. & J. S. RICHARDSON. 1991. Review of oxygen free radicals and brain dysfunction. Int. J. Neurosci. **57:** 1–17.
10. PACKER, L., L. PRILIPKO & Y. CHRISTEN, Eds. 1992. Free Radicals in the Brain. Aging, Neurological and Mental Disorders. Springer. Berlin, Germany.
11. SEMSEI, I. & I. ZS.-NAGY. 1985. Superoxide radical scavenging ability of centrophenoxine and its salt dependence in vitro. J. Free Radic. Biol. Med. **1:** 403–408.
12. ZS.-NAGY, I. 1989. Centrophenoxine as OH· free radical scavenger. *In* CRC Handbook of Free Radicals and Antioxidants in Biomedicine. J. Miquel, H. Weber & A. Quintanilha, Eds. **2:** 87–94. CRC Press. Boca Raton, Fla.
13. NANDY, K. & G. H. BOURNE. 1966. Effect of centrophenoxine on the lipofuscin pigments in the neurons of senile guinea pigs. Nature **210:** 313–314.
14. RIGA, S. & D. RIGA. 1974. Effects of centrophenoxine on the lipofuscin pigments in the nervous system of old rats. Brain Res. **72:** 265–275.
15. ZS.-NAGY, I. 1987. An attempt to answer the questions of theoretical gerontology on the basis of the membrane hypothesis of aging. *In* Advance in Age Pigments Research. E. Aloj-Totaro, P. Glees & F. A. Pisanti, Eds.: 393–413. Pergamon Press. Oxford, England.
16. GEDYE, J. L., A. N. EXTON-SMITH & J. WEDGWOOD. 1972. A method for measuring mental performance in the elderly and its use in a pilot clinical trial of meclofenoxate in organic dementia. Age Aging **1:** 74–80.
17. PÉK, G., T. FÜLÖP & I. ZS.-NAGY. 1989. Gerontopsychological studies using NAI ("Nürnberger Alters-Inventar") on patients with organic psychosyndrome (DSM-III, Category 1) treated with centrophenoxine in a double blind, comparative, randomized clinical trial. Arch. Gerontol. Geriatr. **9:** 17–30.
18. POPA, R., F. SCHNEIDER, G. MIHALAŞ, P. ŞTEFĂNIGĂ, I. G. MIHALAŞ, R. MĂTIEŞ & R. MATEESCU. 1993. Antagonic-Stress superiority versus Meclofenoxate in gerontopsychiatry (Alzheimer type dementia). 5th Cong. Int. Assoc. Biomed. Gerontol. Budapest, Hungary. Abstr.: P-6.
19. HOYER, S. 1982. Cerebral blood flow, electroencephalography and behavior. *In* Geriatrics 1. Cardiology and Vascular System. Central Nervous System. D. Platt, Ed.: 201–226. Springer. Berlin, Germany.
20. HEIDRICH, H., Ed. 1986. Proof of Therapeutical Effectiveness of Nootropic and Vasoac-

tive Drugs. Advances in Clinical and Experimental Nicergoline Research. Springer. Berlin, Germany.

21. BAN, T. A. 1980. Psychopharmacology for the Aged. S. Karger. Basel, Switzerland.
22. HOFFMEISTER, F., S. KAZDA & F. SEUTER. 1981. Cerebrovascular agents in gerontopsychopharmacotherapy. In Psychotropic Agents. Part II: Anxiolytics, Gerontopsychopharmacological Agents, and Psychomotor Stimulants. F. Hoffmeister & G. Stille, Eds.: 493–532. Springer. Berlin, Germany.
23. ARRIGO, A., A. MOGLIA, L. BORSOTTI, M. MASSARINI, E. ALFONSI, A. BATTAGLIA & G. SACCHETTI. 1982. A double-blind, placebo controlled, crossover trial with nicergoline in patients with senile dementia. Int. J. Clin. Pharmacol. Res. 2(Suppl. 1): 23–41.
24. BATTAGLIA, A., G. BRUNI, A. ARDIA & G. SACCHETTI. 1989. Nicergoline in mild to moderate dementia. A multicenter, double-blind, placebo-controlled study. J. Am. Geriatr. Soc. 37: 295–302.
25. SCHNEIDER, F., R. POPA, G. MIHALAŞ, P. ŞTEFĂNIGĂ, I. G. MIHALAŞ, R. MĂTIEŞ & R. MATEESCU. 1993. Antagonic-Stress superiority versus Sermion in gerontopsychiatry. 5th Cong. Int. Assoc. Biomed. Gerontol. Budapest, Hungary. Abstr.: L-16.
26. HARMAN, D. 1988. Free radical theory of aging: current status. In Lipofuscin—1987: State of the Art. I. Zs.-Nagy, Ed.: 3–21. Akadémiai Kiadó. Budapest, Hungary.
27. ZS.-NAGY, I. 1978. A membrane hypothesis of aging. J. Theor. Biol. 75: 189–195.
28. RIGA, S., G. PAMBUCCIAN & S. OERIU. 1972. Changes in lipofuscin pigments of rat central nervous system under -SH groups' releasing substances' influence. 9th Int. Cong. Gerontol. Kiev, U.S.S.R. Session, Abstr., 3: 383.
29. RIGA, D. & S. RIGA. 1992. Anti-stress, anti-impairment, anti-aging drug and its manufacturing method (Antagonic-Stress drug). Romanian patent no. 105891. State Office for Inventions and Trademarks. Bucharest, Romania.
30. ROMANIAN MINISTRY OF CHEMICAL INDUSTRY. 1989. Antagonic-Stress drug. Pharmaceutical Technical Industrial Standard no. 13125. Bucharest, Romania.
31. ROMANIAN MINISTRY OF HEALTH. 1990. Antagonic-Stress drug. Registration Certificate no. 1255; Manufacturing Authorization no. 592. Bucharest, Romania.
32. SCHNEIDER, F., R. POPA, G. MIHALAŞ, P. ŞTEFĂNIGĂ, I. G. MIHALAŞ, R. MĂTIEŞ & R. MATEESCU. 1992. Antagonic-Stress in mild to moderate dementia—a double-blind, placebo-controlled study. 3rd Int. Cong. Clin. Psychopathol. Timişoara, Romania. Abstr. Vol.: 15.
33. AMERICAN PSYCHIATRIC ASSOCIATION. 1987. Diagnostic and Statistical Manual of Mental Disorders. 3rd edition, revised. American Psychiatric Association. Washington, D.C.
34. WORLD HEALTH ORGANIZATION. 1992. The ICD-10 Classification of Mental and Behavioural Disorders: Clinical Descriptions and Diagnostic Guidelines. World Health Organization. Geneva, Switzerland.
35. SPILKER, B. 1984. Guide to Clinical Studies and Developing Protocols. Raven Press. New York, N.Y.
36. SPILKER, B. 1986. Guide to Clinical Interpretation of Data. Raven Press. New York, N.Y.
37. WORLD HEALTH ORGANIZATION. 1991. Evaluation of Methods for the Treatment of Mental Disorders. WHO Technical Report no. 812. World Health Organization. Geneva, Switzerland.
38. GOTTFRIES, C. G. 1990. Classification of dementias. In Progress in Dementia Research. J. M. Orgogozo & C. G. Gottfries, Eds.: 15–24. Parthenon. Park Ridge, N.J.
39. SHADER, R. I., J. S. HARMATZ & C. SALZMAN. 1974. A new scale for clinical assessment in geriatric populations: Sandoz Clinical Assessment-Geriatric (SCAG). J. Am. Geriatr. Soc. 22: 107–113.
40. VENN, R. D. 1983. The Sandoz Clinical Assessment-Geriatric (SCAG) scale. A general-purpose psychogeriatric rating scale (SCAG manual). Gerontology 29: 185–198.
41. YESAVAGE, J. A., M. ADEY & P. D. WERNER. 1981. Development of a geriatric behavioral self-assessment scale. J. Am. Geriatr. Soc. 29: 285–288.
42. HAMOT, H. B., J. R. PATIN & J. M. SINGER. 1984. Factor structure of the Sandoz Clinical Assessment Geriatric (SCAG) scale. Psychopharmacol. Bull. 20: 142–150.
43. BECH, P., M. KASTRUP & O. J. RAFAELSEN. 1986. Mini-compendium of rating scales for

states of anxiety, depression, mania, schizophrenia with corresponding DSM-III syndromes. Acta Psychiatr. Scand. **73**(Suppl. 326): 7–37.

44. HOWARD, J. C. 1989. Clinical interpretation of intelligence assessment. *In* Contemporany Approaches to Psychological Assessment. S. Wetzler & M. M. Katz, Eds.: 157–176. Brunner/Mazel. New York, N.Y.

45. WECHSLER, D. & C. P. SONTE. 1954. The Wechsler Memory Scale. Psychological Corporation. New York, N.Y.

46. OVERALL, J. E. & H. M. RHOADES. 1988. Clinician-rated scales for multidimensional assessment of psychopathology in elderly. Psychopharmacol. Bull. **24**: 587–594.

47. ALLAIN, H., P. MORAN, D. BENTUE-FERRER, J.-P. MARTINET & A. LIEURY. 1989. Pharmacology of the memory process. Arch. Gerontol. Geriatr. Suppl. **1**: 109–120.

48. GOTTFRIES, C. G. 1992. Reappraisal of current therapy in the treatment of age-related cognitive disorders. *In* Treatment of Age-Related Cognitive Dysfunction: Pharmacological and Clinical Evaluation. G. Racagni & J. Mendlewicz, Eds.: 121–129. S. Karger. Basel, Switzerland.

49. MEIER-RUGE, W., Ed. 1993. Teaching and Training in Geriatric Medicine, Vol. 3 (Dementing Brain Disease in Old Age). S. Karger. Basel, Switzerland.

50. ZS.-NAGY, I. & I. SEMSEI. 1984. Centrophenoxine increases the rates of total and mRNA synthesis in the brain cortex of old rats: an explanation of its action in terms of the membrane hypothesis of aging. Exp. Gerontol. **19**: 171–178.

51. ZS.-NAGY, I., K. NAGY, V. ZS.-NAGY, Á. KALMÁR & É. NAGY. 1981. Alterations in total content and solubility characteristics of proteins in rat brain and liver during aging and centrophenoxine treatment. Exp. Gerontol. **16**: 229–240.

52. NANDY, K. 1978. Centrophenoxine: effects on aging mammalian brain. J. Am. Geriatr. Soc. **26**: 74–81.

53. MOSHARROF, A. H., V. D. PETKOV & V. V. PETKOV. 1987. Effects of meclofenoxate and citicholine on learning and memory in aged rats. Acta Physiol. Pharmacol. Bulg. **13**: 17–24.

54. LAZAROVA-BAKAROVA, M. B. & M. G. GENKOVA-PAPASOVA. 1989. Influence of nootropic drugs on the memory-impairing effect of clonidine in albino rats. Methods Findings Exp. Clin. Pharmacol. **11**: 235–239.

55. PETKOV, V. D., D. GETOVA & A. H. MOSHARROF. 1987. A study of nootropic drugs for anti-anxiety action. Acta Physiol. Pharmacol. Bulg. **13**: 25–30.

56. SCHNEIDER, F., C. MEDERLE, R. MĂTIEŞ, G. SĂVOIU, S. GOŢIA, G. MIHALAŞ & A. BUFTEA. 1992. Drug influence of morphological and functional response in contention stress by rats. Fiziologia (Physiology) **2**: 27–29.

57. RIGA, S. & D. RIGA. 1993. Antagonic-Stress: an advanced drug for aging deceleration. I. Brain lipofuscinolytic activity demonstrated by light and fluorescence microscopy. 5th Cong. Int. Assoc. Biomed. Gerontol. Budapest, Hungary. Abstr.: L-58.

58. SUZUKI, J., S. FUJIMOTO, K. MIZOI & M. OBA. 1984. The protective effect of combined administration of anti-oxidants and perfluorochemicals on cerebral ischemia. Stroke **15**: 672–679.

59. CLAUSEN, J., S. ACHIM NIELSEN & M. KRISTENSEN. 1989. Biochemical and clinical effects of an antioxidative supplementation of geriatric patients. A double blind study. Biol. Trace Element Res. **20**: 135–151.

60. FUXE, K., L. F. AGNATI, P. HELDLUND, S. E. ÖGREN, F. BORTOLOTTI, C. CARANI & G. BIAGINI. 1992. Failure of integrative mechanisms in the aging brain. *In* Treatment of Age-Related Cognitive Dysfunction: Pharmacological and Clinical Evaluation. G. Racagni & J. Mendlewicz, Eds.: 1–18. S. Karger. Basel, Switzerland.

61. EYSENCK, H. J. & S. B. G. EYSENCK, Eds. 1991. Improvement of I.Q. and behaviour as a function of dietary supplementation. A symposium. Person. Individ. Diff. **12**: 329–365.

Superiority of Antagonic-Stress Composition versus Nicergoline in Gerontopsychiatry

FRANCISC SCHNEIDER,[a] RODICA POPA,[c]
GEORGETA MIHALAS,[a] PETRE STEFANIGĂ,[a]
ION GHEORGHE MIHALAS,[b] ROSANA MĂTIES,[a]
AND RODICA MATEESCU[a]

[a]Department of Physiology
[b]Department of Biophysics and Biostatistics
University of Medicine and Pharmacy
Eftimie Murgu Square no. 2
Post Office Box 135
RO-1900 Timişoara, Romania

[c]Department of Neurology
Clinical Hospital no. 1 of Timiş District
Ştefan Plăvăţ Street no. 156
RO-1900 Timişoara, Romania

INTRODUCTION

The advancing longevity of the world's population causes a growth in the number of aging people and an increase in morbidity by neurological and mental diseases.[1]

One recognizes the importance of cerebral circulation for ensuring normal conditions of brain metabolism and for neuropsychic functions.[2] Although the brain represents only 2.5% of the weight of the human body, it uses approx. 17% of the cardiac flow capacity. The reduction of the cerebral blood flow as well as of the glucose and oxygen brain metabolism in normal aging (ischemic theory of aging) and the chronic cerebrovascular insufficiency in pathological aging and senile dementia[2–4] are associated with neuronal dysfunctions: cognitive decline and loss, emotional-affective disorders, exhaustion, apathy.

Therefore, cerebral vasodilators (including nicotinic acid) were studied for their favorable actions in gerontopsychopharmacotherapy.[5–7] For the same reason, cerebral activator drugs (cerebral vasodilators, compounds that increase brain glucose turnover, as well as nootropics) are recommended in the treatment of cognitive function impairment, presenile and senile dementia, as one of the four directions of cerebral activation therapy.[8]

One finds nicotinic acid as 5-bromo-nicotinic acid esterified with ergoline in the molecule of the drug Nicergoline (Sermion-Farmitalia, Italy and Biofarm, Romania). Nicergoline (NE) is a cerebrovascular vasodilator and neurometabolic activator,[9] which in the hepatic metabolism is hydrolyzed at the ester linkage with release of nicotinic acid derivative. One also finds nicotinic acid (with fast and prolonged release) in the composition of the drug Antagonic-Stress (AS) (cerebroprotective, antiaging, and antioxidative stress combined formula), a neurometabolic nootropic and cerebral vasodilator.[10]

In comparative studies vs. placebo, both NE[11] and AS[12] have been demonstrated as active in mild to moderate senile dementia.

On the other hand, one is aware of the implication of free radicals in aging processes, mental and neurological disorders[13] and of the fact that the anti–free radical medications—scavengers[14] and antioxidants[15]—are active in aging and in gerontopsychiatry (senile dementia).[15-17] Therefore, we assumed that AS combined formula—with scavengers and antioxidants in its composition, associated with nicotinic acid and with the other neurometabolic activators—achieves a multiple, more intense, and complex intervention in aging processes and in the cognitive loss of the elderly.

As a consequence, the present study proposes a comparative and multiple gerontopsychiatric evaluation of NE and AS, which have previously been demonstrated as active in senile dementia.

SUBJECTS AND METHODS

Type of Study

In conformity with the requirements of clinical studies on drug effectiveness and with the clinical interpretation of these data,[18,19] a double-blind, randomized, comparative and parallel clinical trial was performed. Informed consent was obtained from all participants before the beginning of the investigation.

Characterization of the Patients

TABLE 1 summarizes the general and clinical features of the two groups of treated patients who finished the experiment. Medical and nonmedical dropouts were 8.8% (5.9% and respectively 2.9%).

Senile dementia of Alzheimer's type (SDAT), represented by Category F 00.1— uncomplicated, predominantly depressive, with communication, behavioral, or mo-

TABLE 1. Clinical Characteristics of Patients with SDAT Treated with Nicergoline ($n = 30$) and Antagonic-Stress Composition ($n = 32$)[a]

	Nicergoline	Antagonic-Stress Composition[a]
Age, years (mean ± SD)	68.7 ± 4.8	70.8 ± 5.9
(range)	65–81	65–87
Sex (F/M)	14/16	15/17
Duration of disease		
Years (mean ± SD)	4.2 ± 1.0	4.7 ± 1.1
Range	2–8	2–10
Severity of dementia:		
SCAG item 19 (no. and %)		
Moderately severe	1 (3%)	2 (6.3%)
Moderate	3 (10%)	4 (12.5%)
Mild to moderate	18 (60%)	22 (68.7%)
Mild	8 (27%)	4 (12.5%)

[a]The differences between groups are not significant ($p > 0.05$; ANOVA).

tor skill disturbances and with mixed symptoms—was diagnosed in accordance with ICD-10, 1990[20] and DSM-IV Options Book, 1991[21] guidelines.

Criteria for inclusion were patients of both sexes; age of 65 or over; only university education level; clinical history of cognitive loss for at least 2 years; subjects who for one month before our clinical trial had not had any other treatment (cerebral vasodilators, antihyperlipidemic agents, psychotropics, nootropics, cholinergic agents, anabolic or lipotropic drugs, hepatoprotectants, multivitamins and multiminerals) that could have interfered with the therapeutical effects of the drugs tested.

Criteria for severity were item 19 (overall impression of the patient) of the Sandoz Clinical Assessment-Geriatric (SCAG) scale[22] from intensity 3 (mild) to 6 (moderately severe), but frequently 4 (mild to moderate); the simultaneous presence of the first eight dementia key symptoms of the SCAG scale, with a score of at least 3 (mild) or higher; and a deterioration index over 10 on the Wechsler Adult Intelligence Scale (WAIS).[23]

Criteria for exclusion were inadequate conditions for interview and assessment (severe disturbances of eyesight, hearing, and speech); coexistence of severe somatic diseases; neurological pathology (head injuries, inflammatory diseases of the brain and the meninges, tumors of the brain and of the spinal cord, cerebrovascular and degenerative diseases). Other types of dementia due to nonpsychiatric medical conditions, of the other cognitive impairment disorders, and of other psychiatric diseases of elderly people had already been excluded by diagnostic criteria and by differential diagnosis.

Cerebral Vasodilator–Nootropic Treatments

Prolonged treatments with AS or with NE administered orally and with daily frequency were applied for 3 months.

AS is a neurometabolic and cerebrovascular vasodilator composition, with cerebroprotective, nootropic, antiaging, and antistress actions.[10] The complementarity of its composition and of its pharmaceutical form (gastro- and enterosoluble capsules) ensures controlled release and absorption of the active substances. The retardation of nicotinic acid in enterosoluble capsules ensures its prolonged delivery and vasodilatory action. The composition of a gastrosoluble (blue) capsule is 260 mg meclofenoxate, 150 mg methionine, 90 mg aspartic acid · Mg salt, 10 mg fructose, 8 mg vitamin B-1, 11 mg vitamin B-6, 10 mg nicotinic acid with fast release, and 10.5 mg zinc sulfate. The composition of an enterosoluble (yellow) capsule is 315 mg orotic acid, 10 mg fructose, 80 mg nicotinic acid with prolonged release, 98 mg di-potassium hydrogen phosphate, 20 mg magnesium oxide, 2.5 mg lithium carbonate, and 0.12 mg potassium iodide. The AS active therapeutical dose was of two gastrosoluble capsules and one enterosoluble capsule, three times a day (morning, noon, and afternoon), before meals and with liquid in abundance.

NE (10 mg/capsule) was processed in blue gastrosoluble capsules, while yellow capsules were filled with lactose and then enterically coated by the same procedure as AS. In this way, two blue gastrosoluble capsules with NE and one yellow enterosoluble capsule with lactose, three times daily, represent the NE active dose (60 mg/daily) in dementia[11] and the same conditions as AS pharmaceutical form and administration.

In accordance with the study design, a double-blind, randomized procedure was utilized in the administration of the drugs.

Psychogeriatric Scales and Psychometric Tests

Multidimensional rating instruments: SCAG scale[22] and SASG (Self-Assessment Scale-Geriatric)[24] were used for psychogeriatric assessment. The clinician rated the psychopathological intensity by using the SCAG manual[25] and factor structures of SCAG.[26] The patient self-evaluated the frequency of his psychopathological symptoms by using SASG. Similar subscales (factor structures) of SASG related to SCAG were calculated subsequently.

Digit symbol (coding) of WAIS,[23] Wechsler Memory Scale (WMS),[27] and WAIS[23] were applied for the psychometric testing of attention-concentration, memory, intelligence, and brain impairment.

All patients were tested before and after 3 months of treatment.

Statistics

The results were analyzed using an SPSS/PC + package.

Pre- and posttreatment differences were compared by the analysis of variance (ANOVA).

Final scores AS vs. NE, taking baseline scores as covariates, were compared by the analysis of covariance (ANCOVA).

RESULTS

Assessments in psychogeriatric scales (TABLES 2 and 3) and psychometric tests (TABLE 4) have shown a positive evolution of cognitive, affective, and behavioral functions after 3 months of treatments: for NE from $p < 0.01$ to $p < 0.001$ and for AS $p < 0.001$ significance levels (final vs. baseline intratreatment comparisons).

TABLE 2. Comparative Psychogeriatric Assessment of Nicergoline and Antagonic-Stress Composition: Doctor Evaluation by Sandoz Clinical Assessment-Geriatric (SCAG) Scale and Its Factors[a]

| | Treatment for 3 Months | | | | Significance Level (p) AS vs. NE |
| | Nicergoline (NE) | | Antagonic-Stress (AS) Composition | | |
	Before	After	Before	After	
SCAG total score	66.5 ± 11.5	50.5 ± 8.6[b]	71.2 ± 7.7	46.1 ± 6.5[c]	0.002
SCAG factors					
I. Cognitive dysfunctions	14.9 ± 2.9	11.0 ± 2.1[b]	15.3 ± 2.5	10.3 ± 1.9[c]	0.006
II. Interpersonal relationships	16.1 ± 2.6	11.5 ± 2.4[b]	16.8 ± 3.2	10.3 ± 2.0[c]	0.018
III. Affective disorders	12.6 ± 2.7	9.4 ± 1.9[b]	14.0 ± 2.1	8.4 ± 1.5[c]	0.000
IV. Apathy	12.8 ± 2.7	10.6 ± 1.9[b]	13.1 ± 2.7	9.6 ± 1.7[c]	0.005
V. Somatic dysfunctions	10.1 ± 2.8	8.0 ± 1.9[b]	11.9 ± 1.8	7.5 ± 1.3[c]	0.010

[a]Results are expressed as mean values ± standard deviation (SD). After vs. before treatment comparisons are significant (ANOVA, $p < 0.001$) both for NE ([b]) and for AS ([c]). Final AS vs. final NE intertreatment comparisons (taking the initial scores as covariates, ANCOVA) are shown in the last column.

TABLE 3. Comparative Psychogeriatric Assessment of Nicergoline and Antagonic-Stress Composition: Patient Evaluation by Self-Assessment Scale-Geriatric (SASG) and Its Factors[a]

| | Treatment for 3 Months | | | | Significance Level (p) |
| | Nicergoline (NE) | | Antagonic-Stress (AS) Composition | | |
	Before	After	Before	After	AS vs. NE
SASG total score	65.8 ± 9.5	52.1 ± 9.4[b]	68.4 ± 8.9	47.3 ± 6.5[d]	0.000
SASG factors					
I. Cognitive dysfunctions	15.6 ± 2.9	12.1 ± 2.5[b]	15.7 ± 2.5	11.1 ± 2.0[d]	0.002
II. Interpersonal relationships	14.7 ± 2.6	11.4 ± 2.3[b]	16.2 ± 3.3	10.6 ± 2.1[d]	0.001
III. Affective disorders	11.9 ± 2.4	9.1 ± 1.9[b]	12.1 ± 2.3	7.9 ± 1.6[d]	0.000
IV. Apathy	13.3 ± 2.5	11.1 ± 2.4[b]	13.5 ± 2.6	10.5 ± 1.7[d]	0.000
V. Somatic dysfunctions	10.3 ± 2.7	8.4 ± 1.9[c]	11.0 ± 2.4	7.2 ± 0.9[d]	0.000

[a]Results are expressed as mean values ± SD. After vs. before treatment comparisons are significant (ANOVA) both for NE ([c]$p < 0.01$; [b]$p < 0.001$) and for AS ([d]$p < 0.001$). Final AS vs. final NE intertreatment comparisons (taking the initial scores as covariates, ANCOVA) are shown in the last column.

Therapeutical improvements are the results of the diminution in psychogeriatric symptomatology and in the deterioration index, being at the same time accompanied by the increase (recovery) of cognitive performance. Thus, the prolonged treatments with NE and AS, which decelerate the evolution of the disease in the early stages,

TABLE 4. Comparative Psychometric Evaluations of Nicergoline and Antagonic-Stress Composition Using Digit Symbol of WAIS, Wechsler Memory Scale (WMS) for MQ-Memory Quotient, and Wechsler Adult Intelligence Scale (WAIS) for Intelligence-Intelligence Quotient (IQ) and for Impairment-Deterioration Index[a]

| | Treatment for 3 Months | | | | Significance Level (p) |
| | Nicergoline (NE) | | Antagonic-Stress (AS) Composition | | |
	Before	After	Before	After	AS vs. NE
Digit symbol of WAIS (score)	7.8 ± 1.2	9.6 ± 1.6[b]	7.5 ± 1.6	11.5 ± 2.4[d]	0.000
WMS-MQ	83.2 ± 6.0	100.4 ± 7.9[b]	81.3 ± 9.8	108.6 ± 11.4[d]	0.001
WAIS					
• Verbal IQ	101.8 ± 6.4	109.3 ± 7.4[b]	99.5 ± 11.3	116.2 ± 11.5[d]	0.000
• Performance IQ	91.8 ± 12.0	101.2 ± 14.7[c]	87.8 ± 7.9	111.0 ± 13.5[d]	0.000
• Full IQ	95.8 ± 7.4	106.1 ± 10.9[b]	93.0 ± 8.4	114.2 ± 11.9[d]	0.000
• Deterioration Index	14.3 ± 3.3	9.1 ± 2.8[b]	15.4 ± 4.3	6.7 ± 3.9[d]	0.003

[a]Results are expressed as mean values ± SD. After vs. before treatment comparisons are significant (ANOVA) both for NE ([c]$p < 0.01$; [b]$p < 0.001$) and for AS ([d]$p < 0.001$). Final AS vs. final NE intertreatment comparisons (taking the initial scores as covariates, ANCOVA) are shown in the last column.

become useful in SDAT. Moreover, the intertreatment comparisons (final AS vs. final NE) point out the superiority of using the AS composition in gerontopsychiatry: $p < 0.05$ to $p < 0.001$ significance level.

The reduction of the total score of geriatric psychopathology intensity hetero-assessed by SCAG (1 severity interval = 18.0) went from the superior limit of mild to moderate (72.0–54.0 level) to mild (54.0–36.0 interval): ($-$)25.1 AS vs. ($-$)16.0 NE.

The comparative decreases in the scores of SCAG subscales were:

- in cognitive dysfunctions (1 interval = 4.0): ($-$)5.0 AS vs. ($-$)3.9 NE;
- in interpersonal relationships (1 interval = 4.0): ($-$)6.5 AS vs. ($-$)4.6 NE;
- in affective disorders (1 interval = 3.0): ($-$)5.6 AS vs. ($-$)3.2 NE;
- in apathy (1 interval = 4.0): ($-$)3.5 AS vs. ($-$)2.2 NE;
- in somatic dysfunctions (1 interval = 3.0): ($-$)4.4 AS vs. ($-$)2.1 NE.

The reduction in the total score of geriatric psychopathology frequency self-evaluated by SASG (the same quantification of the scores and levels in scale and subscales as SCAG) went from the superior limit of mild to moderate to mild: ($-$)21.1 AS vs. ($-$)13.7 NE.

The comparative decreases in the factor structures of SASG were:

- in the cognitive subscale: ($-$)4.6 AS vs. ($-$)3.5 NE;
- in the interpersonal subscale: ($-$)5.6 AS vs. ($-$)3.3 NE;
- in the affective subscale: ($-$)4.2 AS vs. ($-$)2.8 NE;
- in the apathy subscale: ($-$)3.0 AS vs. ($-$)2.2 NE;
- in the somatic subscale: ($-$)3.8 AS vs. ($-$)1.9 NE.

The recovery of attention-concentration—increase in WAIS digit symbol scores—was ($+$)4.0 for AS (from weak baseline to medium final level) and ($+$)1.8 for NE (also from weak baseline to medium final level), marking a > 2.5 times improvement for AS vs. NE.

The restoration of memory-learning—increase in MQ of WMS—was ($+$)27.3 for AS, from the inferior limit of mild deficit (81–90) to the superior level of medium memory (91–110) and ($+$)17.2 for NE, also from the inferior limit of mild deficit, but to the middle level of medium memory, showing a > 1.6 times increase for AS vs. NE.

Improvement of cognitive performance (general intelligence)—increase in IQ of WAIS—was ($+$)16.7 at verbal IQ, ($+$)23.2 at performance IQ, and ($+$)21.2 at full IQ for AS vs. ($+$)7.5, ($+$)9.4, and ($+$)10.3 for NE. The efficiency of AS vs. NE was > 2.5 times in performance IQ and > 2.1 times in full IQ.

The restoration of cognitive performance (noted also in cognitive subscales of SCAG and SASG) was demonstrated by the reduction in the WAIS deterioration index, with ($-$)8.7 for AS vs. ($-$)5.2 for NE. Both drugs reduced mental impairment from the 19%–10% interval (possible deterioration) to the 9%–0% level (nonsignificant impairment, physiological deterioration), but AS proved > 1.7 times more efficacious than NE.

DISCUSSION

The baseline psychopathological homogeneity of the two groups was ensured by the diagnostic guidelines, the clinical variables of patients, the criteria of inclusion, severity, and exclusion, as well as by statistical analysis (taking the initial scores as covariates). But illustrative of AS vs. NE is the little higher baseline severity of psychogeriatric symptoms and of the cognitive deficit as well as the higher final improvement of all determinations (in scales, subscales, tests, quotients, and indices).

The multidimensional instruments used in this study are known to possess psychopathologic and psychopharmacologic validity, reliability, and sensitivity both in gerontopsychiatry (organic mental disorders and cognitive impairment disorders) and in assessing the effects of nootropic-geriatric psychopharmaca.[28,29] Therefore, numerous gerontopsychopharmacological agents (ergolid-mesylates,[30] nicergoline,[9] meclofenoxate,[31] and piracetam[32]) were previously assessed with these instruments.

The possible deceleration of SDAT evolution, associated with the improvement in cognitive, affective, behavioral, and somatic functions after prolonged and large dose treatments with NE and AS, is in agreement with recent similar studies[11,12] and could be explained by the multiple actions of these drugs at the neurometabolic and systemic levels.[9,10]

Moreover, the superiority of AS vs. NE in the treatment of brain aging and cognitive loss of the elderly is determined by (1) its multiple composition; (2) the synergism of its components; (3) the antiischemic action of its antioxidants; and (4) its anti–free radical complementary action.

The dependence of normal cerebral electrogenesis, cognitive functions, and behavior on the good and adequate nutrition of the brain was demonstrated by therapeutical proofs with optimal multivitamin and multimineral compositions.[33] These improved brain electrical activity mapping, cognitive performance, intelligence, and behavior.[33] By associating a biologic cerebral vasodilator—nicotinic acid (both fast and prolonged release)—with neurometabolic nootropic agents—meclofenoxate (MF) and orotic acid, sustained in their actions by amino acids, vitamins, and minerals—the AS formula achieves for the brain a multiple metabolic-energetic support as well as a larger area of anabolic and functional activation. Therefore, the advance of AS vs. NE is in harmony with the superiority of multi-therapy vs. monotherapy in SDAT,[34] demonstrated by the dynamic brain mapping investigation. In this case, because age-related brain dysfunctions and disorders do not depend on one mechanism alone, the AS composition represents a well-balanced antiaging multitherapy comprised in a single drug.

The synergism of AS composition was demonstrated both preclinically (aged animals) and clinically (old people) with prolonged and high dose treatments. Two months of treatment with AS[35]—multiple antiaging formula containing also 80 mg/kg wt MF—show a higher brain lipofuscinolytic activity vs. single MF treatment[36] in the same dose and length. Also, 3 months of treatment in SDAT points out the superiority of AS (which, besides the other substances, has in its composition also MF in 1520 mg total daily dose) vs. single MF (same total daily dose) in reducing psychogeriatric symptoms and in improving cognitive functions.[31]

During the aging processes and Alzheimer's dementia, one notices the augmentation of free radical attacks,[13] an increase of lipid peroxidation,[37] and an accumulation of lipofuscin pigments.[38] Also, accelerated aging, lipofuscin increase, and Alzheimer's disease were found in relation with deficiencies in dietary antioxidants.[39] MF and antioxidative compositions oppose these pathogenic processes. MF is acknowledged as a free radical scavenger[14,40,41] active in decelerating the aging rate,[42] as an inhibitor of brain lipofuscinogenesis and cerebral lipofuscinolytic agent,[36,43] as well as active in senile dementia.[16,31] Antioxidative therapy (selenomethionine, zinc, vitamins B-6, C, A, E, and gamma-linolenic acid) significantly reduces the erythrocyte lipofuscin, improves regional blood flow in all brain areas, and decreases the psychogeriatric scores in demential syndromes.[15] In this therapeutical direction, AS[10] is a scavenger as well as an antioxidative and lipofuscinolytic composition—through its conjugated actions of MF,[36] methionine,[44] zinc, and vitamin B-6. It also proves to be an active nootropic drug in SDAT.[12,31]

One knows the complementary therapeutical approach in decreasing free radical formation[45] by increasing the levels of scavenger molecules within the brain or by improving cerebral blood flow, glucose metabolism, and mitochondrial function. NE improves only the last mechanism[9,46,47] in comparison with AS which acts complementarily, by the amelioration of both mechanisms. In this way, MF (which is incorporated into the cell membrane of neurons[42]), methionine, and zinc increase the levels of scavengers within the brain. Also, AS improves the cerebral blood flow (by nicotinic acid and MF[48]), activates the glucose metabolism (by MF,[49] magnesium, and zinc), and finally protects mitochondrial function (by MF[50]).

In conclusion, our study reconfirms the usefulness of different classes of cerebral activators (brain vasodilator—NE,[9] neurometabolic nootropic—MF,[16] or combined formula—AS[12,31]) as a medical-drug direction as part of cerebral activation therapy,[8] currently recommended in the treatment of presenile and senile Alzheimer's dementia.

SUMMARY

Nicergoline (NE)—a cerebral vasodilator with nicotinic acid esterified in its molecule—and Antagonic-Stress (AS) composition—a neurometabolic nootropic, also containing nicotinic acid but with fast and prolonged release—were evaluated in senile dementia of Alzheimer's type (SDAT), mild to moderate intensity (DSM-IV Options Book, 1991 and ICD-10, 1990 criteria).

A double-blind, randomized, comparative, and parallel clinical trial was performed on 62 old people divided into 2 groups and exclusively treated with NE or AS. Psychogeriatric evaluations (Sandoz Clinical Assessment-Geriatric scale, Self-Assessment Scale-Geriatric and their subscales) and psychometric tests (digit symbol of WAIS, Wechsler Memory Scale, and Wechsler Adult Intelligence Scale—WAIS) were made before and after 3 months of treatment.

Prolonged and large dose treatments with NE and AS significantly decreased the psychogeriatric scores, diminished the deterioration index, and improved cognitive performances (ANOVA). Therapeutical effects of AS were significantly higher than those of NE (ANCOVA).

The better actions of AS in senile dementia and for improving cognitive function and behavior are discussed in connection with its multiple neurometabolic composition, the synergism of components, the antiischemic action of its antioxidants, its anti–free radical complementary action (deceleration of the aging rate, brain and erythrocyte lipofuscinolysis, complex antioxidative and scavenger formula), the multivitamin and multimineral supplementation and, finally, with the superiority of multitherapy vs. monotherapy.

REFERENCES

1. HÄFNER, H., G. MOSCHEL & N. SARTORIUS, Eds. 1986. Mental Health in the Elderly. A Review of the Present State of Research. Springer. Berlin, Germany.
2. LASSEN, N. A. & D. H. INGVAR. 1980. Blood flow studies in the aging normal brain and in senile dementia. *In* Aging of the Brain and Dementia. L. Amaducci, A. N. Davison & P. Antuono, Eds.: 91–98. Raven Press. New York, N.Y.
3. LENZI, G. L. & T. JONES. 1980. Cerebral metabolism–to–blood flow relationships with

respect to aging and dementia. *In* Aging of the Brain and Dementia. L. Amaducci, A. N. Davison & P. Antuono, Eds.: 99–102. Raven Press. New York, N.Y.

4. SOKOLOFF, L. 1975. Cerebral circulation and metabolism in the aged. *In* Genesis and Treatment of Psychologic Disorders in the Elderly. S. Gershon & A. Raskin, Eds.: 45–54. Raven Press. New York, N.Y.

5. BAN, T. A. 1978. Vasodilators, stimulants, and anabolic agents in the treatment of geropsychiatric patients. *In* Psychopharmacology: a Generation of Progress. M. A. Lipton, A. DiMascio & K. F. Killam, Eds.: 1525–1533. Raven Press. New York, N.Y.

6. BAN, T. A. 1980. Psychopharmacology for the Aged. S. Karger. Basel, Switzerland.

7. HOFFMEISTER, F., S. KAZDA & F. SEUTER. 1981. Cerebrovascular agents in gerontopsychopharmacotherapy. *In* Psychotropic Agents. Part II: Anxiolytics, Gerontopsychopharmacological Agents, and Psychomotor Stimulants. F. Hoffmeister & G. Stille, Eds.: 493–532. Springer. Berlin, Germany.

8. MEIER-RUGE, W., Ed. 1993. Teaching and Training in Geriatric Medicine, Vol. 3 (Dementing Brain Disease in Old Age). S. Karger. Basel, Switzerland.

9. HEIDRICH, H., Ed. 1986. Proof of Therapeutical Effectiveness of Nootropic and Vasoactive Drugs. Advances in Clinical and Experimental Nicergoline Research. Springer. Berlin, Germany.

10. RIGA, D. & S. RIGA. 1992. Anti-stress, anti-impairment, anti-aging drug and its manufacturing method (Antagonic-Stress drug). Romanian patent no. 105891. State Office for Inventions and Trademarks. Bucharest, Romania.

11. BATTAGLIA, A., G. BRUNI, A. ARDIA & G. SACCHETTI. 1989. Nicergoline in mild to moderate dementia. A multicenter, double-blind, placebo-controlled study. J. Am. Geriatr. Soc. **37:** 295–302.

12. SCHNEIDER, F., R. POPA, G. MIHALAŞ, P. STEFĂNIGĂ, I. G. MIHALAŞ, R. MĂTIEŞ & R. MATEESCU. 1992. Antagonic-Stress in mild to moderate dementia—a double-blind, placebo-controlled study. 3rd Int. Cong. Clin. Psychopathol. Timişoara, Romania. Abstr. Vol.: 15.

13. HARMAN, D. 1993. Free radical involvement in aging. Pathophysiology and therapeutic implications. Drug Aging. **3:** 60–80.

14. ZS.-NAGY, I. 1989. Centrophenoxine as OH· free radical scavenger. *In* CRC Handbook of Free Radicals and Antioxidants in Biomedicine. J. Miquel, H. Weber & A. Quintanilha, Eds. **2:** 87–94. CRC Press. Boca Raton, Fla.

15. CLAUSEN, J., S. ACHIM NIELSEN & M. KRISTENSEN. 1989. Biochemical and clinical effects of an antioxidative supplementation of geriatric patients. A double blind study. Biol. Trace Element Res. **20:** 135–151.

16. PÉK, G., T. FÜLÖP & I. ZS.-NAGY. 1989. Gerontopsychological studies using NAI ("Nürnberger Alters-Inventar") on patients with organic psychosyndrome (DSM-III, Category 1) treated with centrophenoxine in a double blind, comparative, randomized clinical trial. Arch. Gerontol. Geriatr. **9:** 17–30.

17. PACKER, L., L. PRILIPKO & Y. CHRISTEN, Eds. 1992. Free Radicals in the Brain. Aging, Neurological and Mental Disorders. Springer. Berlin, Germany.

18. SPILKER, B. 1984. Guide to Clinical Studies and Developing Protocols. Raven Press. New York, N.Y.

19. SPILKER, B. 1986. Guide to Clinical Interpretation of Data. Raven Press. New York, N.Y.

20. WORLD HEALTH ORGANIZATION. 1990. International Classification of Diseases, 10th revision. Draft of Chapter V(F): Mental and behavioural disorders. Clinical description and diagnostic guidelines. World Health Organization. Division of Mental Health. Geneva, Switzerland.

21. AMERICAN PSYCHIATRIC ASSOCIATION. 1991. DSM-IV Options Book: Work in Progress. Task Force on DSM-IV. American Psychiatric Association. Washington, D.C.

22. SHADER, R. I., J. S. HARMATZ & C. SALZMAN. 1974. A new scale for clinical assessment in geriatric populations: Sandoz Clinical Assessment-Geriatric (SCAG). J. Am. Geriatr. Soc. **22:** 107–113.

23. WECHSLER, D. 1955. Wechsler Adult Intelligence Scale. Psychological Corporation. New York, N.Y.

24. YESAVAGE, J. A., M. ADEY & P. D. WERNER. 1981. Development of a geriatric behavioral self-assessment scale. J. Am. Geriatr. Soc. **29:** 285–288.
25. VENN, R. D. 1983. The Sandoz Clinical Assessment-Geriatric (SCAG) scale. A general-purpose psychogeriatric rating scale (SCAG manual). Gerontology **29:** 185–198.
26. HAMOT, H. B., J. R. PATIN & J. M. SINGER. 1984. Factor structure of the Sandoz Clinical Assessment Geriatric (SCAG) scale. Psychopharmacol. Bull. **20:** 142–150.
27. WECHSLER, D. & C. P. SONTE. 1954. The Wechsler Memory Scale. Psychological Corporation. New York, N.Y.
28. YESAVAGE, J. A. & M. ADEY. 1981. Design aspects of studies of drugs claimed to improve cognitive function in the aged. J. Psychiatr. Treat. Evaluat. **3:** 545–549.
29. SHADER, R. I., J. S. HARMATZ & H.-A. TAMMERK. 1979. Towards an observational structure for rating dysfunction and pathology in ambulatory geriatrics. Interdiscipl. Topics Gerontol. **15:** 153–168.
30. WEIL, C. 1988. Hydergine. Pharmacologic and Clinical Facts. Springer. Berlin, Germany.
31. POPA, R., F. SCHNEIDER, G. MIHALAȘ, P. ȘTEFĂNIGĂ, I. G. MIHALAȘ, R. MĂTIEȘ, & R. MATEESCU. 1993. Antagonic-Stress superiority versus meclofenoxate in gerontopsychiatry (Alzheimer type dementia). 5th Cong. Int. Assoc. Biomed. Gerontol. Budapest, Hungary. Abstr.: P-6.
32. VERNON, M. W. & E. M. SORKIN. 1991. Piracetam. An overview of its pharmacological properties and a review of its therapeutic use in senile cognitive disorders. Drugs Aging. **1:** 17–35.
33. EYSENCK, H. J. & S. B. G. EYSENCK, Eds. 1991. Improvement of I.Q. and behaviour as a function of dietary supplementation. A symposium. Person. Individ. Diff. **12:** 329–365.
34. FÜNFGELD, E. W. 1993. Monotherapy versus multitherapy-combined therapeutical approaches for treatment of senile dementia of Alzheimer's type (SDAT). 15th Cong. Int. Assoc. Gerontol. Budapest, Hungary. Abstr. Vol: 163.
35. RIGA, S. & D. RIGA. 1993. Antagonic-Stress: an advanced drug for aging deceleration. I. Brain lipofuscinolytic activity demonstrated by light and fluorescence microscopy. 5th Cong. Int. Assoc. Biomed. Gerontol. Budapest, Hungary. Abstr.: L-58.
36. RIGA, S. & D. RIGA. 1974. Effects of centrophenoxine on the lipofuscin pigments in the nervous system of old rats. Brain Res. **72:** 265–275.
37. SUBBARAO, K. V., J. S. RICHARDSON & L. C. ANG. 1990. Autopsy samples of Alzheimer's cortex show increased peroxidation in vitro. J. Neurochem. **55:** 342–345.
38. CLAUSEN, J. 1984. Demential syndromes and the lipid metabolism. Acta Neurol. Scand. **70:** 345–355.
39. CUTLER, R. G. 1991. Human longevity and aging: possible role of reactive oxygen species. Ann. N.Y. Acad. Sci. **621:** 1–28.
40. ZS.-NAGY, I. & R. A. FLOYD. 1984. Electron spin resonance spectroscopic demonstration of the hydroxyl free radical scavenger properties of dimethylaminoethanol in spin trapping experiments confirming the molecular basis for the biological effects of centrophenoxine. Arch. Gerontol. Geriatr. **3:** 297–310.
41. SEMSEI, I. & I. ZS.-NAGY. 1985. Superoxide radical scavenging ability of centrophenoxine and its salt dependence in vitro. J. Free Radic. Biol. Med. **1:** 403–408.
42. ZS.-NAGY, I. 1987. An attempt to answer the questions of theoretical gerontology on the basis of the membrane hypothesis of aging. *In* Advance in Age Pigments Research. E. Aloj-Totaro, P. Glees & F. A. Pisanti, Eds.: 393–413. Pergamon Press. Oxford, England.
43. NANDY, K. & G. H. BOURNE. 1966. Effect of centrophenoxine on the lipofuscin pigments in the neurons of senile guinea-pigs. Nature **210:** 313–314.
44. RIGA, S., G. PAMBUCCIAN & S. OERIU. 1972. Changes in lipofuscin pigments of rat central nervous system under -SH groups' releasing substances' influence. 9th Int. Cong. Gerontol. Kiev, U.S.S.R. Session, Abstr., **3:** 383.
45. FUXE, K., L. F. AGNATI, P. HELDLUND, S. E. ÖGREN, F. BORTOLOTTI, C. CARANI & G. BIAGINI. 1992. Failure of integrative mechanisms in the aging brain. *In* Treatment of Age-Related Cognitive Dysfunction: Pharmacological and Clinical Evaluation. G. Racagni & J. Mendlewicz, Eds.: 1–18. S. Karger. Basel, Switzerland.
46. MORETTI, A. 1979. Metabolische und neurochemische Wirkung von Nicergolin auf das

Zentralnervensystem. Übersicht über die experimentellen Untersuchungen. Arzneimit-telforsch. (Drug Res.). **29:** 1213–1223.
47. LEHRL, S. & L. BLAHA. 1981. Untersuchung von Verlaufstypen bei zerebralen Hypoxi-dosen am Beispiel einer Doppelblindstudie mit Nicergolin (Sermion). Therapiewoche. **31:** 3143–3155.
48. HOYER, S. 1979. Effects of centrophenoxine on cerebral circulation in geriatric patients. *In* Geriatric Psychopharmacology. K. Nandy, Ed.: 261–274. Elsevier North Holland. New York, N.Y.
49. OERIU, S., D. WINTER, V. DOBRE & B. BRUHIS. 1973. Glucose transport across blood brain barrier, as related to age and meclofenoxate treatment. J. Pharmacol. (Paris) **4:** 497–503.
50. GLEES, P. & M. HASAN. 1976. Lipofuscin in Neuronal Aging and Diseases. G. Thieme. Stuttgart, Germany.

Index of Contributors

343

Subject Index